Dioptrica nova. A treatise of dioptricks, in two parts. Wherein the various effects and appearances of spherick glasses, both convex and concave, single and combined, in telescopes and microscopes are explained. The second edition.

William Molyneux

Dioptrica nova. A treatise of dioptricks, in two parts. Wherein the various effects and appearances of spherick glasses, both convex and concave, single and combined, in telescopes and microscopes, together with their usefulness in many concerns of humane The second edition.
Molyneux, William
ESTCID: T097131
Reproduction from British Library
On verso facing title page: "I think this book fit to be printed. June the 4th. 1690. John Hoskyns. .. ". With a final advertisement leaf.
London : printed for Benj. Tooke, 1709.
[18],301,[3]p.,plates,table ; 4°

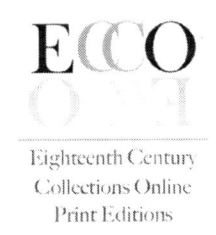

ECCO
Eighteenth Century
Collections Online
Print Editions

Gale ECCO Print Editions

Relive history with *Eighteenth Century Collections Online*, now available in print for the independent historian and collector. This series includes the most significant English-language and foreign-language works printed in Great Britain during the eighteenth century, and is organized in seven different subject areas including literature and language; medicine, science, and technology; and religion and philosophy. The collection also includes thousands of important works from the Americas.

The eighteenth century has been called "The Age of Enlightenment." It was a period of rapid advance in print culture and publishing, in world exploration, and in the rapid growth of science and technology – all of which had a profound impact on the political and cultural landscape. At the end of the century the American Revolution, French Revolution and Industrial Revolution, perhaps three of the most significant events in modern history, set in motion developments that eventually dominated world political, economic, and social life.

In a groundbreaking effort, Gale initiated a revolution of its own: digitization of epic proportions to preserve these invaluable works in the largest online archive of its kind. Contributions from major world libraries constitute over 175,000 original printed works. Scanned images of the actual pages, rather than transcriptions, recreate the works *as they first appeared.*

Now for the first time, these high-quality digital scans of original works are available via print-on-demand, making them readily accessible to libraries, students, independent scholars, and readers of all ages.

For our initial release we have created seven robust collections to form one the world's most comprehensive catalogs of 18th century works.

Initial Gale ECCO Print Editions collections include:

History and Geography
Rich in titles on English life and social history, this collection spans the world as it was known to eighteenth-century historians and explorers. Titles include a wealth of travel accounts and diaries, histories of nations from throughout the world, and maps and charts of a world that was still being discovered. Students of the War of American Independence will find fascinating accounts from the British side of conflict.

Social Science
Delve into what it was like to live during the eighteenth century by reading the first-hand accounts of everyday people, including city dwellers and farmers, businessmen and bankers, artisans and merchants, artists and their patrons, politicians and their constituents. Original texts make the American, French, and Industrial revolutions vividly contemporary.

Medicine, Science and Technology
Medical theory and practice of the 1700s developed rapidly, as is evidenced by the extensive collection, which includes descriptions of diseases, their conditions, and treatments. Books on science and technology, agriculture, military technology, natural philosophy, even cookbooks, are all contained here.

Literature and Language
Western literary study flows out of eighteenth-century works by Alexander Pope, Daniel Defoe, Henry Fielding, Frances Burney, Denis Diderot, Johann Gottfried Herder, Johann Wolfgang von Goethe, and others. Experience the birth of the modern novel, or compare the development of language using dictionaries and grammar discourses.

Religion and Philosophy
The Age of Enlightenment profoundly enriched religious and philosophical understanding and continues to influence present-day thinking. Works collected here include masterpieces by David Hume, Immanuel Kant, and Jean-Jacques Rousseau, as well as religious sermons and moral debates on the issues of the day, such as the slave trade. The Age of Reason saw conflict between Protestantism and Catholicism transformed into one between faith and logic -- a debate that continues in the twenty-first century.

Law and Reference
This collection reveals the history of English common law and Empire law in a vastly changing world of British expansion. Dominating the legal field is the *Commentaries of the Law of England* by Sir William Blackstone, which first appeared in 1765. Reference works such as almanacs and catalogues continue to educate us by revealing the day-to-day workings of society.

Fine Arts
The eighteenth-century fascination with Greek and Roman antiquity followed the systematic excavation of the ruins at Pompeii and Herculaneum in southern Italy; and after 1750 a neoclassical style dominated all artistic fields. The titles here trace developments in mostly English-language works on painting, sculpture, architecture, music, theater, and other disciplines. Instructional works on musical instruments, catalogs of art objects, comic operas, and more are also included.

bibliolife
old books, new life.

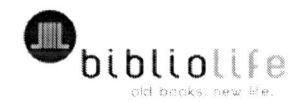

The BiblioLife Network

This project was made possible in part by the BiblioLife Network (BLN), a project aimed at addressing some of the huge challenges facing book preservationists around the world. The BLN includes libraries, library networks, archives, subject matter experts, online communities and library service providers. We believe every book ever published should be available as a high-quality print reproduction; printed on-demand anywhere in the world. This insures the ongoing accessibility of the content and helps generate sustainable revenue for the libraries and organizations that work to preserve these important materials.

The following book is in the "public domain" and represents an authentic reproduction of the text as printed by the original publisher. While we have attempted to accurately maintain the integrity of the original work, there are sometimes problems with the original work or the micro-film from which the books were digitized. This can result in minor errors in reproduction. Possible imperfections include missing and blurred pages, poor pictures, markings and other reproduction issues beyond our control. Because this work is culturally important, we have made it available as part of our commitment to protecting, preserving, and promoting the world's literature.

GUIDE TO FOLD-OUTS MAPS and OVERSIZED IMAGES

The book you are reading was digitized from microfilm captured over the past thirty to forty years. Years after the creation of the original microfilm, the book was converted to digital files and made available in an online database.

In an online database, page images do not need to conform to the size restrictions found in a printed book. When converting these images back into a printed bound book, the page sizes are standardized in ways that maintain the detail of the original. For large images, such as fold-out maps, the original page image is split into two or more pages

Guidelines used to determine how to split the page image follows:

- Some images are split vertically; large images require vertical and horizontal splits.
- For horizontal splits, the content is split left to right.
- For vertical splits, the content is split from top to bottom.
- For both vertical and horizontal splits, the image is processed from top left to bottom right.

I think this Book fit to be Printed.

June the 4th.
1690.
JOHN HOSKYNS. V.P.R.S.

DIOPTRICA NOVA.

A TREATISE OF DIOPTRICKS,

In Two PARTS.

Wherein the

Various Effects and Appearances OF

𝕾𝖕𝖍𝖊𝖗𝖎𝖈𝖐 𝕲𝖑𝖆𝖘𝖘𝖊𝖘,

BOTH

Convex and Concave, Single and Combined,
IN
TELESCOPES and MICROSCOPES,
Together with
Their USEFULNESS in many Concerns of Humane Life,
ARE EXPLAINED.

By WILLIAM MOLYNEUX of *Dublin* Esq;
Fellow of the ROYAL SOCIETY.

Ex Visibilibus Invisibilia.

𝕿𝖍𝖊 𝕾𝖊𝖈𝖔𝖓𝖉 𝕰𝖉𝖎𝖙𝖎𝖔𝖓.

London: Printed for BENJ. TOOKE, at the *Middle-Temple Gate* in *Fleet-street*, MDCCIX.

To the ILLUSTRIOUS
The Royal Society.

THE Design of the ensuing Treatise being the Promotion of a Part of Physico-Mathematical Knowledge in the English Nation; I know not to whom I can more properly present it, than to that noble Body of English Philosophers, whose Foundation by the Royal Charter of King Charles II. is to this very purpose. How far, and how successfully you have hitherto prosecuted the end of this excellent Institution, 'tis needless for me to declare: since the literate World is already so abundantly stored with your learned Labours, and useful Discoveries; whereof I could here recount a List of many Hundreds published by several Members of the Society. But I design not a Panegyrick, but an humble Address for your Favour and Countenance to my present Endeavours: And this I hope for, with the more Assurance, having already seen your favourable Acceptance of many Offerings of this kind, and your ready Incouragement of all such Philosophical Inquiries, as tend to the use of Life, or Advancement of Arts and Sciences.

And on this Occasion I cannot omit expressing my Sence of that excellent Method of Experimental Philosophy, which now, by your Example and Incouragement, does so universally prevail, and is so highly advanced all over Europe, and other Parts of the World.

'Tis wonderful to consider, how the Schools were formerly overrun with a senseless kind of Jargon, which they call'd Philosophy;

and

DEDICATION

and which men studied with the greatest Labour and Assiduity, that they might attain the name of Wise and Learned. This certainly was the greatest Cheat was ever imposed on the mind of Man: But why say I, imposed? Men drew it on themselves, and run their own Heads into the Noose: and when they had intangled themselves in a thousand ridiculous Disputes about empty Questions, they vainly thought they had attained the Perfection of Philosophers; whilst they had no Ideas in their Minds answerable to those Noises they made with their Tongues; but took more pains to deceive both themselves and others, than is requisite for the Propagation of true Knowledge. And indeed we may well imagine, that, had the former Ages of the World been at half that Labour and Study for the Advancement of real Knowledg, which they spent in promoting verbose Stuff; Mankind by this time might have been by many Degrees more wise, and consequently more happy even in this Life; for Wisdom only makes men so.

But in this last Age the generous Undertakings of the Philosophick Societies of Europe (to whom your Institution has shewn the way, and been an illustrious Example) have dissipated these dark Mists, and have abdicated this kind of empty Stuff, which had crept into even Natural Disquisitions, and like a Leprosie had quite over-run the whole Body of Philosophy, deforming its Beauty, and ruining its Strength. Men are not satisfied now with noisy Words, and nothing else, but require more solid Foundations of Knowledge, and believe no farther than they can find good Proofs.

This great Change, which Philosophy or the Prosecution of Knowledg in general has received of late years, is manifest in all its Parts; but in none more than in natural Enquiries. To these you have given a clearly new Turn, wholly different from the Methods, by which they were formerly prosecuted in the Schools. And how advantageously the Change has been made, will be evident to any that considers the one and t'other Method.

The

To the ROYAL SOCIETY.

The Commentators on Aristotle, (who was certainly himself a most diligent and profound Investigator of Nature) have rendred Physicks an heap of froathy Disputes, managing the whole Knowledge of Body and Motion, of Animals, Plants, and Minerals; of Celestial, Aerial and Terrestrial Bodies; by Hypothetical Conjectures, confirm'd by plausible Arguments of Wit and Rhetorick, ordered in a Syllogistical form; and answering Objections in like manner: But never studied to prove their Opinions by Experiments. By which Method they were as ignorant of the Properties and Affections of Natural Bodies, as if they were not at all the Subject of their Disquisitions. And yet these were the great Dictators of Physicks for many Ages in our Colleges and Schooles; and no one was accounted worthy the Name of a Philosopher, that would not on their Authority Jurare in verba. He that could Dispute and distinguish, about Sympathy, Antipathy, occult Qualities, Antiperistesis, and a Thousand such other fantastick Terms, was reputed a great Proficient, and deeply vers'd in Natures Secrets: tho all the while perhaps he knew not any one of the admirable Phænomena of the Magnet, or was not at all versed in the History of any one Branch in Nature. They'd rumble out indeed the Definition and Divisions of Comets, but knew nothing of the Laws of their Motions, or other Affections. They'd tell you the Tides depend on the Influence of the Moon; and when you proceed farther, and ask, what is this Influence? They'll yet give you a Word for it, and say, 'tis an occult Quality: If you inquire, what an occult Quality is? They'r at a Stand, and having no farther hard Word here to fly to, are forced to confess 'tis a Quality they know nothing of. Had they not better at first have plainly confest, they know not the Cause of the Tides? no surely; For tho this had been more becoming modest Philosphers, it would not so well captivate the Vulgar, and gain to themselves the Repute of deep Knowledge.

Yet this verbose Philosophy is that, which for many Generations prevail'd in the World: This it is, which is injoyn'd to be read and studied in our Colleges and Academies, by the Statutes and Charters thereof;

> Consult Magirus, Eustathius, Zanardus, Col. Complutensis Com. &c the common Natural Philosophy Books read in our Colleges.

DEDICATION

thereof: which in this Particular, to the apparent Hindrance of the Advancement of real and useful Knowledge, do yet remain unaltered in our Universities: wherein the first years of young Students may be imploy'd with much more Advantage by prosecuting other Methods. And, My thinks, it were now full time (after so happy a Reformation of our Errors in Religion, and purging our Seminaries of Learning from the Fopperies and Superstition of a false Worship) to begin a Reformation of our Human Literature, by establishing more useful Methods of Education, especially for the Employment of our more tender years.

But tho this weighty Undertaking has hitherto been deferr'd in them (the Reason whereof I leave to the Consideration of the learned and reverend Heads of our Universities) yet the strong Wits of many in this last Age have broken all these Fetters; And have happily advanced the true Method of prosecuting Knowledge upon solid Foundations.

This is manifest in every Branch of Learning. Logick has put on a Countenance clearly different from what it appeared in formerly: How unlike is its shape in the Ars Cogitandi, Recherches de la Verite, &c. from what it appears in Smigletius, and the Commentators on Aristotle? But to none do we owe for a greater Advancement in this Part of Philosophy, than to the incomparable Mr. Locke, Who, in his Essay concerning Humane Understanding, has rectified more received Mistakes, and delivered more profound Truths, established on Experience and Observation, for the Direction of Man's mind in the Prosecution of Knowledge, (which I think may be properly term'd Logick) than are to be met with in all the Volumes of the Antients. He has clearly overthrown all those Metaphysical Whymsies, which infected mens Brains with a Spice of Madness, whereby they feign'd a Knowledge where they had none, by making a noise with Sounds, without clear and distinct Significations.

Natural

To the ROYAL SOCIETY.

Natural Philosophy *is now prosecuted by Observation, Experiment, and History thereof. And indeed if we consider it rightly, there is really no other sort of Natural Philosophy, but this only. For by* Natural Philosophy, *or* Physicks, *do we mean any thing else, but the Knowledge of the Properties and Affections of Natural Bodies? And is this to be obtain'd any otherwise, than by Experiment and Observation? Can any Man Dispute me into the Knowledge of the* Magnet's *Attraction, Direction and Variation; or of the Phænomena of the Mercurial Baroscope without Tryal and Experiment? Can any Arguments prove that a little Sulphur, Nitre, and Charcole should produce such a quick and strong Blast as Gunpowder; before they be actually put together and tryed? Men might have disputed to all Eternity, before their Gibberish could discover the Use of that ordinary despicable Substance,* Iron-Ore: *To which, for ought I see, (as a most ingenious Author has observ'd) we are beholding for all the Politure and Plenty, all the Learning, State, and Magnificence of the World, beyond the Rudeness, Wants, and Ignorance of the ancient savage* Americans: *Whose Natural Endowments and Provisions equal those of the most flourishing and polite Nations; But they wanted the Advantagious Uses of this contemptible Mineral. So that he, who first discovered the Use of that one poor Mine; or* Tubalcain, *that first taught the way of working in Iron, may be deservedly celebrated as the Father of Arts, and Author of most of the Conveniences of Human Life.*

I know some will say, that by Natural Philosophy *is meant not only the Knowledge of the Properties and Uses of Natural Bodies; but also the Assigning the true Reasons or Causes of these Properties. But in this Particular we are to proceed with great Caution. I know the Mind of man is of that inquisitive, prying Nature, that upon any Appearance offer'd to the Senses, it immediately falls to the search after the Cause producing this Effect. But indeed in Natural Disquisitions, 'tis generally (I may say almost alwayes) to no purpose. We may make plausible Conjectures, and some sort of feasible Guesses; but others perhaps may make others, and these also equally*

B

DEDICATION

equally probable. But these deserve not the Name of Natural Philosophy; they serve only for Chat and Diversion. For the omnipotent Contriver of the Universe has order'd Natures Operations to be performed by such fine Springs, secret Motions, and inexplicable Ways, that Man in this Life may well despair of attaining the intimate Knowledge thereof, and must therefore content himself with the Contemplation of plain matter of Fact, in which he cannot be deceived. But yet, that we may not wholly suppress this inquisitive Humour, but may only keep it within just Bounds: It will be granted, That whatever immediate Cause can be assigned to an Effect; and it can be proved so to be by some convincing Experiments; and these be often repeated, and diligently examin'd, and found to agree and conspire together; we may be allow'd to found thereon an Hypothesis or Supposal of this Cause, but no more. We must not positively establish it as the undoubted, adequate Cause; for this we may miss after our most diligent Inquiry. However the Experiments we use and demonstrate to sense, for the establishing our Hypothesis, shall be allowed as unquestionable Verities; and shall be embraced as so many Steps of Advancement in the Knowledge of Nature.

But of the Uncertainty of Assigning Natural Causes I shall give but one Instance, and that perhaps as strong as any we shall meet with in Philosophy. We are apt to think, that the Cause of the Suspension of the Mercury in the Torricellian Experiment is undoubtedly the Gravitation of the Air: And we prove it by a most convincing Experiment, for putting the Baroscope into the Pneumatick Engine, exhaust the Air, and the Mercury immediately subsides. But when we consider it a little farther, we shall find, That hereby we have obtain'd little more certain Knowledge, than plainly the matter of Fact of this latter Experiment, and not the adequate Cause of the first Experiment enquired after. For we can only conclude from hence, that the Equipoise of Liquors is the Cause of the Mercury's Suspension: But what is the Cause of this Equipoise of Liquors, or the Cause of the Gravitation of any Liquors, or any Bodies? That is, What is the Cause of Gravity in general is clearly unknown to us,

and

To the ROYAL SOCIETY.

and consequently the ultimate Cause of the Mercury's Suspension is not hereby discovered. 'Tis true indeed, by this Experiment we have most probably arriv'd at the Knowledge of one Link more in the Chain of Natural Causes; but this is not conclusive; this puts not an end to the Enquiry: For so if one looking at a Pendulum Clock should enquire, Why the Pendulum does not cease by degrees from vibrating? And he were answered, That it is kept in motion by the next immediate Wheel that beats on the Pallats. And this were offer'd to be proved by Experiment, for stop the motion of this Wheel, and the Pendulum soon ceases: Would he not presently be satisfied, and go away secure, that he had discovered the Cause of the Continuation of the Pendulum's Motion? And yet certainly he has mistaken one single Link for the whole Chain. For if he proceeded farther, and had enquired, What moved this Wheel? He would find, the next Wheel, and so onwards to the Weight or Spring. But here he's at a Loss; for what moves them, is absolutely unknown.

As to most other Reasons in Natural Philosophy, that usually pass as satisfactory, and are received as Accounts of Nature's Proceedings: We shall generally find them little more, than farther Illustrations of the Matter enquired after in some different Words. Thus if it be asked, What is the Reason the Sun casts a shadow from some Bodies, viz. those we call opaque, and none from others, viz. Transparent Bodies? 'Tis answer'd, Because by the opaque Body the Rays of the Sun are stopt in their Progress, and hindred from enlightning that Part of the Ground or Floor that is behind the Body: In the Transparent Body the Rays pass freely. This would be taken by several as deep Reasoning; and yet is really no more than Tautology, as if we should say, the Sun casts a Shadow, Because he casts a Shadow. But it gives no Account of the Opacity of one Body, and Transparency of another, which truly the Question requires. If we ask, How Fire burns? 'Tis answered, by exciting a violent Motion in the Parts of the Combustible Matter: Which indeed is no more than the same thing in different Words. But how Motion is excited or communicated by one Body to another, is absolutely inexplicable. Yet these

DEDICATION

Kind of Verbal Reasons do generally pass in Talk, and serve to amuse as well as the best.

Since therefore we cannot expect to arrive at the intimate Knowledge of Natures Operations: Let us apply our selves to know as much of Her, as we may be certain of. And this only is in Matters of Experiment and Tryal, wherein by the infallible Guidance of our Sences, we cannot be deceived. For tho, Experimentum periculosum, be an ancient Aphorism, yet we must consider of what Experiments it was pronounced, viz. of those in Medicine and Diseases. It agrees not to all, when diligently enquired into, and often repeated. But when we meet with any Experiment that is thus fallacious, we are not to rely on it, yet of this we may be sure, and lay it down as a discover'd Certainty, that sometimes it hits, sometimes it misses; and in this Truth we cannot be deceived, seeing we have so often found it.

But I have lanch'd out thus far, before I was aware: I must recover my self, and beg Pardon both for this Digression, and for telling you Things which you very well know already, at the same time when I offer you a Petition. But my Desire of propagating this useful Method of Philosophy will excuse my Fault, and at the same time will recommend me the more to your Favour, who are the great Patrons thereof, and in Account whereof your Name is deservedly celebrated all over Europe.

Permit me therefore to lay this Offering at your Feet, it being the Explication of one of the most noble Instruments of Experimental Philosophy. Not that I think thereby to add any think considerable to the vast Treasure of Curiosities you already possess: But that I may have an Opportunity of declaring to the World, how much I am

April 17
1690

Your Devoted

Humble Servant,

WILLIAM MOLYNEUX.

ADMONITION TO THE READER.

BEFORE the Reader proceed to the following Sheets, I desire he may take notice;

First, That he is not to expect *Geometrical Strictness* in several Particulars of this Doctrine. I say, in *several* Particulars; For many there are, which will bear the most *precise Exactness* Kepler, Cavallerius, Herigon, Dechales, Honoratus Faber, Gregorius, Barrow, and other Authors have taken this Liberty; as being more desirous of shewing in gross the Properties of Glasses and their Effects in Telescopes, than of affecting a *Nicety*, which would be of little Use in Practice. Thus we shall find in what follows, that many Lines are supposed *equal*, which strictly taken are really not so, but yet are so very little different, that for all use, and ease of Demonstration, they may be taken as *equal* Thus also we suppose very small *Angles* and their *Sines* to be *proportional*; which *precisely* is not so, but is so to the smallest and most insensible Difference. Thus likewise, we sometimes consider not the *Glasses Thickness*, but suppose it of the *least Thickness imaginable*, or of no Thickness at all; which yet is false, but does hardly prejudice any Demonstration. For *Dioptricks* being a part of *mixt Mathematicks*, conversant about *material Lines* (or Rays of Light) and the refractive Power of a *corporeal* Glass, cannot be delivered with that Ἀκρίβεια *Geometrica* requisite in *abstracted Mathematicks*.

Secondly, The Reader will find some *Corollaries* and *Scholiums* hereafter delivered, which of themselves more properly might have constituted Propositions. But these did not occur so readily in the course of the Work, And therefore I chose rather to add them as *Corollaries* than

ADMONITION

than change the number of Propositions and Citations. Of this kind are *Corol. ad Prop.* 8. *Corol. ad Prop* 15. *&c.*

Thirdly, I have presumed to intitle this Work *Dioptrica Nova*, as being indeed almost *wholly new*. Very little being borrowed from others, but what is requisite to shew the former Methods of Authors in demonstrating their Propositions, and to keep up the Consecution and Series of the Propositions of this Book. Besides, I can say, that the *Geometrical Method* of calculating a Rays Progress, which in many particulars is so amply delivered hereafter, is *wholly new*, and never before publish'd. And for the first Intimation thereof, I must acknowledg my self obliged to my worthy Friend Mr. *Flamsteed. Astron. Reg.* who had it from some unpublished Papers of Mr. *Gascoignes*.

Lastly, I declare, That if in any thing hereafter delivered, I have made any Mistakes, or not so clearly expressed my self upon Intimation thereof, I shall be most ready to *retract*. And therefore if in any thing I have *slip'd*, or made a *false Step*, I desire the ingenious and candid Reader either to inform me thereof, and upon Conviction, I shall *submit*; or else that he would freely pardon the Error; *Humanum est*.

Tho I had begun, and made some Progress in this Work in *Latin*, yet I thought it convenient (at least for the present) to alter my Design: There being nothing in *this Part of Mathematicks* ever yet publish'd in *English*. And I am sure there are many ingenious Heads, great Geometers, and Masters in Mathematicks, who are not so well skill'd in *Latin*.

If Forreigners may think this Work deserves their Perusal; in time perhaps I may satisfie them.

And because I have studied to be as plain as possibly I could, I have chosen rather to be *prolix* in many Particulars, than leave any Ambiguity to the most ordinary Mathematician. And therefore in demonstrating, I often repeat several Steps tho the least altered; that all things may lye as plain as possible. And on this Account I hope, the curious and profound Geometers will pardon me; I know they are used to what is *concise* and *closely* put together, much expressed in a little But this Method suits not every Reader: And I have chosen to accommodate mine to the plainest Capacities

Lastly, in this practical kind of Mathematicks, I desire the Reader to have frequent recourse to Experiments, for these illustrate the Theory and make many things clear, which otherwise will pass obscurely.

I

To the READER.

I use the common Notes of Algebra, with two or three new ones introduced by *Branker* or Dr. *Pell*, such as

÷ Signifies *Divided by*, ÷ 2 signifies *Divided by* 2.

2̄ With a Line over it signifies the absolute Number 2.

✶ Is the Note of Multiplication or drawing into.

In the Demonstrations the larger and lesser Margins or Columns are of the same use as is expressed in Dr. *Pell*'s *Algebra*. To which I refer the Reader.

April 17. 1690.

WILL. MOLYNEUX.

DIOPTRICKS.

Tab. pag. 1

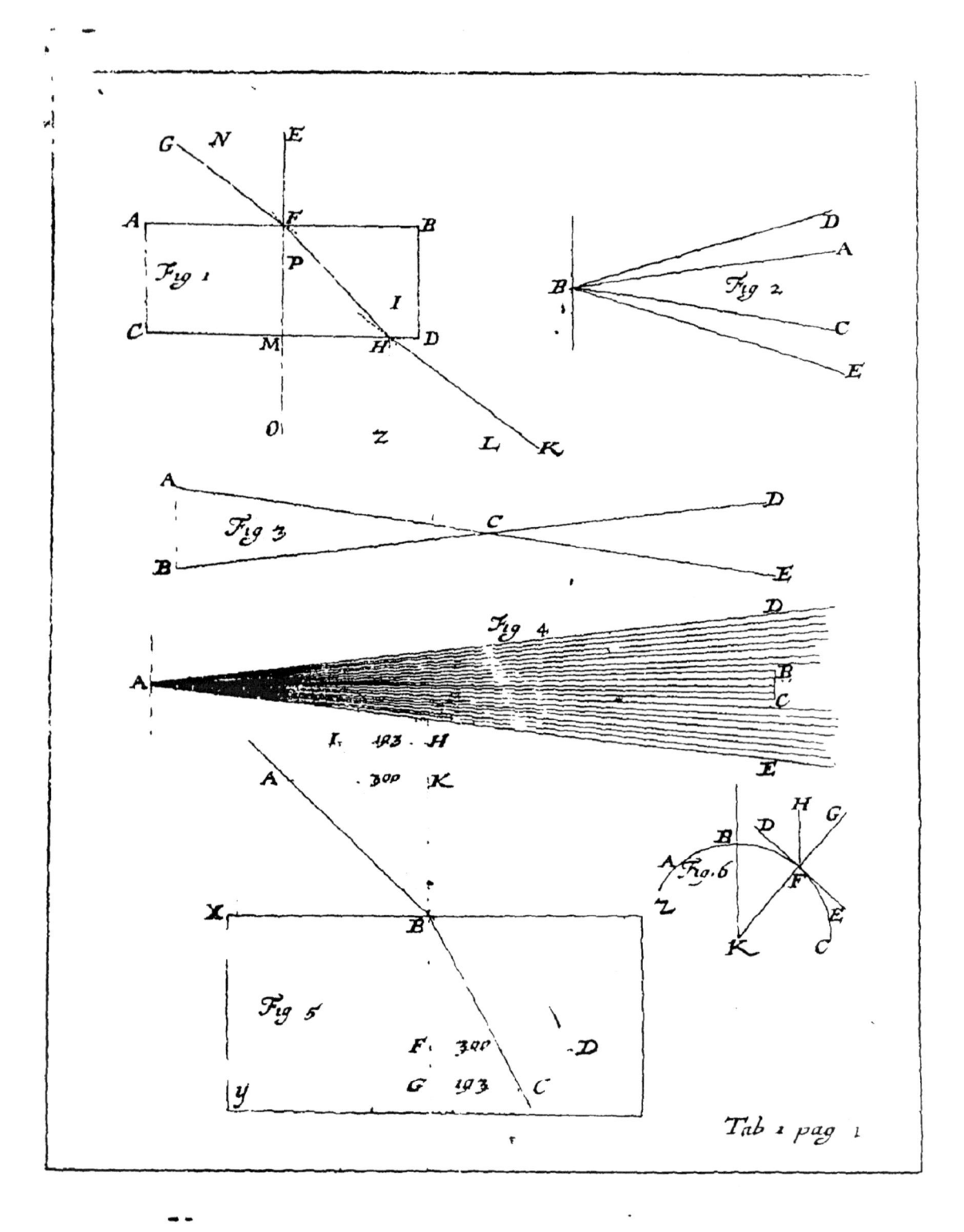

DIOPTRICKS.

Definitions.

I. *Tab.* 1. *Fig.* 1. ABCD is a Body of Glass, EFM is perpendicular to AB: suppose GF a Ray of Light falling inclined on the Glass AD, the Point F is called the *Point of Incidence.*

II. The Angle EFG comprehended between the Perpendicular and the Ray, is the *Angle of Incidence* (with *Barrow*, &c.) tho by many Dioptrick Writers 'tis called the *Angle of Inclination*; and its Complement AFG, is usually by them called the *Angle of Incidence*. But I shall use the Terms *Inclination* and *Incidence* promiscuously, always designing thereby the *Angle comprehended between the Perpendicular* EF *and the Ray* GF.

Experiments.

I. GF is a Ray of Light falling inclined on the Glass ABCD, this Ray coming out of a *Rare Medium*, as Air, into a *Dense Medium*, as Glass, does not proceed on its direct Course in a streight Line towards I, but at the Point of Incidence F 'tis bent or refracted *towards* the Perpendicular FM, and becomes the refracted Ray FH.

II. At H is its Point of *Incidence* again, from Glass a *Dense Medium* to Air a *Rare*, and in this Passage, 'tis refracted *from* the Perpendicular HZ, so that instead of proceeding directly strait in FHL, 'tis refracted from the Perpendicular HZ, and becomes HK: So that if the Surface AB be parallel to the Surface DC, the Ray becomes again as if it had not been refracted; for now HK runs parallel to GF. The natural Reason of this Refraction is variously assigned by divers, and is properly of a Physical consideration, and what is offered therein, is little more than Hypothetical Conjecture. I shall not therefore mix Guesses with Demonstration: The Matter of Fact is manifest from Ten Thousand repeated Experiments, and this is sufficient to my purpose. But yet there is such an ingenious Hypothesis concerning this Matter, published in the *Acta Eruditorum Lipsiæ, Anno 1682. Mens. Junii*, pag 185. by the Learned and Ingenious *G. G. Leibnutzius*, that I cannot omit inserting it in the Second Part of this Work, *Chap.* 1.

III. The Ray that falls perpendicular (as suppose EF a Ray) passes unrefracted, but all inclined Rays are refracted.

Definitions.

Ta 1 Fi.1.   III. The Angle IFH, and KHL comprehended by the Ray directly prolonged, and the refracted Ray is the *Angle of Refraction*.

IV. The Angle HFM or ZHK comprised between the refracted Ray and Perpendicular is the *refracted Angle*.

V. *Diverging Rays* are those that spread and separate the farther from each other, as they flow farther from the Object.

Ta.1.Fi.2   *Tab.* 1. *Fig.* 2. B is a radiating Point, AB, DB, CB, EB, are diverging Rays.

VI. *Converging Rays* are those that approach nigher each

Ta 1.Fi 3   other, till they cross, and then become *Diverging*. *Tab.*1.*Fig.*3. A, B, are two Radiating Points in the Object AB, the Rays CA, CB, do *Converge*, till they cross in C, and then they become *Diverging* DC, EC.

VII. *Parallel*

VII. *Parallel Rays* are those that flowing from one and the same Point of a *remote* Object pass at the same distance, as to sense: But this is not to be strictly taken, for then the Rays flowing from one and the same Point of an Object, cannot be *parallel*, for they always *diverge*: Yet when an Object is at such a great distance, and that parcel of Rays which is considered, is so small, that their Divergence is little or nothing considerable, these Rays are said to be parallel. *Tab.* 1. *Fig.* 4. A is a Point in an Object sending forth its diverging Rays AD, AB, AC, AE; let BC be the breadth of the Pupil or breadth of an Optick Glass: Here if the Point A be so remote, and BC be so small, that the Parcel of Rays BAC, do insensibly run parallel, then these are said to be parallel Rays.

VIII. Those radiating Points or Objects are said to be *remote*, whose distance from the Eye or Glass is so great, that the breadth of the Pupil or Glass, in respect thereto, is inconsiderable.

IX. Those radiating Points or Objects are said to be *nigh*, when there is a sensible proportion between the Pupils or Glasses breadth, and the distance; so that the Rays flowing from any single Point thereof do not run parallel to each other, but diverge considerably in respect of the Pupils or Glasses breadth.

Experiments.

V. *Tab.* 1. *Fig.* 5. ZXY is a Body of Glass, HBG is perpendicular to ZX, AB is a Ray falling on this Glass, and the Angle of Inclination or Incidence is HBA=DBG. *Kepler* tells us, that under 30 deg. of Inclination from Air to Glass, the Angle of Refraction DBC is $\frac{1}{3}$ of the Inclination, therefore the refracted Angle CBG is $\frac{2}{3}$ of the Inclination. Wherefore we lay down the following Proportions, as confirmed by *Kepler's* Experiments, and usually retain'd by most Optick Writers.

∠ Inclination DBG : refracted ∠ CBG :: 3 : 2
∠ Inclination DBG : ∠ Refraction DBC : 3 : 1
∠ Refraction DBC : refracted ∠ CBG : 1 : 2

V. But suppose the Ray CB to proceed from Glass to Air, at B 'tis refracted *from* the Perpendicular BH, and becomes BA; here the Inclination is CBG=HBI, and then

∠ Incidence HBI : refracted ∠ HBA : 2 : 3
∠ Inclination HBI : ∠ Refraction IBA : 2 : 1
∠ Refraction IBA : refracted ∠ HBA : 1 : 3

These Propositions in the 4th. and 5th. Experiments we shall retain in the following Demonstrations, for the Ease and Plainness thereof. But in Calculation we shall observe the Proportion that follows in the 6th. Experiment.

VI. But the most Learned and Ingenious Mr. *Isaac Newton* of *Cambridge* discovered by most accurate Experiments, that these Proportions of *Kepler* were not sufficiently exact: For *Des Cartes* first found, that Refractions were not to be measured by the Proportion of Angles, but by the Proportion of Sines. See his Dioptricks *Cap.* 2. *Sec.* 7. And therefore Mr. *Newton* apply'd himself to discover the Proportion of the Sines, and found, *That from Air to Glass, the Sine* AK *or* DF *of the Angle of Incidence* ABK *or* DBG: *is to the Sine* IH *or* CG *of the refracted Angle* CBG *or* IBH :: *As* 300 *to* 193. (*or near, as* 14 *to* 9.) *And on the contrary, that from Glass to Air, the Sine of the Incidence : Is to the Sine of the refracted Angle* :: *as* 193 : *to* 300, *or as* 9 *to* 14. But the same Mr. *Newton* in his Dissertations concerning *Colours* and *Light*, publish'd in the *Philosophical Transactions*, has at large demonstrated, that the Rays of Light are not all *Homogeneous*, or of the same sort, but of different Forms and Figures, so that

that some are more refracted than others, tho they have the same or equal Inclinations on the Glass: And therefore there can be no constant Proportion setled between the Sines of the Incidence and of the refracted Angles. But the Proportion that comes nearest Truth, for the middle and strong Rays of Light, is nearly as 300 to 193, or 14 to 9.

VII. As the Sine of the Angle of any one Inclination: To the Sine of its refracted Angle :: So is the Sine of any other Inclination: To the Sine of its refracted Angle. Therefore by Experiment, finding the Proportion of the Sines of any one Inclination, and of its correspondent refracted Angle, this Proportion will hold in any other Inclination or Incidence. See *Des Cartes Diopt. Cap. 2 Sec. 7. Mersenni Optic. Lib. 7. Prop. 12. Dechales Dioptr. Lib. 1. Prop. 1, 2, &c.* See also *Cap. 1. Sec. 4. Part 2.*

Wherefore the Incidence or Inclination of a Ray being given, 'tis easie finding the refracted Angle, for the Proportion is, as 300: To 193 :: (or as 14 to 9) So the Sine of the Incidence: To the Sine of the refracted Angle, from Air to Glass.

Or Mechanically thus, A B K being the given Angle of Incidence, by a Sector make the Sine thereof K A or D F 300 parts (or 14) and take 193 (or 9) of the same parts, and make therewith C G or H I the Sine of the refracted Angle; then draw B C, this is the progress of the Ray A B after it enters the Glass.

VIII. *The Progress of Light through different Mediums is reciprocal* That is, Tab. 1. Fig. 1 Suppose the luminous Point Ta. 1 F. 1 G in Air, to send from it the Ray G F upon the Glass A D; this Ray by the Glass is refracted into F H within the Glass. Let us now imagin the Point H within the Glass, to be a luminous Point, sending out from it self the Ray H F: This Ray upon its Emersion from Glass into Air, instead of proceeding

ceeding directly to N, is refracted into F G. And so likewise supposing the Luminous Point G, to send its Ray G F, which after a double Refraction on each Surface of the Glass proceeds first in F H, and afterwards in H K; if we conceive K a Luminous Point, sending its Ray K H on the Glass; this Ray after a double Refraction on the two Surfaces of the Glass shall be refracted first into H F and then into F G; taking the same reciprocal Progress in both Cases.

And this is not so properly proved from Experiment (tho that also does abundantly and most exactly confirm this Truth) but 'tis manifest and self-evident from the very Nature of the thing. For whatever physical Reason there is, which causes the Ray G F proceeding from Air into the Glass A D to be refracted from its direct Course F I into F H; the same reason there must needs be to cause the Ray H F, proceeding from the Glass A D into the open Air, to be refracted from its direct Course F N into F G. For doubtless the Refraction proceeds from the Disparity of the Mediums (but how or in what manner 'tis needless to enquire in this place). Now the difference of the Mediums on their two determining Surfaces, or at the Point of Incidence F, continues the same, let the Ray proceed from which of them soever. For there is as great a reciprocal Difference between Glass and Air, as between Air and Glass, and consequently the Refraction must needs be reciprocal. *Vid.* Barrow, *Lect. Opt.* 3. *Sect.* 3.

Definitions.

X. Whatever Line is perpendicular as to the Tangent of any Curve Line at the point of Contact, is said to be perpendicular to the same Curve. *Tab.* 1. *Fig.* 6. D E being a Tangent to the Arch of a Circle A B C, and F G being perpendicular to D E at the point of Contact F, the Line F G is also perpendicular to the Curve A B C.

XI. A

Tab. 2 pag. 7

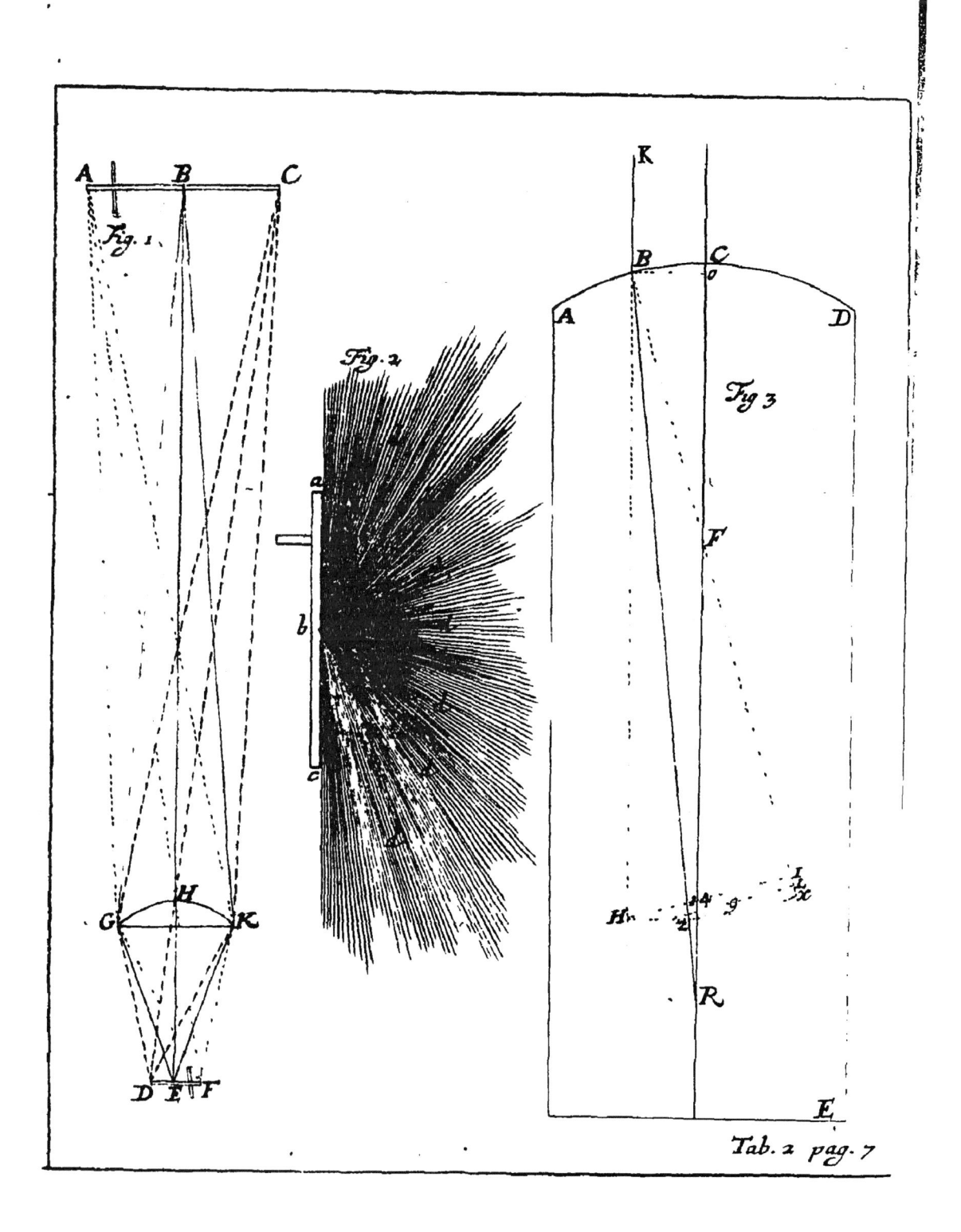

XI. A Line that is inclined to the Tangent of any Curve, is inclined to the Curve; and the Angle of Inclination to the Curve, is the same with the Angle of Inclination to the Tangent. F H is inclined to the Curve A B C, by the Angle H F G, according to which Angle the same Line H F is inclined to the Tangent D E.

XII. K being the Centre of the Circle A B C, draw B K parallel to H F, the Arch B F measures the Inclination of the Line H F to the Curve A B C, or to the Tangent D E: For the Angle B K F is equal to the Angle H F G. (*Pr.* 29. 1. *Eucl.*

XIII. The Rays that proceed from the *middle* Point of an Object, when the Glass is exposed directly before it, are said to fall *directly* on the Glass, but the Rays that flow from the *Collateral* Points of an Object, are said to fall *obliquely* on the Glass. *Tab.* 2. *Fig.* 1. A B C is a *distant* Object, sending *parallel* Rays from each of its Points on the Glass G K, exposed *directly* before it. Here the Rays flowing from the Point B, are said to fall *directly* on the Glass, as B G, B H, B K. But the Rays flowing from the Point A, or any other *Collateral* Point, are said to fall *obliquely* on the Glass, as A G, A H, A K. And here 'tis to be noted, that the Point B is said to be *directly* exposed to the Glass, when the Axis of the Glass E H B *directly* produced, meets this Point B: But all other Points in the Object are *Collateral* Points; for tho they may be *directly* exposed to some other Points in the Glass, yet *direct* and *collateral*, are here to be understood only in respect of the Glass's *Axis* or *Vertex*. Or in short, that Point in an Object is said to be *direct*, the *Axis* of whose Cone of Rays is coincident or the same with the *Axis* of the Glass; that Point in an Object is said to be *oblique* or *collateral*, the *Axis* of whose Cone of Rays falls *obliquely* to the *Axis* of the Glass. *Vid. Def.* 17. 18.

XIV. Suppose

XIV. Suppose the Glass G K exposed in the Hole of a Shutter in a dark Room, and that thereby the Object A B C were represented on a white Paper in F E D (how this is done we shall see hereafter) From each Point of this Object there falls a parcel of Rays on the Surface of the whole Glass, thus from the Point B, there falls B G, B H, B K. This parcel of Rays is called *A Cone of Rays*, having its Vertex in the Point of the Object B, and its Base on the Glass.

XV. To this Cone of Rays there is another Correspondent on t'other side the Glass G E K, which has its Base likewise on the Glass, and its *Vertex* in a correspondent Point E of the Representation.

XVI. Both these Cones together (that is B G E K) are called *A Pencil of Rays*.

XVII. Each Pencil of Rays has one Ray amongst the rest, which is called its *Axis*. The *Axis* of the direct Pencil BGEK is the Ray B H E, which falls perpendicularly on the Glass, and passes through it unrefracted But the Axis of any of the oblique Pencils, as A G F K is some certain Ray, as A H F, which, tho it fall obliquely, and consequently is refracted by the Glass, yet being refracted *from* the perpendicular at its Egress from the Glass, as much as it was refracted *towards* the Perpendicular, at its Ingress into the Glass; it may be taken as not refracted at all, but that part of this Axis which is before the Glass (*viz.* A H between the Object and Glass) and that part of it which is behind the Glass (*viz.* H F between the Representation and the Glass) do run parallel to each other, or rather in one Right Line, that part of it only which is within the Glass, being bent out of its strait Course. And that in each oblique Pencil of Rays (for of the direct Pencil 'tis manifest) there is such a certain Ray thus affected, shall appear more fully hereafter. And here we are to distinguish between the *Axis of a Pencil of Rays*, and the *Axis of the Glass*. See Def. 18.

The

The Pencils of Rays from various Points are expressed differently in the Schemes (*viz.* by Lines or small Points) for better Illustration, and easier distinguishing their Progress.

XVIII. *Tab.* 2. *Fig.* 3. A E is a Body of Glass, whose Surface A C D is the Segment of a Sphere, the Centre whereof is F. K B a Ray falling on the Glass; through the Centre F draw CFR parallel to K B, C F R is the *Axis*, and the Point C the *Pole* or *Vertex* of the Glass: Or more generally thus, The *Axis* of a Glass is that *Right Line*, which, being produced both ways, falls on the *Centres* of the *Two* Spherick Surfaces (if the Glass be a double Convex, or double Concave) or which being produced both ways, falls on the *Centre* of the *Spherick* Surface, and perpendicular to the plain Surface, (if the Glass be a Plano-Convex, or Plano-Concave.) So that the Axis of a *Convex-Glass* passes perpendicular to the *thickest* part of the compleat Glass; and of a *Concave* to the *thinnest* part of the compleat Glass. Why *Compleat* is added, *vid.* Second Part, *Chap.* 4. *Sect.* 4. The *Poles* of a Glass are those two Points in the Glass through which the *Axis* passes. [Tab 2. Fig 3]

'Tis needless to define what is meant by a Convex or Concave-Glass, *&c.* for every one knows this already.

XIX. The Ray K B falling on the Convexity A C D, parallel to the Axis C R, and being refracted to B R; so that now it runs no more parallel, but crosses the Axis in R: the Point R is called the *Point of Concourse, or of Convergency, or the Focus.*

1. *Supposition.*

That from every Physical Point in an Object Rays of Light are diffused in direct Lines through the Hemisphere round it. *Tab.* 2. *Fig.* 3. Thus the Point *b* in the Object *a b c* projects from it the Rays *b d*, *b d*, *b d*, wherever they are not hindered by some Opaque Body intervening. And these Rays are [Ta 2. Fi 2]

C   strait

strait Lines, whilst they pass through a Diaphanous Uniform *Medium*. But here we are to conceive a radiating or luminous Point, not in a strict *Mathematical* Sense, but in a *Physical*, considering it as the least part imaginable in an Object.

2. *Supposition.*

That the *Axis* of the Eye, Glass, or Glasses, exposed before an Object be *Perpendicular* to the Plane of the Object, or that the Eye, Glass, or Glasses exposed before an Object, are supposed *directly* exposed thereto.

3. *Supposition,* or *Admonition.*

Because in many Authors of Opticks, much Perplexity and Error arises from their confused mentioning of Rays, and applying to them the Epithets of *Diverging*, and *Converging*, and *Crossing*; without expressing clearly whether they mean Rays from *one* and the *same* Point in an Object, or from *Different* Points. Therefore we are to consider in the ensuing Doctrin, whether the Name Rays do relate to those from *one* and the *same* Point, or from different Points. And that this may be the more easie, I do generally express the Rays from the same Point to be *such*, that is, I call them Rays from the same Point.

PROP. I. PROBL.

Tab. 2. Fig. 3. *A E is a Body of Glass, whose Surface A B C D is the Segment of a Sphere, the Centre whereof is F. K B is a Ray of Light parallel to the Axis C F R. There being given C F the Radius of the Convexity, and B O the Distance*

[11]

Distance of the Ray from the Axis; 'tis required to find the Point R, wherein this Ray, after one sole Refraction at the Point of Incidence B, crosses the Axis CR.

Produce K B at pleasure to H, and draw B F X at pleasure.

1. In the Right Angled Triangle B O F, we have given B O and B F, whence we may find the Angle BFO=HBF, which is the Incidence.

2. Then say, as 300 : to 193 :: (or as 14 to 9) so the Sine H I of the Incidence H B F : to the Sine Z L of the refracted Angle R B F, then HBF—RBF=HBR=BRF, which is the Angle of Refraction.

3. In the Triangle R B F, all the Angles and one of the Sides B F are known, whence we may find F R; *Which was required.*

Example.

F B = F C = 2 Inches, or 20000 Parts, an Inch being 10000. B O = ½ an Inch, or 5000 such Parts. The Angle of Incidence or Inclination B F O = H B F will be found 14° 29'. And the refracted Angle F B R shall be 9° 15'. Wherefore BRF=HBR= 5° 14'. Whence the Line F R is found 35341. Then RF+FC=35341+20000=55341=CR.

Corollary.

From this Calculation 'tis manifest, That in this Case the Point of Concourse R is distant from the Pole of the Glass C, almost a Diameter and half of the Convexity: For a Diameter and half is 60000, and CR is 55341, which wants only about ⅟ of 60000.

Scholium

Scholium 1.

This Proposition is the 34th. of *Keplers Dioptricks*, and in him and other Opticians, 'tis usually thus expressed and demonstrated.

The Rays that are parallel to the Axis, and fall so on the Convex Surface of a Glass, and at their Ingress are refracted, and so pass forward in Glass only, are united with the Axis at the distance of almost a Diameter and half of the Convexity, supposing the Glass to be a Portion of no more than about 30 degrees of its Convexity, or (which is the same thing) supposing the Inclination of the most extreme Ray to be but 15 degrees.

This Limitation of 15 degrees Inclination is added, because above 15 degrees Sines and Angles are not proportional, but under 15 degrees they are nighly proportional, a double Angle having a double Sine, a treble Angle a treble Sine, &c.

Ta 2 Fi 3. Wherefore they thus demonstrate this Proposition. *Tab. 2. Fig. 3.* BFC=HBF is the Inclination, HBR=BRF is the Angle of Refraction, RBF the refracted Angle. But by *Experiment* 4. RBF the refracted Angle : is to BRF the Angle of Refraction :: as 2 to 1. Therefore the Sines of these Angles, being under 15 degrees, shall be as 2 : to 1. But in plain Triangles the Sines of the Angles and the Sides subtending these Angles are proportional; therefore the Side RF is double FB or FC. Wherefore RC is thrice FC, or equal to three Semidiameters. *Which was to be demonstrated.*

Scholium 2.

But a neater way of Expressing and Demonstrating this Proposition is thus.

When

Tab. 3. pag. 12

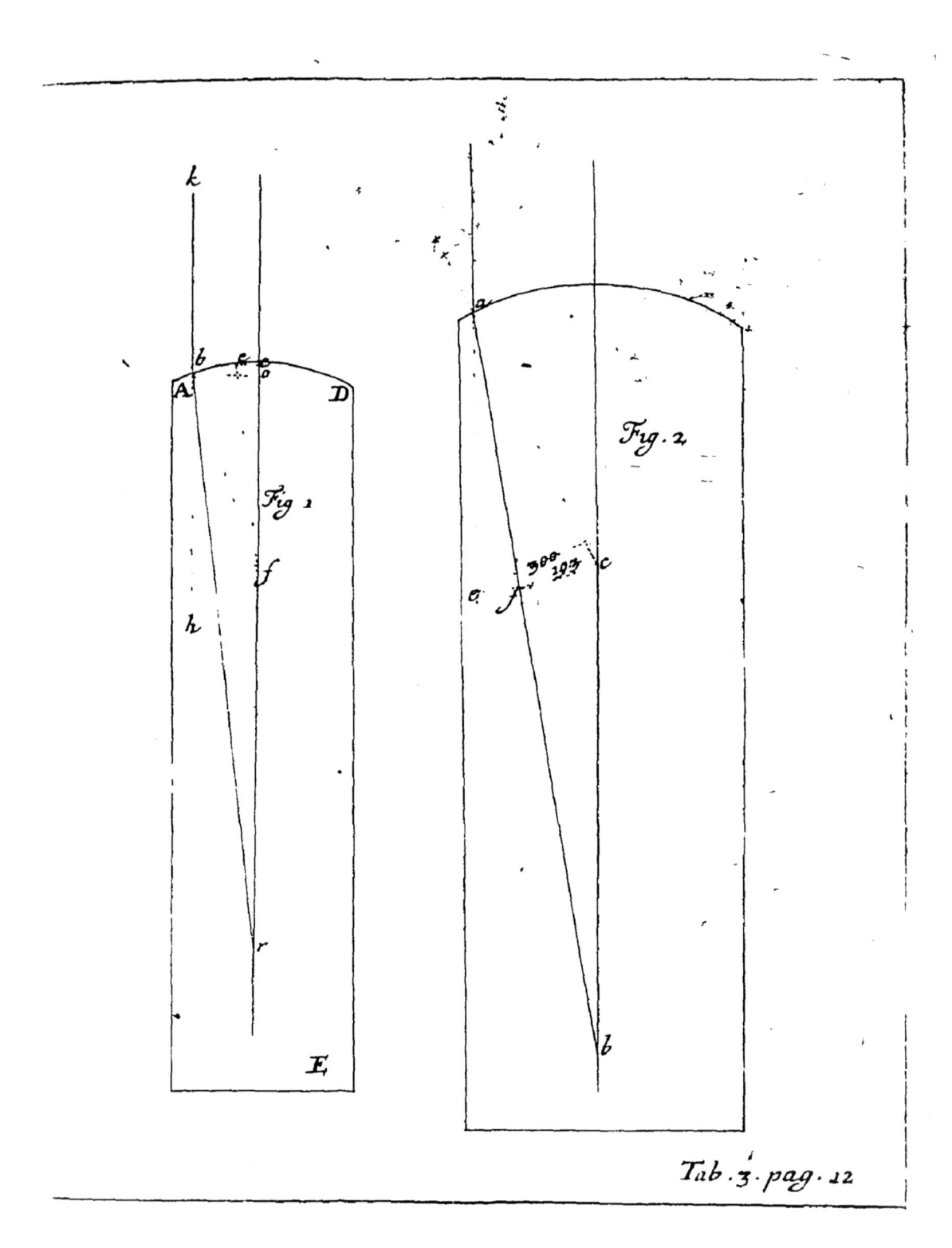

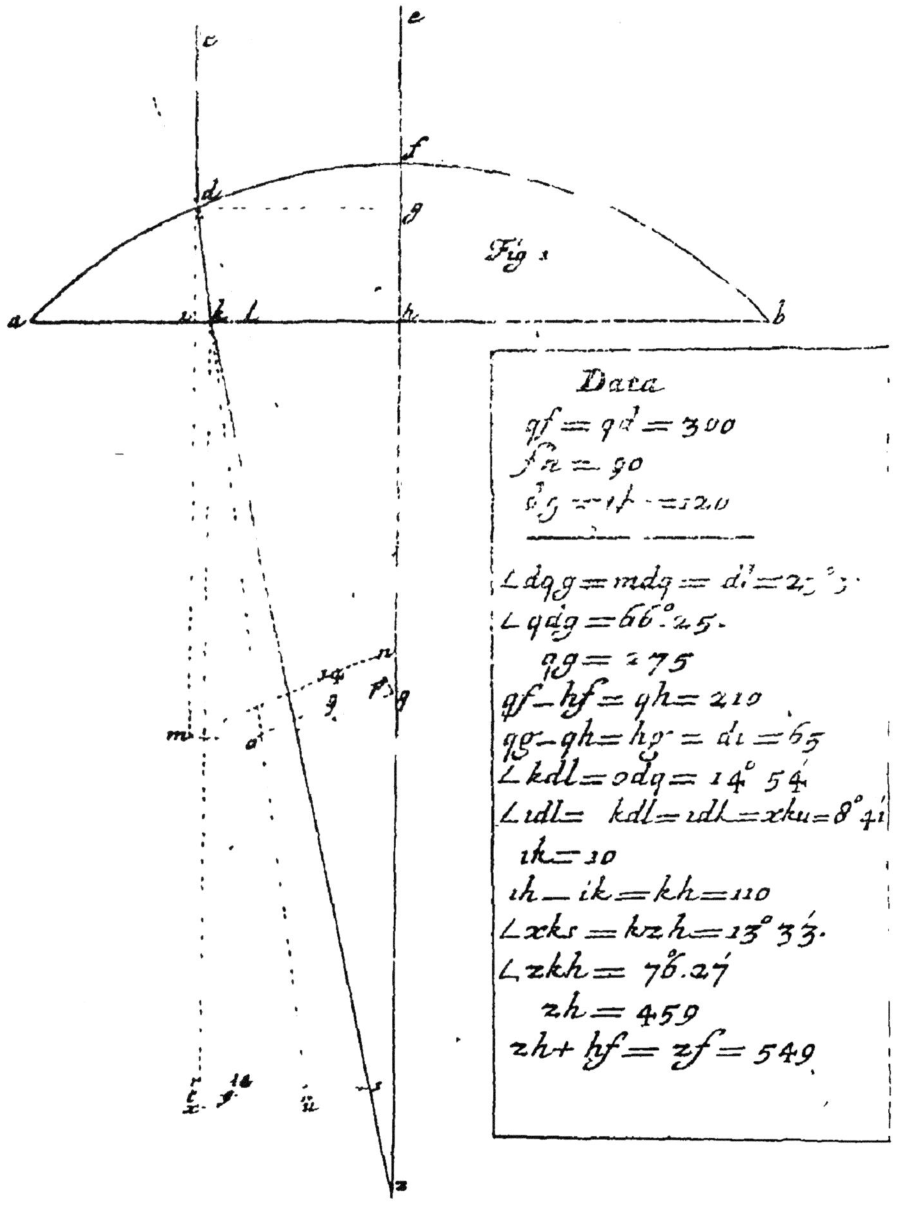

Data

$qf = qd = 300$
$fn = 90$
$dg = if = 120$

$\angle dqg = mdq = di = 25°3'$
$\angle qdg = 66°25'$
$qg = 275$
$qf - hf = qh = 210$
$qg - qh = hg = di = 65$
$\angle kdl = odq = 14°54'$
$\angle idl = kdl = idl = xku = 8°41'$
$ik = 10$
$ih - ik = kh = 110$
$\angle xks = kzh = 13°33'$
$\angle zkh = 76°27'$
$zh = 459$
$zh + hf = zf = 549$

Fig 1

Tab 4 pag 13

[23]

When a Ray falls on a Spherick Glass, and afterwards it being but once refracted, crosses the Axis. It shall be, as the Sine of the Angle of Refraction : to the Sine of the Angle of Inclination :: so the Radius of the Glass's Sphere . to the refracted Ray.

Tab. 3. *Fig.* 1. Let bec be the Convex Surface of the Glass ADE, kb a Ray of Light, f the Centre of the Convexity, bfc the Angle of Inclination, bo the Sine of the Inclination, br the refracted Ray meeting the Axis in r, $bbr=brc=$ to the Angle of Refraction; draw fe parallel to br, then efc is equal to brc, and ec is the Sine of the Angle of Refraction. And by reason of the similar Triangles bro, efc, it shall be $ec . bo . : ef : br$. Which was to be demonstrated. Ta.3 F. 1.

Wherefore supposing that from Air to Glass, the Sine of the Angle of Inclination : be to the Sine of the refracted Angle :: as 300 : to 193 : then the Sine of the Inclination shall be : to the Sine of the Angle of Refraction :: as 300 : to 300 — 193 = 107. Because the Angle of Refraction is equal to the difference between the Angle of Inclination and the refracted Angle. And Sines and Angles being (in these small Angles) proportional. It shall be, As 107 : 300 :: so Radius of the Convexity : to the Concourse of the refracted Ray with the Axis.

It shall also be, As 107 : 193 :: so the Radius of the Convexity : to the Concourse of the refracted Ray beyond the Centre of the Sphere.

For *Tab.* 3. *Fig.* 2. 1 | $eac : fac :: 300 : 193$ Ta 3 Fi 2.
Dividing the First 2 | $eac - fac : fac :: 300 - 193 : 193$
That is   3 | $eaf . fac :. 107 \; 193$
    Moreover,   4 | $eaf = fbc =$ Angle of Refraction.
From 3 and 4   5 | $fbc . fac :: 107 : 193$
But in the △ abc 6 | $fbc : fac ::$ Rad.$= ac : cb$
From 5 and 6   7 | $107 . 193 :: ac : cb =$ To the Concourse of the Ray beyond the Centre of the Sphere c. Which was to be demonstrated.

PROB.

Prop. II. Probl.

A Plano-Convex Glass a f b *Tab.* 4. *Fig.* 1. *being exposed to a distant Object with its Convex side towards it, and receiving the Ray* c d *parallel to the Axis* e z, *'tis required to determin the Point of Concourse* z, *from these Data,* f h *the Glasses thickness,* q f *the Radius of the Convexity, and* d g *the distance of the Ray* c d *from the Axis* e z.

The same Problem is proposed from the same *Data,* for the plane Side towards the Object.

But first for the Convex-Side to the Object: The Mechanical Construction is thus, *Tab.* 4. *Fig.* 1. Produce the Ray c d through the Glass at pleasure to m. And from d the Point of Incidence draw the Line d q to the Centre of the Convexity; this is the Perpendicular, and the Angle q d m the Incidence or Inclination. On d as a Centre at any distance strike the Arch m o q, in which make m n the Sine of the Angle of Incidence, to o p the Sine of the refracted Angle, as 14 to 9 (or o p 9 such parts as m n is 14, which is easily done by the Sector) the Line d k o shall be the Line in which the Ray would proceed, if the Medium of Glass were continued so far.

But because in this Line at k the Ray emerges from the plain Surface of the Glass a dense Medium into Air a rare Medium, from k raise k x perpendicular to the plain Surface a h b, and on k, as a Centre at any distance strike the Arch x u s, then the Angle x k u is the Incidence of the Ray passing from Glass to Air.

Making therefore t u the Sine of this Angle, to r s the Sine of the second refracted Angle from the Perpendicular as 9 to 14, the Line drawn from k through the Point s, and produced to the Axis at z, shews the Progress of the Ray in the Air after its Emersion from Glass: Wherefore the Point z is determined in the Axis.

Trigo-

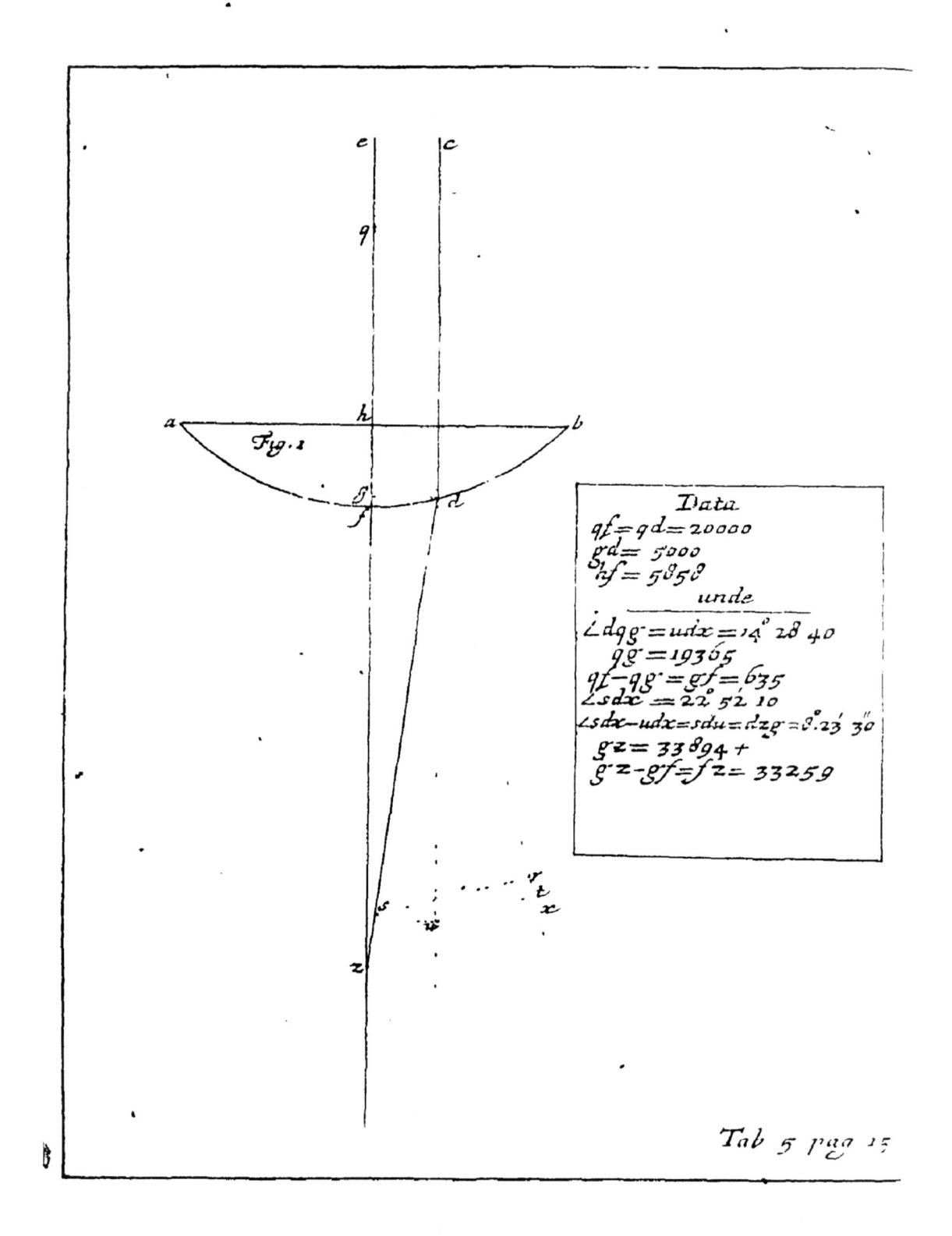

Fig. 1

Data
$qf = qd = 20000$
$gd = 5000$
$hf = 5858$

unde

$\angle dqg = udx = 14° 28' 40''$
$qg = 19365$
$qf - qg = gf = 635$
$\angle sdx = 22° 52' 10''$
$\angle sdx - udx = sdu = dzg = 8° 23' 30''$
$gz = 33894 +$
$gz - gf = fz = 33259$

Tab 5 pag 15

Trigonometrical Calculation.

But this Point z, or the Measure of the Line fz may be found more accurately by Calculation thus. In the Triangle qdg Right Angled at g are given qd and dg, to find the Angle of Incidence dqg, and the Side qg. Then $qf - hf = qh$, and $qg - qh = hg = di$.

First then, because the Ray passes at d from a rare Medium into a dense, it shall be refracted towards the Perpendicular dq. Wherefore the Analogy is, As $14 : $ to $9 :: $ so the Sine of the Angle of Incidence dqf ($= mdq$) : to the Sine of the refracted Angle odq (that is kdl). But mdq ($= idl$) $- kdl = idk = xku$, dm and kx being parallel :) And this is the Angle of Incidence as the Ray passes from Glass to Air.

Secondly, In the little Right Angled Triangle idk, the Side di, and the Angle idk are known, whence the Side ik may be found, then ih ($= dg$) $- ik = kh$.

Thirdly, Because at k the Ray emerges from a Dense into a Rare *Medium*, it shall be refracted from the Perpendicular kx; and the Analogy shall be, as $9 : $ to $14 :: $ so the Sine of the Angle of Incidence xku : to the Sine of the Second refracted Angle xks ($= hzh$, kx, and hz being Parallel.)

Fourthly, In the Right Angled Triangle khz, the Side kh, and all the Angles are known, whence the Side hz, and consequently fz ($= fh + hz$) the Distance of the Point of Concourse from the Pole of the Glass f is discovered.

When the plain Side is turned to the Object, the Method is the same, only shorter, for *Tab.* 5. *Fig.* 1. in the Right Angled Triangle qdg, we have qd and dg to find $dqg = udx$, the Incidence, and the Side qg: Then $qf - qg = gf$. Next, As 9 . to 14 : (or as 193 to 300 ::) so the Sine of udx : to the

[16]

Ta.4.F.1 the Sine of sdx. But $sdx - udx = sdu = dzg$. Then in the Right Angled Triangle dzg we have dg, and the Angles to find gz. And $gz - gf = fz$. Which was to be found.

Scholium.

In the little Tables inserted in *Tab.* 4. and *Tab.* 5. I have given Examples at large of the Calculation of the Progress of the Ray cd, which I presume is pretty truly wrought: But if perhaps any Errors do intervene, they are easily corrected.

By these Tables we may perceive, that the Point of Concourse z is distant from the Pole of the Glass f about a Diameter of the Convexity, but not fully so much.

'Tis also to be noted in *Tab.* 4. *Fig.* 1. That the Point of Concourse z, shall be less or more removed from the Pole f, according as we give the Glass less or more thickness. For 'tis manifest, that the farther we let the Ray run in the *Medium* of Glass, after it enters it at d, before it emerges into Air at k, the farther the Point of Concourse z shall be protracted from *Ta.6.F.1* f. For we may imagin the *Medium* of Glass continued below the Diameter of the Convexity, and then 'tis evident that the Point of Concourse z shall be much more below it. But it can be no more below it than a Diameter and half. By the First Proposition hereof.

This our Second Proposition is usually found in Dioptricks thus expressed and demonstrated.

Parallel Rays falling on a Plano-Convex-Glass, are united with the Axis about the distance of a Diameter of the Convexity from the Pole of the Glass, if the Segment be but 30 *Degrees.*

Demon-

Tab 6 pag. 16

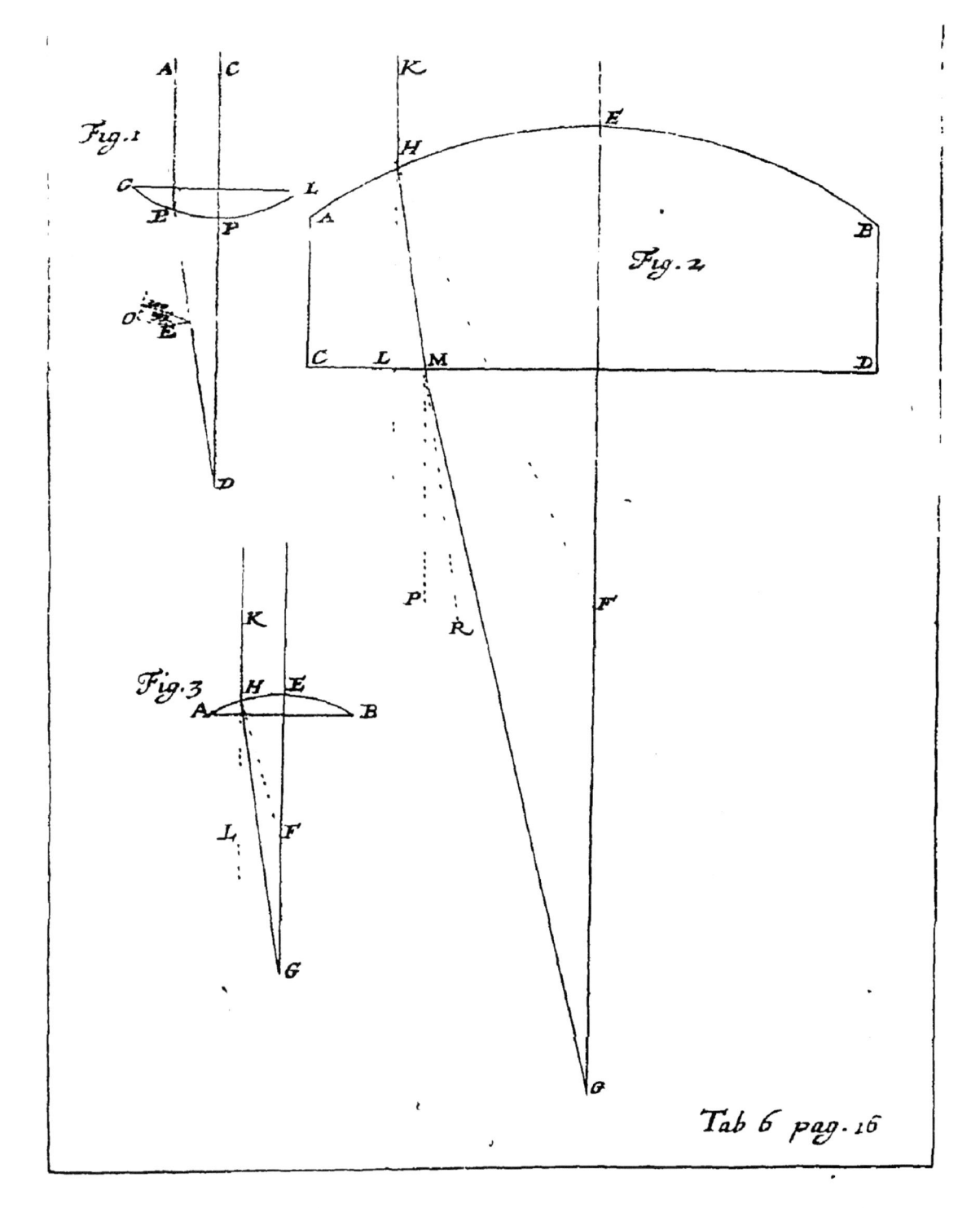

Demonstration.

First for the plain Side towards the Object. *Tab.*6. *Fig.*1. A B is a Ray of Light falling on the Glass G L parallel to the Axis C D. C is the Centre of the Convexity G P L. Joyn C B; the Angle of Incidence or Inclination is B C D, the Angle of Refraction is E B D or B D C

Wherefore in the Triangle B C D, the Angle B C D being double the Angle B D C (For by *Kepler*'s Experiments, which are follow'd by most Authors, from Glass to Air, the Angle of Incidence : is to the Angle of Refraction :: as 2 : to 1.) the Side B D shall be double the Side B C; the Angles and Sides or Sines under 15 Degrees being proportional; but D P is almost equal to B D (for the Thickness and Breadth of the Glass, in Optick Glasses especially in Glasses of Long *Foci*, are inconsiderable), therefore D P is double C P. *Which was to be Demonstrated.*

Secondly, for the Convex-side towards the Object. *Tab.*6. *Fig.*2. A B C D is a Plano-Convex Glass (I have here expressed it of this thickness, to shew the Angles and Progress of the Ray more plainly, tho really this great Thickness hinders the Exactness of the Demonstration; for the Glass is to be supposed of the most inconsiderable Thickness) F is the Centre of the Convexity. K H is a Ray falling thereon, parallel to the Axis E G. This Ray, (after it has suffered a Double Refraction, one at its Ingress from Air into Glass at H towards the Perpendicular H F, by which it becomes the Refracted Ray H M, and another Refraction at its Egress from Glass to Air at M from the Perpendicular P M, by which, instead of going forward towards R, it becomes the Refracted Ray M G) at G crosses the Axis, so that G E is the Diameter of the Convexity A E B.

For the Incidence or Inclination of the Ray K H is L H F, of which Angle there is taken off ⅓ L H M, for the Angle of Refraction from Air to Glass is ⅓ of the Incidence (by *Exper.* 4.) If therefore the Ray had proceeded onwards in Glass towards R, it had crossed the Axis at a Diameter and half (by the foregoing Proposition), but at its egress into Air at M, it is again refracted from the Perpendicular P M by the Angle R M G = ¼ P M R. The Angle of Refraction R M G from Glass to Air, being ¼ the Incidence P M R (by *Exper.* 5.) But P M R is equal to L H M. Wherefore the first Angle of Incidence LHF by this Double Refraction, has lost first ⅓ of it self L H M, and again ¼ of this Third R M G. But ⅓ and ¼ of ½ is equal to ½, wherefore the Angle of Incidence is diminished by its Half.

Ta.6.F.3. Let us therefore consider the Glass A B, *Tab. 6. Fig. 3.* without respect to its Thickness, or to the Refraction the Ray suffers at its egress on the lower side of the Glass into Air. But let us imagin, that by the first Refraction, the Ray were brought nigher the Perpendicular H F by half the Angle of Incidence L H F, and we shall find, that then the Ray shall cross the Axis at G, so that G E shall be the Diameter of the Convexity. For L H G or G H F is equal to ½ L H F or HFE the Incidence; but H F E is equal to G H F + H G F (32. 1. *Eucl.*) therefore G H F and H G F are equal, each of them being ½ H F E, and consequently their opposite Sides H F and G F are equal. Wherefore G E is the Diameter of the Convexity A E B. *Which was to be Demonstrated.*

Corollary.

In Plano-Convex Glasses, As 300 — 193 = 107 : To 193 :: So Radius of the Convexity · To the refracted Ray taken to its Concourse with the Axis; which in Glasses of large Spheres and small Segments is almost equal to the Distance of the Focus taken in the Axis. *Tab. 6. Fig. 1.*

Tab. 7

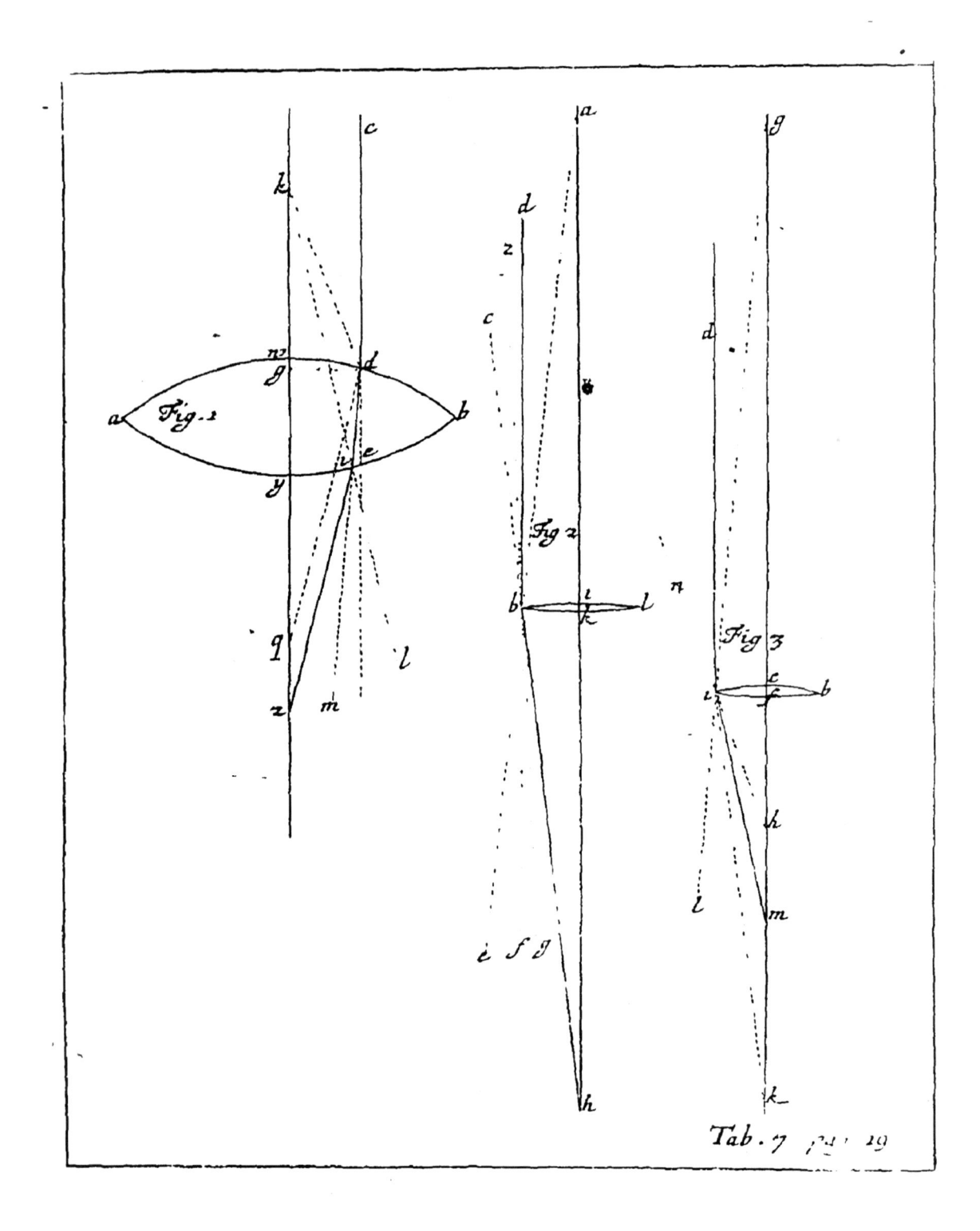

Demonstration.

The Inclination = A B C = O B E = B C D = 19;.
Refracted Angle = O B D = ;oo
Angle of Refraction = E B D = B D P = O B D — O B E
= ;oo — 19; = 107.

In the △ BDC : s ∠BDC : s ∠BCD :: Rad. = BC : BD.

That is,

107 : 19; ∵ : BC : BD = PD in Glasses of large Spheres. *Which was to be Demonstrated.*

PORP. III. PROBL.

In a Double Convex-Glass a b, *Tab.* 7. *Fig.* 1. *of equal or unequal Convexities, Let the Centres of the Spherical Surfaces be* k *and* q, c d *a Ray falling parallel to the Axis* k q z, *and being Refracted at its Ingress at* d, *and at its Egress at* i; *'Tis required to determin the Point of its Concourse with the Axis at* z, *from these Data, the Radii* k y, q w, *of the Convexities, and* g d *the Distance of the Point of Incidence from the Axis.*

This is so easily done by Scale and Compass from what foregoes, that I shall not insist on a farther Explication thereof, but shall shew the more certain Method of tracing the Progress of this Ray by Calculation.

Produce c d directly to e, and d i to m. We have k y + q w — w y = k q.

First therefore in the Right-angled Triangle q d g, g d and q d being given, we may find the ∠ g q d = q d e and the side q g. Then k q — q g = k g.

Secondly, In the Right-angled Triangle k g d, there being given k g and g d, we may have the ∠ g k d = k d c, and the side k d.

Thirdly,

Thirdly, As $300 : \text{to } 193 :: \text{ so } S. \angle qde : \text{to } S. \angle qdi$.

Fourthly, $qde - qdi = edi$. And $180° - kdc - edi = kdi$.

Fifthly, In the Triangle kdi, the Angle kdi and the Sides ki, kd, being known, we have the Angle $kid = mil$. And the Angle ikd. Then $gkd - ikd = qki$.

Sixthly, As $193 : \text{to } 300 :: \text{ so } S. \angle kid . \text{to } S. \angle zil$, then $zil - qki = kzi$.

Lastly, In the Triangle zki, ki and all the Angles being known, we find kz, from which subtracting ky, there remains zy, which was required.

If by this Method we calculate the Progress of a Ray through a Double Convex-Glass of equal Convexities, and the Thickness of the Glass be little or nothing in comparison of the Radius of the Convexity; and the Distance of the Point of Incidence from the Axis be but small, we shall find the Point of Concourse to be distant from the Glass about the Radius of the Convexity nearly.

This our Third Proposition in most Dioptrick Writers is usually thus expressed.

Parallel Rays falling on a Double Convex-Glass of equal Convexities on both sides, are united with the Axis, about the Distance of the Radius of the Convexity from the Pole of the Glass, if the Segment be but 30 Degrees.

But their Demonstrations of this Proposition are usually perplexed enough, by reason of the smallness and multiplicity of Angles, which are expressed in their Figures, as also by the Thickness of the Glass, which they are forced to represent, and yet is to be neglected in their Demonstrations. I shall give as short a Demonstration as I can, after their Method, as follows.

Tab 7. Fig. 2. Let a be the Centre of the Convexity bkl, h the Centre of the Convexity bil, db a Ray of Light produced directly to f parallel to the Axis ah. abe is a Right Line, and hbc is a Right Line. The first Angle of Inclination

tion is $cbd = bbf = ebf$, and the perpendicular is bb. By the first Refraction the Ray is deflected from its straight course bf and becomes bg, approaching the perpendicular bh by the Angle fbg, which is $\frac{1}{3}$ of the Inclination ebf. Produce gb directly to z. Now the Angle of Incidence on the lower Convexity bkl from Glass to Air is $abz = ebg$, and the Perpendicular is ab or be: Wherefore the Ray instead of going forwards in bg is now, by its Emersion into Air, refracted from the Perpendicular be, by the Angle gbh, which is therefore to be equal to $_2$ the second Angle of Incidence ebg. by Exper. 5. and that gbh is equal to $\frac{1}{3} ebg$, I thus demonstrate;

By the Supposals in the Prop. and Common Geometry.	1. $ebf = fbh$
By the Fig. — — — — —	2. $gbh = fbh - fbg$
From 1 and 2 — — — —	3. $gbh = ebf - fbg$
Doct. Refract. Exper. 4. — —	4. $fbg = \frac{1}{3} efb$
From 3 and 4 — — —	5. $gbh = ebf - \frac{1}{3} ebf = \frac{2}{3} ebf$
Moreover by the Scheme —	6. $\frac{1}{2} ebg = \frac{1}{2} ebf + \frac{1}{2} fbg$
4 ÷ 2 ———————	7. $\frac{1}{2} fbg = \frac{1}{6} ebf$
From 6 and 7 — — —	8. $\frac{1}{2} ebg = \frac{1}{2} ebf + \frac{1}{6} ebf = \frac{2}{3} ebf$
From 5 and 8 ———————	9. $gbh = \frac{1}{2} ebg$
	Which was to be Demonst.

Therefore it follows that the Ray by this second Refraction proceeds in hh, crossing the Axis in h the Centre of the Convexity. *Which was to be demonstrated.*

See the Demonstrations of this Proposition *Kepleri* Dioptri. Prop. 39 *Herigon.* Prop. 15. *Dechales* Pr. 21. lib. 13. *Hon. Faber* Prop. 43. Sec 8. *Cherubin de Orleans la Dioptr. Oculair,* Prop. 2. *Zahn Telescop.* Fund 2. Syntag. 1. Cap. 4. Prop. 8.

Of Glasses of unequal Convexities.

As for double Convex Glasses of unequal Spheres on each Side, the foregoing Method of Calculation determines the Point

[22]

of Concourse exactly in them also: But the shorter Rule laid down by most Optick Writers, is this.

As the Sum of the Radii of both Convexities : to the Radius of either Convexity :: So the double Radius of the other Convexity : to the Distance of the Focus. Vid. Corol. Pr. 16.

Demonstration.

T. 7 F 3.   T. 7. F. 3. Let the Axis of the Glass ib be gk, di a Ray of Light Parallel thereto, g the Centre of the Convexity ifb, h the Centre of the Convexity icb, gil and hin are right Lines. The first Angle of Inclination is $din = ihc$, and by the first Refraction the Ray is deflected into ik, crossing the Axis in k, so that kc is equal to $3cb$. The second Angle of Incidence from Glass to Air on the Surface ifb is the Angle lik : I say kim being made $\frac{1}{2}$ of lik, the Ray crosses the Axis in m, and it shall then be (according to the Rule) $gh : 2fg :: cb : mc$. Which I thus Demonstrate.

In the △ kim	1	$\angle kim : \angle k \cdot km : mi = mf$ in large Spheres.
Double the Antecedents	2	$2 \angle kim = lik : \angle k :: 2km : mf :: km : \frac{1}{2}mf = \frac{1}{2}mc:$
Divide the second Step.	3	$\angle lik - \angle k = \angle g . \angle k :: km - \frac{1}{2}mc : \frac{1}{2}mc.$
Then in △ gik it shall be	4	$\angle g : \angle k :: ik = kc : ig = fg.$
From 3 and 4	5	$kc : fg :: km - \frac{1}{2}mc \cdot \frac{1}{2}mc$
Compound the 5th.	6	$kc + fg : fg :: km : \frac{1}{2}mc$
Double the Consequents	7	$kc + fg \cdot 2fg :: km \cdot mc.$
Compound the 7th.	8	$kc + 3fg \cdot 2fg :: km + mc = kc = 3cb : mc$
That is otherwise	9	$3cb + 3fg : 2fg :: 3cb \cdot mc.$
Divide the Ant. by 3.	10	$cb + fg = gb : 2fg :: cb : mc.$

Which was to be Demonstrated.

Vid. *Cherubin* Dioptr. Ocul. pag. 61, 62. Hon. *Faber* Synop. Opt. Prop. 43. Sec. 8, 9. *Dechales* Prop. 23, 24. *Zahn* Telescop. Fund. 2. Cap. 9. Prop. 38.

But

Tab 8 pag 23

[23]

But this Rule will need but little farther Demonſtration, if we conſider, that it holds even in double Convexes of equal Convexities; for in them, as the Sum of the Radii of both Convexities: to the Radius of the Convexity :: ſo the double Radius of the Convexity: to the Diſtance of the Focus. And 'tis the ſame in Glaſſes of unequal Convexities, for theſe refract in the ſame Proportion to their Curvities as the other.

Wherefore from theſe three foregoing Propoſitions we lay theſe down as General Rules, *That the Point of Convergency for Parallel Rays falling on a Plano Convex-Glaſs, is diſtant about the Diameter of the Convexity. On a double Convex of equal Convexities, 'tis about the ſemi-Diameter of the Convexity. And on a Double Convex of unequal Convexities, the Rule for finding it is what we have laid down before.*

Scholium.

Before I proceed, it will be requiſite here to note, *That the Rays which fall nigher the Axis are not united thereto ſo near the Pole of the Glaſs, as thoſe that fall farther from it*; and the difference of the Points of Concourſe is not ſo great, when the Convex ſide of a Plano-Convex Glaſs is turned to the Object, as when the Plain ſide is towards the Object.

For this obſerve *Tab.* 8. *F.* 1, 2, 3. in each of which, the Radius of the Convexity *c v* is 2 Inches, or 20000 Parts (an Inch being 10000 Parts) the Arch *r v r* in the firſt and ſecond Figures is a Quadrant, and conſequently the Thickneſs of the Glaſs *v z* in each is 5858, being the verſed Sine of 45° to the Radius 20000. But in the double Convex *Fig.* 3. the thickneſs of the Glaſs *v z* is ⅘ of an Inch or 8000 ſuch Parts *a b* in each is a Ray falling on the Glaſs Parallel to the Axis *c v*, at the diſtance of ⅒ of an Inch or 1000 ſuch Parts as *c v* is 20000 *d e* a like Ray falling ½ or ½ of an Inch, or 5000 ſuch

Ta 8 F, 1, 2, 3.

Parts

Parts diſtant from the Axis, *i* is the Point wherein the Ray *a b* meets the Axis, *b* the point in which *d e* croſſes the Axis. Here I call *b i the Depth of the Focus*, which we ſee is greater in the ſecond Figure, wherein the plain ſide is towards the Object, than in the firſt *Fig.* wherein the Convex Surface is towards the Object. For Proof of this, let the Angles of Incidence be to the refracted Angle (according to *Kepler*) as 3 to 2, Expreſſed in the firſt Column of the following Table; or let the Sines of the Incidence be to the Sines of the refracted Angles, as 300 to 193 (according to Mr. *Newton*) as is expreſſed in the ſecond Column of the Table. Then by the foregoing Method of Calculation, delivered in the ſecond and third Propoſitions, we ſhall find as in the following Table.

	1ſt. Column. 3 : 2 . Inclin Ref.	2d. Column. 300:193 Inc Ref.
For the Plano-Convex with the Convex Side to the Object Tab. 8. Fig. 1.	$v\,i = 4.1930$ $v\,b = 4.1230$ $b\,i = 700$	$v\,i = 3.4762$ $v\,b = 3.4112$ $b\,i = 650$
For the Plano-Convex with the plain ſide to the Object Tab. 8. Fig. 2.	$v\,i = 3.9910$ $v\,b = 3.7140$ $b\,i = 2770$	$v\,i = 3.5957$ $v\,b = 3.3259$ $b\,i = 2698$
For the Double Convex of equal Convexities Tab. 8. Fig. 3.	$v\,i = 1.841$ $v\,b = 1.685$ $b\,i = 156$	$v\,i = 1.762$ $v\,b = 1.653$ $b\,i = 109$

From this Table 'tis manifeſt, firſt that the Ray *a b*, which falls nigher the Axis *v c*, is not united thereto ſo near the Pole of the Glaſs *v*, as the Ray *d e*, which falls farther from the Axis; for *a b* is united to the Axis at the Diſtance *v i*, and *d e* is united to the Axis at the Diſtance *v b*, but *v i* is greater than *v b*.

Secondly,

Tab. 9 pag. 25

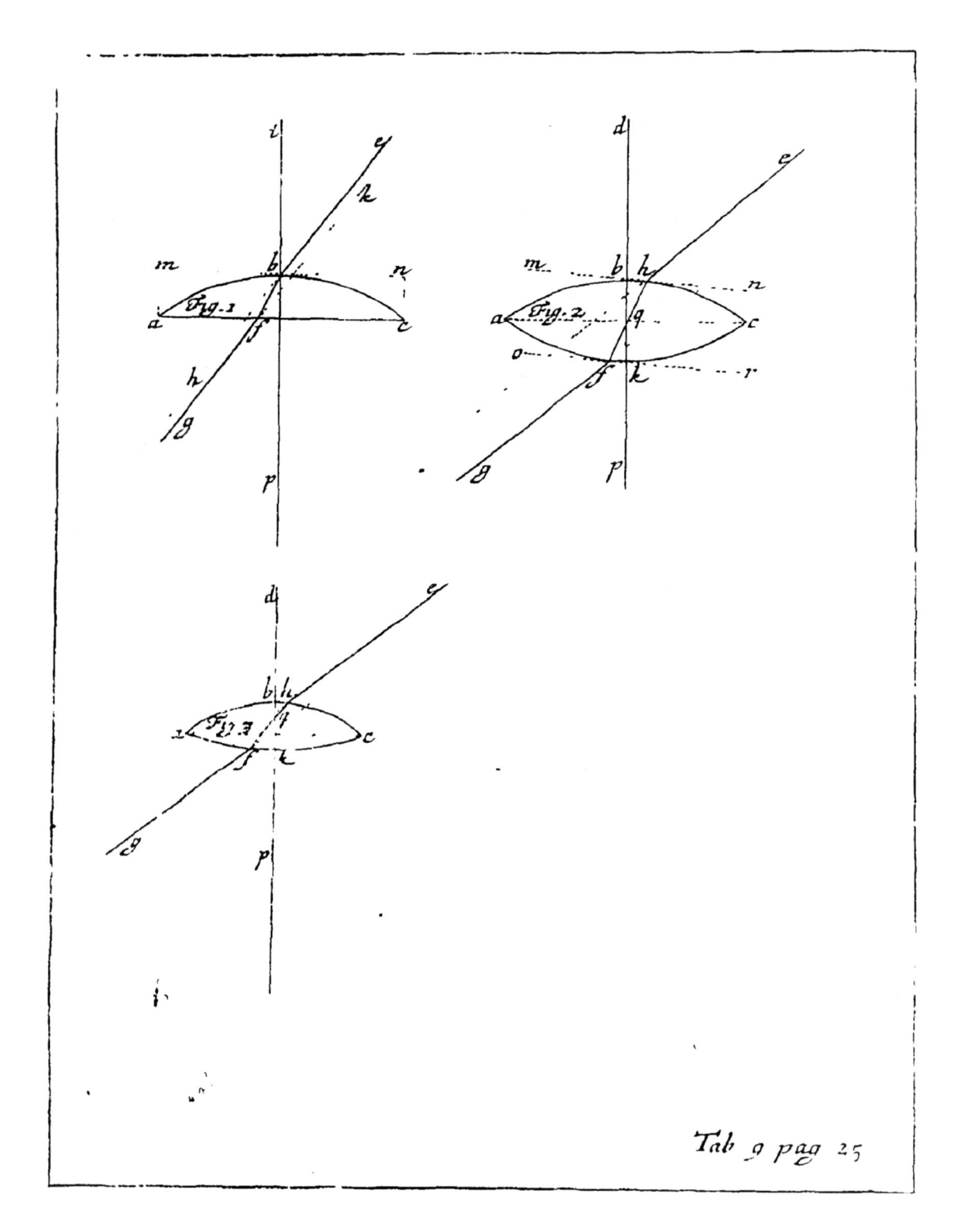

Secondly, 'Tis evident that the *Focal Depth h i* is not so great in a Plano-Convex Glass, when the Convex Side is towards the Object, as in *Fig. 1. Tab. 8.* as when the plain Side is towards the Object, as in *Fig. 2. Tab. 8.* for by the Table *h i* is in the former but 650, but in the latter posture 'tis 2691, that is more than four times greater.

Whence I deduce this, that in viewing an Object by a Plano-Convex Glass, 'tis best turning the Spherical Side to the Object, and so likewise for burning by such a Glass, 'tis best turning the Convex Side towards the Sun.

OF OBLIQUE RAYS.

Premises to the Fourth Proposition.

Hitherto I have consider'd only the *Direct* Rays. I come now to the Consideration of *Oblique* Rays: And for this we must have Recourse to our foregoing 13th. and 17th. Definitions; as also to the first and second Experiments: By the 13th Definition, we know what *Oblique* Rays are: And by the 17th Definition, we learn that in every Parcel of *Oblique* Rays, flowing from the same Point of an Object upon a Glass; there is one certain Ray, which may be called the *Axis*, and that this *Axis* is as it were not at all refracted. But for a farther Declaration hereof, *Tab. 9. Fig. 1.* Let *a b c* be a Plano Convex Glass, with the Convex Side towards the Object, *d b* the Axis of the *Direct* Cone of Rays, *e b* a Ray of the *Oblique* Cone, falling on the Vertex of the Glass at *b*, I say, this is the Axis of an *Oblique* Cone, and after its Double Refraction; first at its Ingress at *b*, and then at its Egress at *f*, it becomes *f g* Parallel to *e b*. This is Evident, if we imagine the Ray *e b* to fall on the Plane Glass *a m n c*, for 'tis refracted the same way in one Case as in t'other. Wherefore the Ray *e b f g*, is as it were strait, as *e b h* or *k f g*, so

Ta 9. F. 1.

E   likewise

likewise we may imagine the Plane Side of this same Glass *a c* turn'd towards the Object, then *p b d* is the Axis of the *Direct* Cone, and *g f* the Axis of an *Oblique* Cone. We see therefore that a Plano-Convex Glass, being exposed with its *Convex Side* to the Object, the Rays that fall from the several Points of the Object, whose *Ingress* is at the Glasses *vertex b*, are the *Axes* of the respective Cones. But the *Plane Side* being towards the Object, the Rays from the several Points, which have their *Egress* at the Glasses *vertex b*, are the Axes of the respective Cones. And that amongst the Infinite Rays that proceed from a *Collateral* Point of an Object, and form an *Oblique* Cone, falling on the Plano-Convex Glass, there is some one certain Ray, that falls on the Vertex, and has its *Ingress* at *b*, Or (if the Plane Side be towards the Object) has its Emersion at *b*, is manifest from this Reason only, that the Rays compounding such a Cone, are spread over the *Whole* surface of the Glass, and are as it were *Infinite* or *Indefinite*.

Ta 9 F 2   In like manner, *Tab. 9. Fig. 2. a b c k* is a Double Convex of Equal Convexities, *d b k p* the Axis of the *Direct* Cone of Rays, *e h* a Ray of an Oblique Cone, which at its Ingress at *h* is refracted into *h f*, in such manner that it makes the Arches *b h*, *k f*, equal, then at its egress it becomes *f g*, Parallel again to *e h*, as if it had not been at all refracted, but had passed directly forward, or through a Plane Glass. This also will be manifest, if at the Point of Incidence *h*, and at the Point of Emersion *f*, we draw the Tangents *m n*, *o r*, for these Tangents are Parallel when *h b* and *f k* are equal Arches; and the Ray *e h* is no otherwise refracted by the Convex Glass, than if it had fallen on the Plane Glass *m n o r*.

And that amongst the Infinite Rays that proceed from a Collateral Point of an Object, and form an *Oblique* Cone, falling on the Double Convex *a b c k*, there is some one certain Ray, that has its Incidence so, that after its Refraction at

its

its Ingress, it may proceed so in the Glass, as to cut off equal Arches *b h*, *k f*, may be easily conceived; because the whole surface of the Glass is occupy'd by each Cone from each Point; so that the Point *h* (for instance) cannot miss of having amongst the rest its Ray, which must necessarily be so refracted.

What has been said concerning a Double Convex of Equal Convexities *Tab.* 9. *Fig.* 2. may be accommodated to a Double Convex of unequal Convexities *Tab.* 9. *Fig.* 3. For as in *Fig.* 2. the Arches *b h*, *k f*, are to be equal (the Convexities being Equal) so in *Fig.* 3. the Arches *b h*, *k f*, are to be *Similar*, that is to say, *b h* is to be as many degrees of its Circumference, as *k f* is of its Circumference. Thus suppose in the same *Fig.* 3. The Arch *a b c* to be struck with a Radius of two Inches, and the Arch *a k c* to be struck with the Radius 4 Inches; these Radii being to each other as 2 to 1, *k f* must be to *b h* as 2 to 1, for then they shall be of equal degrees, each in its own respective Circumference, for here likewise in this third *Fig.* the Tangents at *h* and *f*, run Parallel to each other. *Ta 9 F. 3.*

The Axes of all the Radious Cones, falling on a Plano-Convex with its Convex Side to the Object, Cross each other in the Vertex of the Convex surface, at their *Ingress* into the Glass, as in *Tab.* 9. *Fig.* 1. at *b*, but if the Plane Side be turned towards the Object, they Cross in the Vertex of the Convex surface at their *Egress* from the Glass, as in the same *Fig.* 1. at *b*. *Ta 9 F. 1*

The Axes of all the Radious Cones, falling on a Double Convex of Equal Convexities, Cross each other in the Middle or Centre of the Glasses Axis. Thus in *Tab.* 9. *Fig.* 2. *d b p* is the Line, which produced, would pass through the Centres of the two Convex surfaces; this Line I call the *Axis of the Glass*, let *b q* be equal to *k q*, then *q* is the Point *Ta 9 F. 2.*

E 2 wherein

[28]

wherein the Axes of all the Radious Cones Cross each other.

The Axes of all the Radious Cones, falling on a Double Convex of unequal Convexities, Cross each other in a Point within the Glass in its Axis, which divides the said Axis in the Proportion, that the Radius of one Convexity has to the Radius of t'other. *Tab. 9. Fig. 3.* Let the Radius of the Convexity *a k c* be to the Radius of the Convexity *a b c*, as 2 to 1. Let *b k* the Axis of the Glass be divided in *q*, so that *k q* may be to *b q* as 2 to 1, then *q* is the Point wherein the Axes of all the Radious Cones Cross each other.

Ta 9 F 3

The same may be understood of Concave Glasses.

And this is sufficient for explaining what I mean by the *Axis of an Oblique Cone of Rays*.

I come now to the Fourth Proposition.

PROP. IV.

The Parallel Rays that proceed from each Collateral Point of an Object, and fall Obliquely on a Glass, are united with their Axis at the same Distance, as the Direct Parallel Rays are united with their Axis, viz. By a Plano Convex about the Distance of the Diameter, by a Double Equal Convex about the Distance of the Radius; and by a Double Unequal Convex, as is before determin'd.

I have hitherto proposed the Properties of Glasses Problematically, to be Demonstrated or rather traced out by a Geometrical Calculation of the Rays Progress. This Method, as 'tis the most Artificial, so 'tis the most Legitimate and Exact, and *wholly New* and *Distinct from that of other Optick Writers.* I shall first observe the same Method in this Proposition, proposing it Problematically thus, *Tab. 10. Fig. 1. e f c* is a Plano Convex Glass, with the Convex Side towards the Object.

Tab 10 Fig 1

Let

Tab. 10 pag. 28

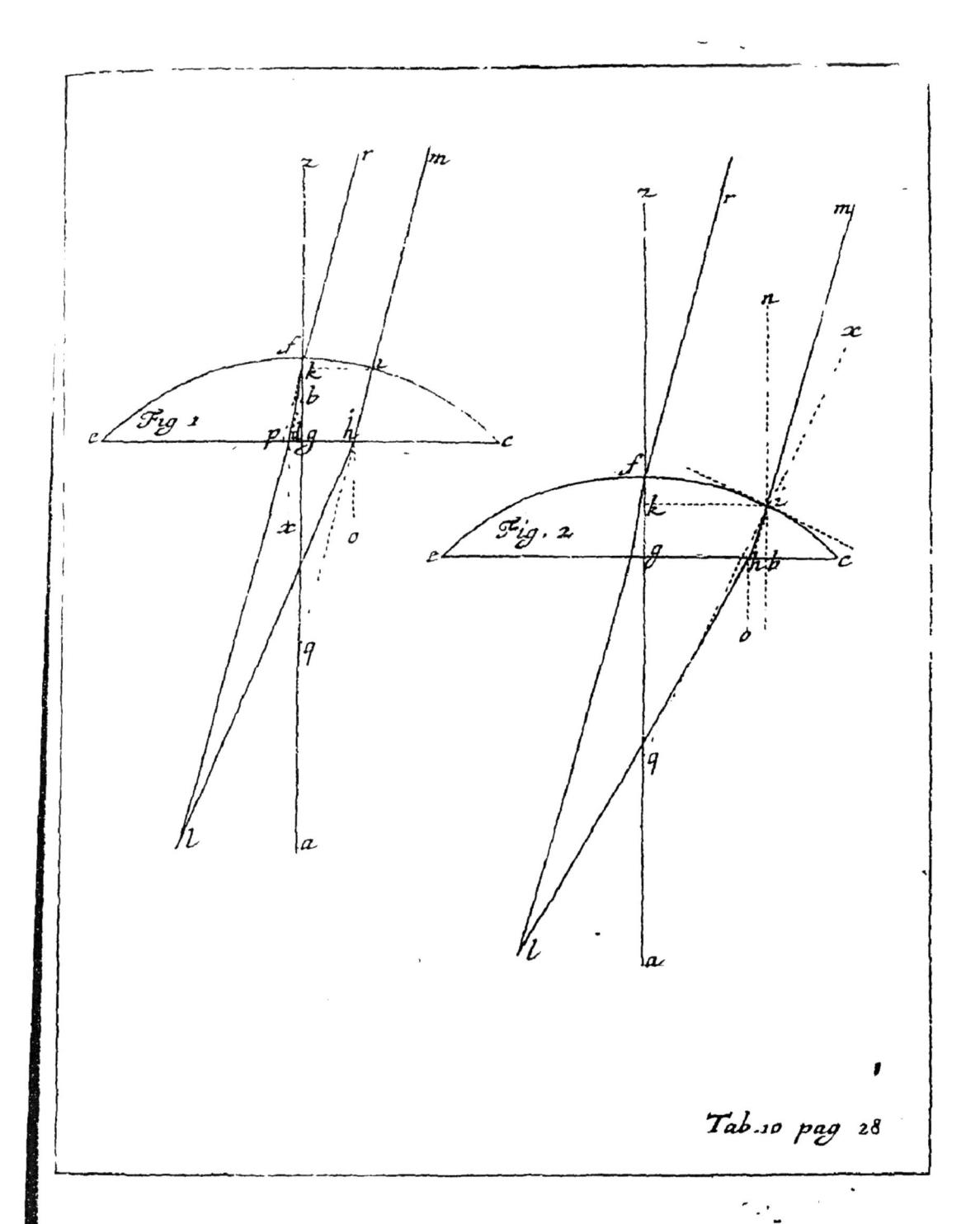

[29]

Let there be given qf the Radius of the Convexity (as in the Table after the foregoing *Scholium*) 20000, and fg the Glasses thickness 5858, $zfqa$ is the Axis of the Glass it self, or of the Direct Cone of *Rays*, the Point of whose Concourse is in a, so that fa (as we have found in the foregoing Propositions) is 34112. Let rf be the Axis of an Oblique Cone of Rays, falling on the Vertex f, and making the Angle of Incidence rfz ($=xdl$) of any given Quantity (as in this Example suppose 14°. 28'. 40".) Let us suppose another Ray mi Parallel to rf, and its Point of Incidence i at such a Distance from the Axis zfa, that being produced directly forwards, it may pass through the Centre q of the Convexity; that is to say, let us suppose kqi to be equal to zfr. Thus I propose it for ease of Illustration, for the Calculation may as truly be performed by supposing the Ray mi at any other Distance, as I shall declare presently.

From these things given, 'tis required to find the Point l in the Axis, where the Ray mi crosses it. For the Discovery whereof we proceed thus.

Draw ik Perpendicular to zq, then in the Right-angled Triangle kqi, we have qi, and the Angle kqi to find kq and ki; then $qf - fg = qg$. And $kq \cdot ki :: qg \cdot gh$.

Produce rf to p, then in the Right-angled Triangle fgp, we have fg, and the Angle $gfp = rfz$ to find the Side pg; or thus, the Triangles gfp, gqh are Similar, then $gq \cdot gh .: gf : gp$. Say then, as 300 : to 193 :: so S. $\angle gfp$: to S. $\angle gfd$.

In the Right-angled Triangle fgd, we have fg, and the $\angle gfd$, to find the Side dg, then $dg + gh = dh$.

Draw ho and dx Perpendiculars to ec, say then, as 193 : to 300 :. so S. $\angle ohq = gqh$. to S $\angle ohl$. But $90° - ohl = dhl$. And $90° + xdl$ or $zfr = hdl$.

Lastly,

[30]

Lastly, In the Triangle bdl, we have the two Angles dbl and bdl, and the Side bd to find the Side dl; which was required.

I have said before, that the same Calculation may be performed for any other Ray Parallel to rf, falling at any distance ki from the Direct Axis $zfqa$; supposing with the former Data (instead of the Angle fqi) (*Tab.* 10. *Fig.* 1.) the Distance ki (*Tab.* 10. *Fig.* 2.) be given. For then in *Tab.* 10. *Fig.* 2. draw nib Parallel to zq, and produce qi to x, then $nim = rfz$. In the Right-angled Triangle qki, having ki and qi, we get the Angle $kqi = nix$, and the Side kq. And $nix - nim = mix =$ to the Angle of Incidence. And $qf - qk = fk$, $fg - fk = kg = ib$, by which in the several small Triangles within the Glass, we may find the Angle of the Rays Incidence from Glass to Air, as in the immediate foregoing Example, and so onwards in like manner.

T 10 F. 2

I shall propose one Case more in this Doctrine of *Oblique Rays*, and that is in *Tab.* 11. *Fig.* 1. where the Plane Side of the Glass is turn'd towards the Object. And that we may trace a Ray in this Case by Calculation, and find out a proper Ray for our purpose, we are to work a little backwards, thus, $qf = qh$ the Radius of the Convexity is given 20000, fg the thickness of the Glass is given 5858, And $qf - gf = qg = 14142$. Let df be a Ray within the Glass, whose Ingress is at d, so that dg is given 1000, and its Egress is at the Glasses Vertex f: In the Right-angled Triangle dgf, we have two Sides given to find the Angle dfg. Let kd be Perpendicular to ec, and produce fd directly to x: Then say, as 193 : to 300 :: so Sine of the Angle $kdx = dfg$ · to Sine $\angle kdr$. And $kdr - kdx = xdr$. Wherefore rd is a Ray of Light falling on the Glass at d obliquely by the Angle kdr, which after its Immersion into the Glass proceeds onwards, and Emerges at the Vertex of the Glass f. This Ray at its

Tab. 11 Fig. 1

Emer-

Tab. II pag. 30

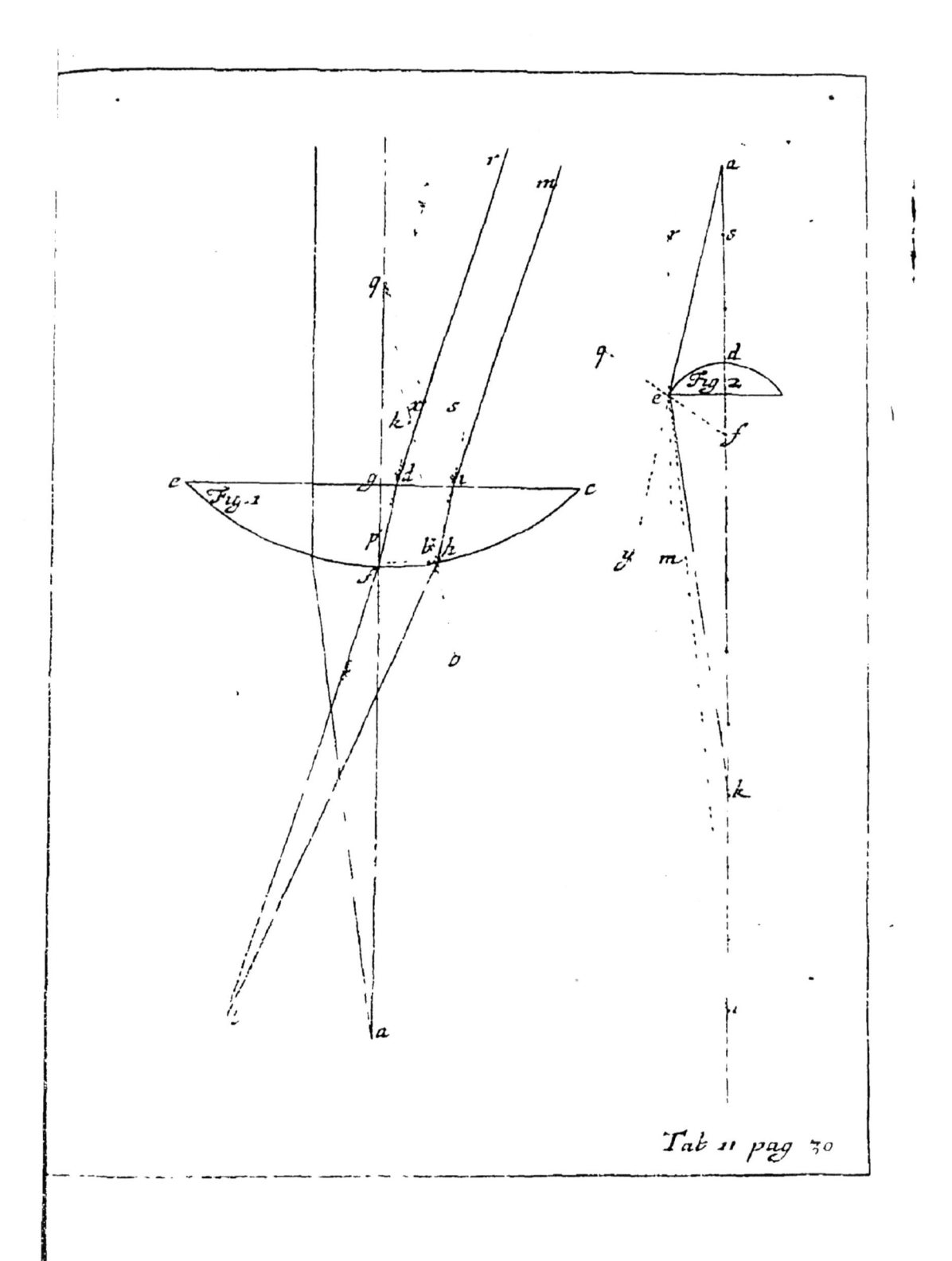

Emerſion at f ſhall again run Parallel to rd, by what foregoes; wherefore the Angle lfa is equal to the Angle kdr.

And thus much for the backward Operation, which we have Inſtituted to find a proper Ray to work with, that is, to find the Axis of an Oblique Cone, and its Angle of Inclination.

Let mi be another Ray Parallel to rd, and falling on the Glaſs at i, ſo that gi, may be given 5000. 'Tis required to determine the Point l, where the Ray mi, after a Double Refraction at its Ingreſs at i, and at its Egreſs at h, meets the Axis $rdfl$.

Produce rd directly to p, and mi to b, and make si Perpendicular to ec, Seeing therefore that mi is Parallel to rd, the refracted part ih, ſhall be Parallel to the refracted part df, and the Angle xdr $(=pdf)$ ſhall be equal to bih, and the Angle kdr is equal to sim. Joyn fh.

Then in the Right-angled Triangle qgi, we have qg and gi to find the Angle $gqi=qis$, and the Side qi: But $qis+sim=miq$, and $180°-miq=qib$. And $qib+bih$ is equal to qih.

Therefore in the Triangle qih we have the Sides qi and qh, and the Angle qih, to find the Angles iqh and qhi. But $gqi-iqh$ is equal to gqh or fqh.

Then in the Iſoſceles Triangle fqh, we have fq and qh equal to each other, and the Angle fqh to find the Side fh, and the Angle $fhq=qfh$.

Produce qh directly to o, then as 193 : To 300 :: So Sine Angle qhi: To Sine of the Angle ohl. But $180°-ohl-fhq=fhl$. Alſo $180°-qfh=hfa$. And $hfa+lfa=hfl$.

Laſtly, In the Triangle hfl, we have fh and all the Angles to find the Side fl, which was required.

Common Demonstration.

<small>Tab 12
Fig 1</small>   I shall now Demonstrate this Proposition the usual Way. *Tab.* 12. *Fig.* 1. *a g b* is a Plano-Convex, let the Plain surface *a b* be first turn'd to the Object: And let the two Parallel Rays *c d*, *e f*, fall Obliquely on the Plane surface *a b*, I say, that these Rays shall be united in *l*, so that *h l* shall be near equal to the Diameter of the Convexity, which we'll suppose *g k*.

Seeing the Angles *e f b*, *c d b*, are equal, these two Rays have equal Angles of Inclination, and consequently shall have equal Correspondent Angles of Refraction within the Glass, and therefore the refracted Rays *d h*, *f g*, shall also be Parallel within the Glass. And because from the same Point in the Object, that transmits these two Rays *c d*, *e f*, there proceed Infinite Rays, which falling on the Glass, and being refracted therein, do occupy the whole Glass; some one of these Rays after its first Refraction, being produced backwards, shall pass through the Centre of the Convexity *i*. Let *h d* be this Ray produced directly both ways to *i* and *l*: Seeing therefore *h d* is Perpendicular to the surface *a g b*, at *h* it suffers no Refraction in its Egress from the Glass. Wherefore let us consider the other refracted Ray *f g*, and what Refraction it suffers at the Point *g* on its Egress from the Glass: Here the Angle of Inclination is *f g i* equal to the Altern *g i h*; Let us suppose the refracted Angle *k g l*, which (by Experiment V) ought to be $\frac{1}{3}$ more than the Inclination *f g i* = *g i h*. Wherefore in the Triangle *i g l*, *l i* : *l g* :: S. ∠ *l g i* = S. ∠ *l g k* : S. ∠ *l i g*. But in these small Angles, as the Sines, so the Angles, and therefore if the Angle *l g k* be $\frac{1}{3}$ more than the Angle *l i g*, the Side *l i* is $\frac{1}{3}$ more than the Side *l g* or *l h* (for *l g* and *l h* are insensibly equal in Glasses of small Segments of large Spheres)

Tab. 12 pag. 32

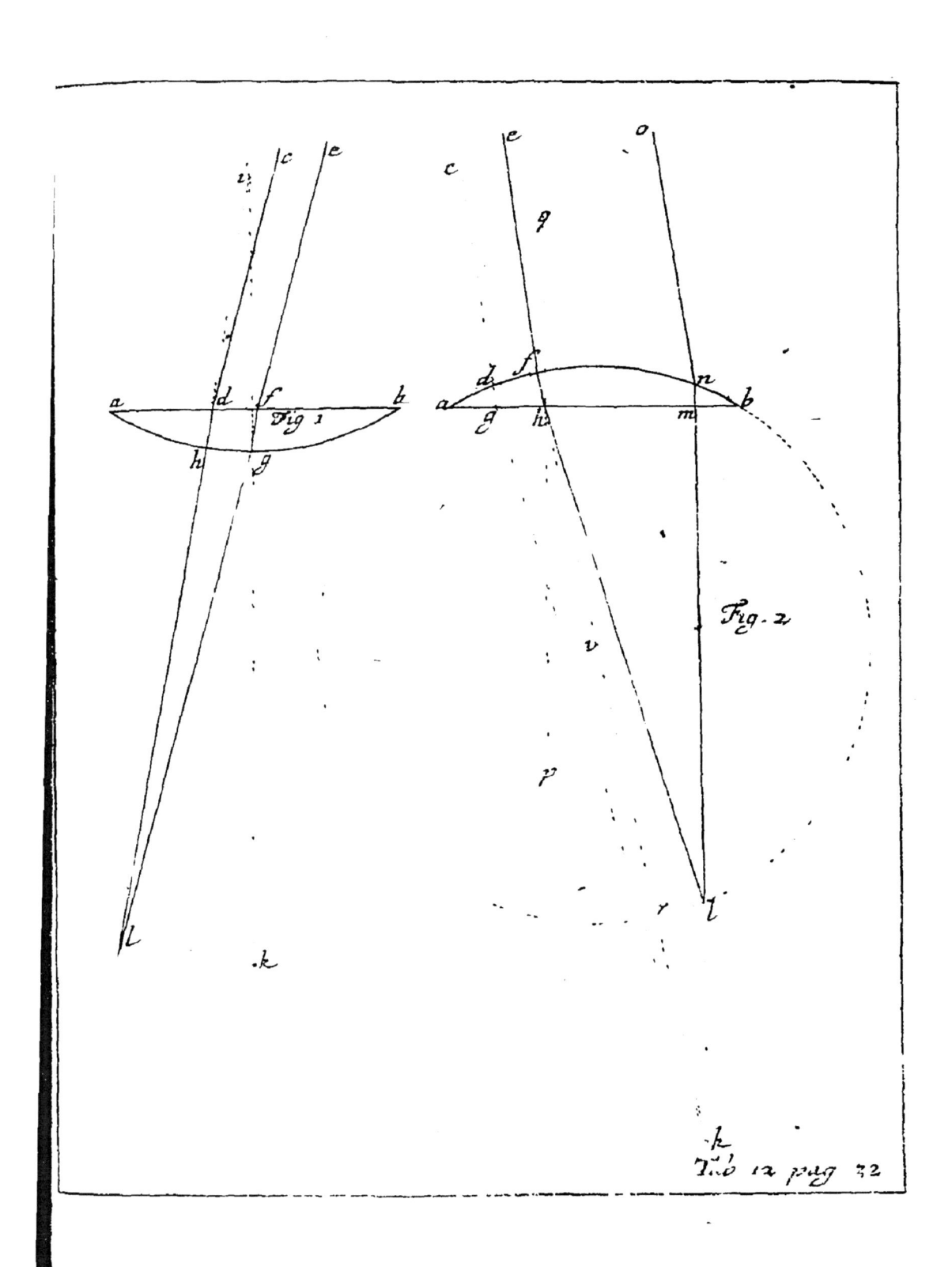

Tab 13. pag 33

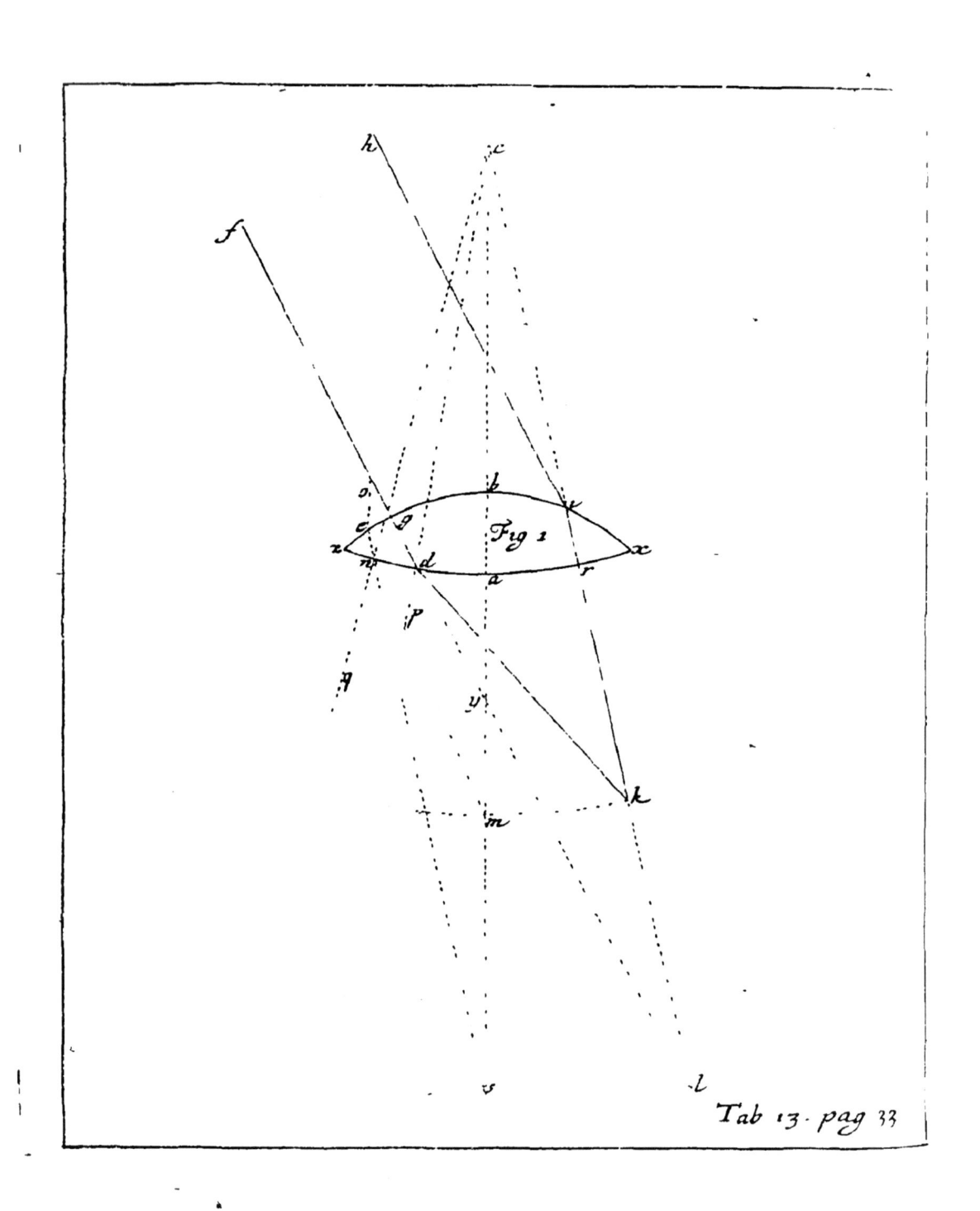

Spheres) wherefore hi being the Semidiameter, hl shall be the Diameter. *Which was to be Demonstrated.*

Secondly in *Tab.* 12. *Fig.* 2. Let the same Glass ab be turned with its Convex-Side to the Object, and thereon let the Parallel Rays cd, ef, fall obliquely to the Axis. These Rays shall be united together behind the Glass almost at the distance of the Diameter of the Convexity.

For amongst the parallel Rays that fall on the Glass, let us conceive one ef, that after its first Refraction at f, passing in the Glass in the Line fh, and being produced directly, would pass through the Centre of the Convexity i. If we conceive the Medium of Glass continued, we know that these two Rays ef, cd, would be united in k at the distance of a Diameter and half from the Glass (by *Prop.* I.). From the point k draw kn perpendicular to the plane surface of the Glass ab, and let the Ray no be drawn parallel to ef, cd; this Ray no shall also, by its first Refraction, be directed towards the Point k; and because within the Glass the Ray nm is perpendicular to the plain Surface ab, it shall proceed unrefracted through mlk. I shall now shew that fh by its second Refraction at its egress at h is refracted to l. Draw hl, and through h draw qhp perpendicular to ab. The Angle of Inclination within the Glass is $fhq = phk = hkl$. And now I shall prove that the Angle khl is ½ the Angle of Inclination phk or hkl. In the Triangle hkl, s. $\angle hkl$: s. $\angle khl$ :: hl . kl (or kr, for they are nearly equal), but hl is almost double kl or kr, therefore the Angle hkl is almost double khl. *Which was to be Demonstrated.* And therefore the parallel Oblique Rays have the Point of Concourse at the distance of a Diameter almost from a Plano Convex Glass. *Which was to be Demonstrated.* Vid. *L'Optique de Pierre Ango Livre* 3. *Sec.* 69. &c.

Thirdly, In *Tab.* 13. *Fig.* 1. zx is a double Convex, c is the Centre of the Convexity zax, y the Centre of the Convexity zbx,

$z b x$, $c y s$ the Axis of the Glass. 'Tis evident by what foregoes, that whatever Rays fall on this Glass parallel to the Glass's Axis are united thereto, at the distance of the Focus, (*viz.* about the Semidiameter in equal Convexities) as suppose at *m*. Wherefore let us consider two other Rays, parallel between themselves, but oblique to the Glass's Axis *c s*, such as *f g*, *h i*, I say these likewise, after a Double Refraction do concur about the distance of the *Principal Focus* (for so I call the Focus of the Rays parallel to the Glass's Axis.)

Seeing there are infinite parallel Rays, that fall thus obliquely on the Surface $z b x$, most certainly there must be one amongst the rest, which so falls thereon, that being produced directly, shall pass through the Centre *y* of the Convexity $z b x$: Let us conceive *f g* to be this Ray, so that *f g y* is a Right Line; let it be produced to *l*, so that *y l* may be equal to double *g y*.

From the Point *l* to *c* the Centre of the Convexity $z a x$ draw the Right Line *l c*, and where this Line cuts the Surface $z b x$, as in *i*, let the Ray *h i* fall parallel to *f g*. 'Tis evident, that by the first Refraction the Ray *h i* suffers on the Convexity $z b x$, it will concur with the Ray *f g* in *l* at the distance of a Diameter and half, for now *f g d y l* may be considered as the principal Axis.

Let us suppose the principal Focus of this Glass to be at *m*. From the Centre *c* strike the Arch *m k* cutting *c l* in the Point *k*. The Ray *h i* shall be refracted at *i*, but the refracted Ray *i r* (seeing it is perpendicular to the Surface $z a x$ by Construction) shall proceed unrefracted directly to *k*; but the Ray *f g d* being refracted in the Point *d* shall proceed refracted, and shall be united with the Ray *i k* in *k*. Which I thus prove,

From *c* draw the Line *c d p*, the Angle *p d y* is equal to the Angle of Inclination *g d c* in the Glass; and therefore if *d k*

be

be truly the refracted Ray, the Angle pdy ought to be double the Angle ydk, and that it is so I thus prove.

Let us suppose the Ray oe Parallel to the principal Axis cs, this Ray by the first Refraction it suffers at e is directed to the Point s, so that bs is a Diameter and half, or triple by, and therefore equal to gl. The same Ray oe being refracted at e to n, and at n suffering a second Refraction is brought to concur with the Axis cs in m, the principal Focus by Supposition. In which Case, the Angle of Inclination in the Glass shall necessarily be enc, which is equal to qns, and the Angle of Refraction shall be snm; and therefore the former qns shall be double the latter snm. But I say, as qns is double of snm :: so pdl is double of ldk. Which I thus prove,

In the Triangle ncm	1	$s. \angle cnm = s \angle qnm : s \angle nmc :: cm = ck : nc = cd$
Also in the Triang. dck	2	$s. \angle cdk = s \angle pdk : s \angle dkc :: kc : cd$
From 1 and 2	3	$s \angle qnm : s \angle nmc :: s \angle pdk : s \angle dkc$
Then Sines and Angles being proportional	4	$qnm \cdot nmc :: pdk : dkc$
By the Scheme	5	$qnm = qns + snm$. Also $pdk = pdl + ldk$.
From 4 and 5.	6	$qns + snm : nmc :: pdl + ldk : dkc$
Alternando 6.	7	$qns + snm : pdl + ldk :: nmc : dkc$
Moreover in $\triangle nms$.	8	$s. \angle smn = s. \angle nmc . s. \angle snm :: ns = dl : ms = kl$
Also in Triang. dkl	9	$s. \angle dkl = s. \angle dkc \cdot s. \angle ldk : dl \cdot kl$
From 8 and 9	10	$s. \angle nmc : s. \angle snm :: s. \angle dkc : s. \angle ldk$
Sines and Angles prop.	11	$nmc : snm :: dkc : ldk$
Alternando 11	12	$snm \cdot ldk : nmc : dkc$
From 7 and 12	13	$qns + snm : pdl + ldk :: snm : ldk$
Alternando 13	14	$qns + snm : snm :: pdl + ldk : ldk$
Dividendo 14	15	$qns \; snm :: pdl : ldk$

F 2 From

From which 15th Step it follows, that if *q n s* be double of *s n m* :: so *p d l* is double of *l d k*. *Which was to be Demonst.*

Note, In this Demonstration we assume *n s* and *d l* to be equal, and *m s* and *k l* to be likewise equal, whereas they are not so exactly, for the Thickness and Breadth of the Glass causes some little difference, but in Glasses of small Segments and large Spheres, and where the Rays do not fall very obliquely, this Difference is so very inconsiderable, that in a Demonstration relating to a Physico-Mathematical Matter, they may well be considered as equal.

Scholium.

But tho the Proposition expresses, that the Parallel Rays which proceed from each collateral Point of an Object, and fall *obliquely* on a Glass are united with their Axis at the same distance, as the direct Parallel Rays; yet this is to be understood with some Limitation. For if the Rays fall *very obliquely*, their Union with the Axis is not so exact, but they are scattered and the Focal Depth is very great. As will appear by Calculation.

Of the Representation of outward Objects in a Dark Chamber; by a Convex Glass.

From what has been hitherto laid down results that admirable Appearance, and Effect of a Convex-Glass duly placed in a small Hole in a Dark Chamber; Which therefore we shall here consider, *Tab.* 14. *F.* 1. A B C is a distant Object, which we are now to consider as very remote, so that tho the Figure, for want of Room in the Paper, expresses the Rays flowing from every single Point, as very much diverging; yet we are to imagine, that the Rays (for Instance) from the Point A run as it were Parallel to each other; the distance of the Object

B H

Tab 14. pag 36

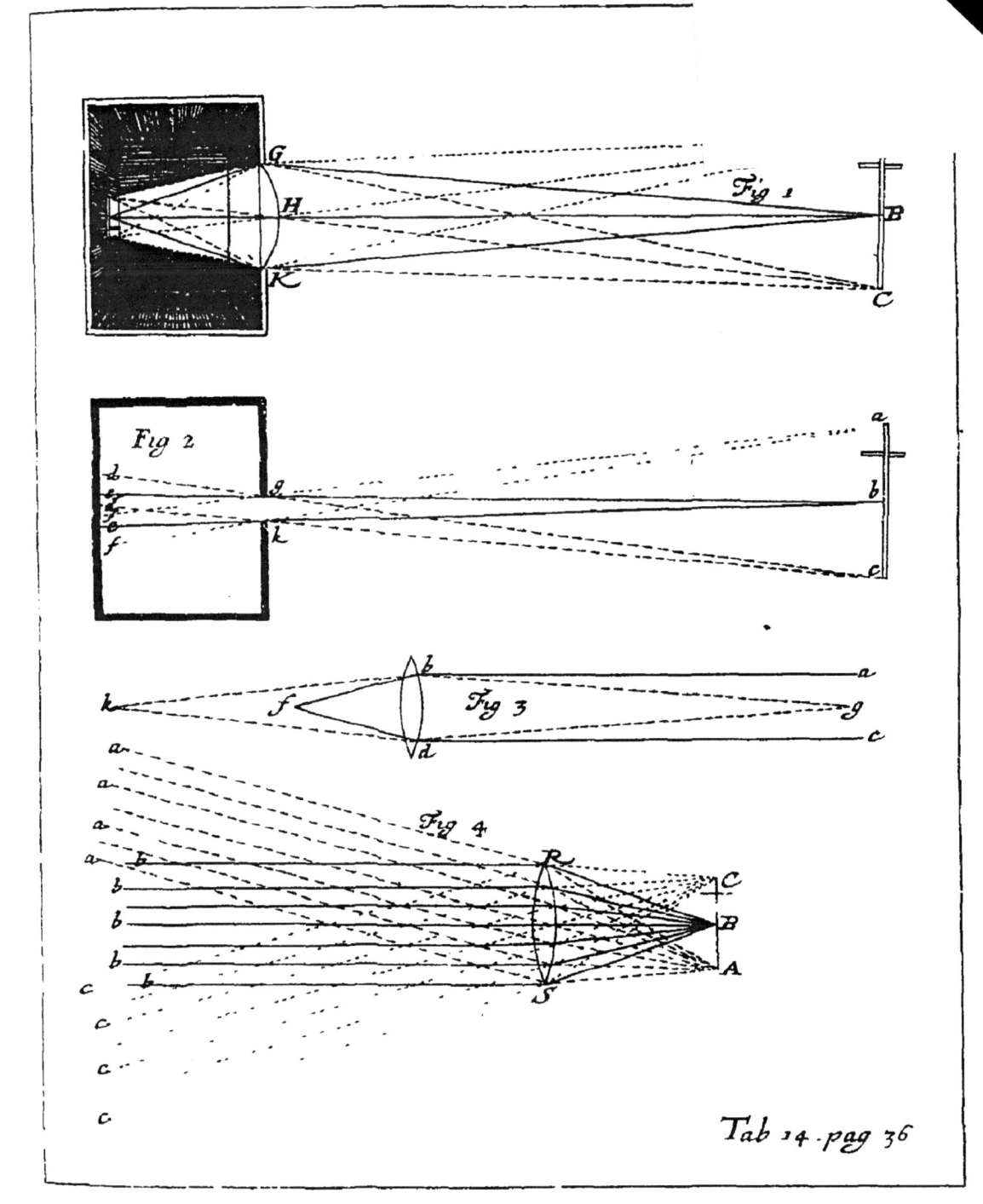

being supposed vastly great, in Comparison to the Glasses Breadth G K (But after the 5th. Proposition following, this Advertisement of the great distance of the Object will be needless, as therein shall appear) G H K is a Plano-Convex-Glass, receiving on its Surface a Cone of Rays from each single Point of the Object, but here for avoiding Confusion in the Scheme, we have only expressed the Cones flowing from the uppermost, middle, and lower Point of the Object, that is, from A, C, and B; and in each of these Cones neither have we expressed any more Rays than the Axis of the Cone (as for instance) A H, and the two extreme Rays of the same Cone A G and A K.

First therefore for the Rays that flow from the Point A. By what forgoes we know that the Axis of this Cone A H, after it has passed the Glass proceeds directly towards F, as if it were not at all refracted; and that the Rays A G, A K, are united with this Axis in a Point (suppose at F) distant from the Glass about the Diameter of its Convexity (the Glass being a Plano Convex) and what is said of the Rays A G, A K, being united with their Axis, must be conceived of all the Rays that make up the whole Cone flowing from this single Point A. and they are all united likewise with the Axis in the Point F, forming another correspondent Cone G F K, having its Base on the Glass, and its Vertex in the Point F, making the Pencil of Rays F G A K F.

And so likewise, what is declared of the Point A, and the Rays that flow from it, and of their being united together in F, may be easily conceived of the Rays flowing from the middle Point B, and their being united in E; and may be also understood of the Rays flowing from C, and their union in D, and so of the Rays proceeding from any other Point in the Object A B C, and their being united in a correspondent Point in F E D. And this F E D we call the *Distinct Base, Focus,* or *Burning Point.* 'Tis called the *Distinct*

ſtinct Baſe, becauſe therein is a *Diſtinct* Repreſentation of the Object. And ſuppoſing the Glaſs G K in the Hole of a dark Room, ſo that the Repreſentation F E D may be diſturbed by no other luminous Rays from outward Objects, and a Paper were placed at D E F, there to receive the Image, we ſhould thereon ſee the Object moſt livelily painted in its exact Shape and Colours. 'Tis called the *Focus*, or *Burning Point*, becauſe the Glaſs being expoſed to the Sun, it there collects the Rays from each Point of the Sun's Body, and paints its Image there moſt vividly, exciting a violent Heat, even to the inflaming of combuſtible Bodies.

But whereas in a *Scholium* after the Third *Propoſition*, it is obſerved, that the Rays falling nigh the Axis are not united thereto ſo near the Glaſs, as the Rays that fall farther from the Axis. And conſequently that all the Rays from one Point in the Object, do not unite in a correſpondent Point in the *Diſtinct Baſe*, but that (as we have noted before) the Focus has ſome Depth, and conſiſts not in an Indiviſible Point. Yet this hinders not the Repreſentation in the *Diſtinct Baſe* to be very lively and exact. For tho all the Rays from each Point are not united in an anſwerable Point in the Image, yet there are a ſufficient quantity of them to render the Repreſentation very perfect. And tho ſome Rays from other adjacent Points may a little intermix with thoſe from its neighbouring Parts, yet theſe are ſo few, that they make no great diſturbance.

N B Moreover in a *Scholium* following the Fourth *Propoſition*, 'tis obſerved, that when the Incidence of the oblique Rays is very oblique, that then their Concourſe with their Axis is not ſo very regular. From hence it proceeds, that the Repreſentation in the *Diſtinct Baſe* is not ſo clear and exact towards the Extremes, as towards the Middle.

As for the reaſon of this ſurprizing Appearance in a dark Chamber, wherein there is a ſmall Hole armed with a Con-
vex-

[39]

vex-Glass; it will be manifest, if we consider, that from every Point in the inverted Representation on the Paper, the Rays proceed to the Eye that looks at it, exactly in the same manner, as from the Object it self. For let us imagin the Point A to be *Blue*, B to be *Yellow*, and C *Red*. Because all the Rays flowing from A are separated by themselves, and fall in the Image on the Point F, where no other Rays intermix with them to disturb them, they must needs there represent *Blue*. For passing through the Glass, it being a Diaphanous Colourless Medium, does not at all alter them (notwithstanding the Appearance of the *Prisme*,) and the Point F in the Paper being enlightened only with Rays of *Blue* Light, and of it self being *White*, indifferent to all Colours, or rather indeed of no Colour, must needs represent *Blue*, and so E *Yellow*, and D *Red*. As to the *Shape* of the Object, it must needs be expressed exact likewise, for every Physical Point in the Object sending out a Cone of Rays falling on the Glass, and these being formed into another Correspondent Cone on the other side the Glass, determining their Vertices in Correspondent Points of the Image, the Eye must necessarily perceive on the Paper the lively Image of the Object, being it is affected in the same way by *This*, as by the Object it self. For from the Object it self the Eye receives only a Cone of Rays from each of its Points, and so it receives a Cone of Rays from each Point in the Image on the Paper; each Point in the Image on the Paper being enlightened by the Rays it receives through the Glass, and consequently the Paper, being an Impolite Surface, reflects these Rays into the whole circumjacent Medium. *Vid. Schol. Prop.* 52. *Gregorii Optic. Promot.*

And now that I am on the Consideration of this Appearance, it may not be improper to consider the Effect of a Plain small Hole without a Glass in a dark Room. *Tab.* 14. *Fig.* 2. Tab 14. Fig 2. represents a dark Chamber, in whose side there is a small Hole

g k

gk, ¼ an Inch wide; *abc* is a distant Object. Now because there is no Glass in the Hole *gk*, the Rays from each Point of the Object pass through the Hole directly strait, and represent on the Wall within, at *d e d f e f*, a faint and confused Image of the Object: Because here by the narrowness of the Hole, the Rays from some Points are hindred from intermixing with the Rays from some other Points; as here the Rays from the Point *a* do not intermix on the Wall with the Rays from the Point *c*; for we see *dd* do not intermix with *ff*. But then the Representation is confused, for tho some Rays are hereby hindred from intermixing with some other Rays, yet other Rays from nigh adjoyning Points do intermix with their neighbouring Rays, as here the Rays from *a*, and those from *b* are blended together in *fe*, and so those from *c* and *b* in *de*. And if the Hole be made so narrow as to hinder this communication of Rays in a great measure (for 'tis absolutely impossible to hinder it altogether) then the opening admits so few Rays from each Point, that the Image is obscure and imperceivable.

There is another Particular relating to this Appearance in a dark Chamber, which seems not so clearly treated of in those Optick Writers which I have consulted. Particularly *Zahn* in his *Ocul. Artif. Fund.* 1. *Synt.* 3. *Cap.* 2. *Sec.* 8. gives no satisfactory Account thereof. The Matter is thus, in *Tab.* 14. *F.* 1. if the Image D E F in the dark Chamber be received on a *Speculum* or Looking-Glass instead of a White Paper, the Eye perceives a most dilute and faint Image on the *Speculum*: But if the *Speculum* be placed any where between G K and D E F, and a Paper placed as far distant from the *Speculum* before it, as the distinct Base D E F is behind the *Speculum*, then the *Speculum* shall reflect on the Paper the distinct Image of the Object.

The dilute and very faint Image, which the Eye perceives on the *Speculum* in the first Case, proceeds from the Imperfect Politure of the *Speculum*; For if it were a most exquisitely

Tab 14 *Fig* 2

smooth

smooth Surface, even that faint Image it self would not appear. But as 'tis impossible by the Industry of Man to procure such, and all Mirors partake in some measure of a little Roughness, therefore it is that we have that dilute Image. And the reason we have no such vivid Representation from a Speculum (considered as a perfectly polish'd Surface) as from a Paper, as also the reason of the appearance in the second forementioned posture of the Speculum, does so depend on the Doctrine of Reflection or Catoptricks, that I shall pass it over in this place, it being manifest to any one meanly versed in that Doctrine. *Vid. Schol. Prop.* 52. *Gregorii Optic. Promot.*

Of Nigh Objects, or Diverging Rays.

We have hitherto considered the Radiating Points of *Distant* Objects both *Direct* and *Oblique*, the Rays from each single Point whereof do proceed as it were Parallel. I come now to the Consideration of *Nigh* Objects or *Diverging* Rays, and for these let us look back on the 5th, 6th, 7th, 8th, and 9th Definitions.

When the Rays from each Point of an Object run as it were *Parallel*, we may imagin that they may be *sooner* or *easier* brought together, than when they *Diverge* considerably, by coming from a *nigh* Object. And that therefore a Convex Glass unites the *Parallel* Rays *nigher* to it self, than *Diverging* Rays. *Tab.* 14. *Fig.* 3. ab, cd are Parallel Rays flowing from one Point of a distant Object, these are united by the Convex-Glass bd in its Focus at f. Let bg, dg be Diverging Rays flowing from the Point g, these are united in the Point k, farther from the Glass than the Point f.

For we may conceive (to omit the farther Proof of this by Geometrical Calculation), that the Parallel Rays have not so great a Reluctancy to be brought together, as the Diverging

ing Rays; and therefore the Refractive Power of the Glaſs has not ſo much to do to bring *thoſe* together, as to bring *theſe*. And conſequently it performs the *Firſt ſooner* than the *Latter*, or in a *ſhorter* ſpace, after the Ray's Emerge from behind the Glaſs. And this the *more*, according as the Object *g* approaches *nigher* and *nigher* to the Glaſs, till at laſt it be ſo nigh, that the Rays, after they have paſſed the Glaſs, become *Parallel* or *Diverging*, as I ſhall ſhew in the following Propoſitions.

Definitions.

The Focus wherein the Parallel Rays of a *Diſtant* Object are united, I call the *Focus*, ſimply without any Addition, ſometimes the *Abſolute Focus*, or *Solar Focus*.

The Focus wherein the Rays from a *Nigh* Object, or the Diverging Rays are united, I call the *Reſpective Focus*.

The foregoing Precepts, which I have given for calculating the Progreſs of a Ray through a Spherical Glaſs, are abundantly ſufficient to find the Point of Union of Rays from Nigh Objects, or of Diverging Rays; The Diſtance of the Object or point of Divergency from the Glaſs (together with the foregoing Data) being given. I ſhall not therefore inlarge thereon, but Inſtead thereof I ſhall give theſe following ſhort Rules in this Matter.

Prop. V.

In Convex-Glaſſes, When a Nigh Object is Placed more Diſtant than the Focus, The Rule for Determining the Diſtinct Baſe, or Reſpective Focus is This,

As the *Difference*, between the *Diſtance of the Object*, and *Focus*:
Is To the *Focus*, or *Focal Length* ::
So the *Diſtance of the Object from the Glaſs*:
To the *Diſtance of the Reſpective Focus or Diſtinct Baſe from the Glaſs.*

Demonstration.

In *Tab.* 11. *Fig.* 2. Let *e d* be a Plano-Convex Glaſs, whoſe abſolute Focus we know is about a Diameter of the Convexity, Let *s d* be this Diameter. *a* is a Radiating Point, *f* the Centre of the Convexity, *f e* the Radius of the Convexity produced directly to *q*. *a e* a Ray falling on the Glaſs, produced directly to *y*. Here we ſee the Angle of Inclination, or Incidence of the Ray *a e* is *q e a*.

Let it then be made —— | 1| *a s : s d :: a d : d k*

I ſay *k* is the reſpective Focus of the Ray *a e*.

Let *k l* be made = ½ *k d*. I ſhall firſt Demonſtrate, that by virtue of the firſt Refraction which the Ray ſuffers at its entrance on the Convex-Side of the Glaſs at *e*, 'tis directed as if it proceeded ſtrait towards *l*.

For to the Conſequents of the Analogy in the firſt ſtep add their Halfs, and it ſhall be —— | 2| *a s : s f :: a d : d l*

And compounding the 2d — | 3| *a f : s f :: a l : d l*

Here we ſee *s f* is equal to three Semidiameters of the Convexity, that is, to thrice *f e*.

The Angle of Refraction is *y e l*, if therefore we prove that *y e l* is ⅓ of *q e a* the Angle of Incidence, it will be manifeſt, that by the firſt Refraction the Ray is directed towards *l*.

In order to the Proof hereof, we lay down these Suppositions.

1. In the Triangle ael we suppose le and ld equal, because we suppose the Glass of the least Thickness imaginable, and the Segment of a large Sphere.

2. We suppose likewise, that the Angles of Incidence are all very small, that so Sines and Angles may be proportional. Tho we could not express this truly in the Figure.

Wherefore, for the Demonstration of the forgoing Position, in the Triangle ael it is ——— $\quad 4\ al : le = ld :: s\angle ael : s\angle a$

But the Angle ael is the Complement of the Angle yel to $180°$ Therefore the Sine of the Angle ael is equal to the Sine of the Angle yel.

Wherefore the 4th Step runs thus $\quad 5\ al . ld :: s.\angle yel : s.\angle a$

But in these small Angles, as the Sines are, so are the Angles. Therefore the 5th stands thus — $\quad 6\ al : ld :: \angle yel : \angle a$
Then from 3 and 6 it follows — $\quad 7\ \angle yel : \angle a :: af : sf = 3\ ef$
Then in the 7 Triple the Antecedent on this side, and subtriple the Consequent on the other side, and it will be ———— $\quad 8\ 3\angle yel : \angle a :: af : ef$

Moreover, in the $\triangle aef$ it is — $\quad 9\ af : ef :: s\angle aef : s\angle a$
But the Sine of the Angle aef is equal to the Sine of the Angle qea, being Complements to $180°$.

Where-

Wherefore the 9 may stand thus $\quad$ 10 $af : ef :: s\angle qea : s\angle a$

But Sines and Angles in these small Angles being proportional, it follows from the 8th and 10th. Steps, That

$\quad$ 11 $3\angle yel : \angle a :: \angle qea : \angle a.$

Wherefore from the Analogy in the 11th, it is evident, that the Angle of Inclination or Incidence qea is thrice the Angle of Refraction yel, seeing three times the Angle yel, and the Angle qea, bear the same Proportion to the same Angle a. And this was the first thing to be proved; and consequently the Ray ae by its first Refraction at its Point of Incidence is directed towards the Point l

It remains to be Demonstrated secondly, that the Ray, at its Eruption on the plain side of the Glass into Air, is refracted into ek.

For the Proof of this draw rem Parallel to the Axis. Now the Angle of Incidence from Glass to Air shall be mel, the Angle of Refraction lek, which we shall prove to be half the Angle of Inclination mel, or we shall prove that the Angle mek is thrice the Angle of Refraction lek. Which being Demonstrated, 'tis certain the Ray is refracted into ek.

For the Demonstration hereof we retain the Series of our former Steps, and in the Triangle lek we have it

$\quad$ 12 $le = ld : lk :: s.\angle ekl : s\angle lek$

But $s.\angle ekl$ is equal to $s.\angle ekf$ being Complements to 180°. Therefore the 12th. Analogy may stand thus

$\quad$ 13 $ld : lk :: s\angle ekf : s\angle lek$

And the Angle ekf is $= \angle mek$

Wherefore $\quad$ 14 $ld : lk \cdot s\angle mek \cdot s\angle lek$

Now the Angles being as the Sines, and lk being by Construction the third Part of ld, it follows from the 14th Step, that

that the Angle *l e k* is the third Part of the Angle *m e k*. Wherefore the Angle *l e k* is the Angle of Refraction agreeable to the Angle of Inclination *m e l*. *Which was to be Demonstrated.*

Example of this Rule.

Of this Rule I shall give this short Example. Let the Focus of a Glass be 48 Inches; the Distance of the Object 156, their Difference is 108. Then 108 : 48 :: 156 : 69 = to the respective Focus.

By this Rule we may view very nigh Objects with long Telescopes, converting them as it were into Microscopes, only by lengthning them. But of this more hereafter.

Also from hence I shall deduce a Method of measuring distances at one Station: but hereof also more hereafter.

Prop. VI.

An Object being placed in the Focus of a Convex-Glass, the Rays from each Point thereof, after passing the Glass become Parallel.

Tab 14 Fig 4

Tab. 14. F. 4. A B C is an Object placed in the Focus of the Glass R S. The Rays from each Point of this Object flow upon the Glass, as here we have expressed those from the Points A B C; I say the Rays from each of these Points after passing the Glass become Parallel, those from A being *a a a*, from B *b b b*, from C *c c c*. For let us imagine a distant Object to send its Parallel Ray, *a a a* from its upper Point, *b b b* from its middle Point, *c c c* from its lower Point: These (by what foregoes) shall be formed by the Glass into the distinct Base A B C. Let us now conceive this distinct Base, A B C, to be made the Object; and the Case is most plain, that its Rays must needs be remitted back again in the same manner as they were received

Tab 15 pag 47

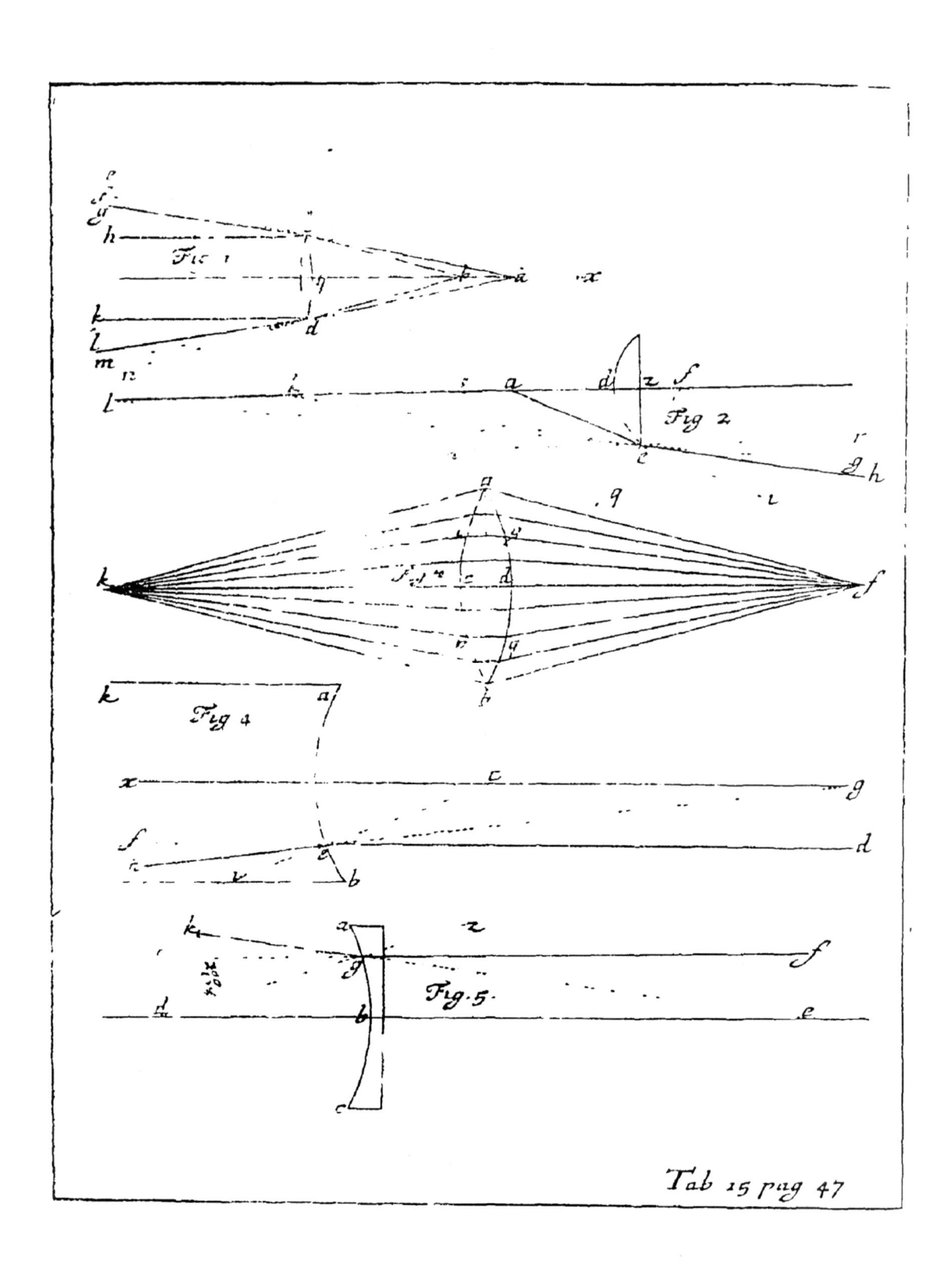

ceived from the distant Object on the side *a b c*, that is, Parallel. For the Progress of a Ray is reciprocal. *per Exp.* 8. *Vid. Prop.* XXVII.

Prop. VII.

If an Object be placed nigher a Convex Glass than its Focus, the Rays from each single Point thereof after they have passed the Glass, do proceed onwards diverging; But do not diverge so much as before they entred the Glass.

For if it be as much as the Glass can do, by its refractive Power to reduce to a Parallelism the diverging Rays from an Object placed in its Focus; it must needs be more than it can do, to reduce to a Parallelism the Divergency of the Rays, from an Object placed nigher to it than its Focus; The Divergence in this latter Posture being much greater than in the former, and consequently not so easily reduced by the refractive Power of the Glass. In *Tab.* 15. *Fig.* 1. *c d* is a Convex-Glass in whose *Focus* at *a* there is a radiating Point, from which proceed the Rays *a c f*, *a d m*, which meeting with the Glass, instead of going onwards to *f* and *m*, are reduced thereby to *c h*, *d k*, Parallel to each other. *b* is another radiating Point nigher the Glass than its Focus *a*, we may plainly perceive the Rays *b c*, *b d*, diverge more than the Rays *a c*, *a d*. Wherefore *b c*, *b d*, instead of proceeding directly onwards to *e* and *n*, are reduced to *c g*, *d l*; But *c g* and *d l* do yet diverge, but not so much as *b c*, *b d*.

Tab. 15. *Fig.* 1.

Definition.

Imaginary Focus.

In the same Figure, draw *g c*, *l d*, directly to Cross in *x*, I call *x* the *Imaginary Focus*; which is determined by the following Proposition.

Prop.

Prop. VIII.

In Convex-Glasses when an Object is placed nigher the Glass than the Focus, the Rule for finding the Imaginary Focus is this,

> *As the Difference between the Distance of the Object from Glass, and the Glasses Focus:*
> *Is to the Glasses Focus ::*
> *So the distance of the Object from the Glass:*
> *To the Distance of the Imaginary Focus from the Glass.*

Demonstration.

In *Tab.* 15. *F.* 2. Let *e d* be a Plano-Convex-Glass, whose absolute Focus is a Diameter of the Convexity, let *s d* be this Diameter; *a* is a radiating Point, *f* the Center of the Convexity *f e* ($= f d$) the Radius of the Convexity produced to *q*, *a e* a Ray falling on the Glass produced directly to *ι*.

We here suppose the Thickness of the Glass to be inconsiderable, and also, that the Breadth of the Glass is so little, that the Angles of Incidence shall be so small, that Sines and Angles may be proportional.

Let it then be made according to the Rule, *a s* : *s d* :: *a d* . *d k*. I say *k d* is the Distance of the Imaginary Focus of this Ray *a e*, after it has passed the Glass. That is, it shall be refracted, and proceed onwards in *e h*, as if it came directly from the Point *k*, *k e h* being a strait Line.

Let *k l* be made $=$ *k d*. I shall first Demonstrate, that by virtue of the first Refraction the Ray suffers at its Entrance on the Convex Side of the Glass at *e*, 'tis refracted so as if it proceeded directly from *l*, that is to say, 'tis refracted into *e g*, *l e g* being a Right Line.

'Tis

'Tis first manifest, that the Angle of Incidence is qea; if therefore we prove, that the Angle of Refraction $ieg = lea$ is $\frac{1}{3}$ of qea, we shew hereby, that by the first Refraction, the Ray is broken as if it proceeded directly from l.

That we may prove this, add to the Consequents of the foresaid Analogy their Halfs, — — — —

1	$as : sd :: ad : dk$
And it shall be — — — — — 2	$as : sf :: ad : dl$
Inverting, and Dividing this Second — — — — — — 3	$sf - as : sf :: dl - ad : dl$
That is by the Scheme — — — 4	$af : sf :: al : dl$
Moreover in the Triangle aef it is 5	$af : ef :: s\angle fea : s\angle eaf$
But $s\angle fea$ is $= s\angle qea$ being Complements to $180°$ — — — — 6	$af : ef :. s\angle qea : s\angle eaf$
And in these small Angles, Sines and Angles being proportional, the 6th shall be — — — 7	$\angle qea . \angle eaf :: af : ef$
Subtriple the Antecedent on this side, and triple the Consequent on t'other — — — — — — 8	$\frac{1}{3}qea : eaf :: af : 3ef = sf$
Then from the 4th and 8th Steps it follows — — — — — 9	$\frac{1}{3} qea : eaf :: al : dl$
Moreover in the Triang. ela it is 10	$la : le = ld .: s\angle lea : s\angle lae$
But $s\angle lae = s\angle eaf$ being Complements to $180°$ — — — 11	$la : ld .: s\angle lea : s\angle eaf$
And Signs and Angles being proportional — — — — — — 12	$al : dl :: \angle lea : \angle eaf$
From the 12th and 9th Steps 'tis manifest that — — — — 13	$\frac{1}{3} qea : eaf :. lea : eaf$

Wherefore from the 13th Step 'tis evident that $\frac{1}{3} qea$ is equal to lea, they having the same Proportion to the same Angle eaf.

H   Which

[50]

Which was the first thing to be proved: and consequently 'tis manifest that the Ray ae, by its first Refraction at its Incidence on e, is refracted into eg, as if it came directly from l, leg being a Right Line.

It remains to be Demonstrated secondly, that the Ray upon its Eruption on the plain side of the Glass into Air is refracted into eh, as if it proceeded directly from k, keh being a Right Line.

Draw mer Parallel to the Axis lf. Now the Angle of Incidence from Glass to Air is $ger = mel = eta$. — The Angle of Refraction is $geh = lek$, which I shall prove to be half the Angle of Inclination mel; Or I shall prove that the refracted Angle $mek = reh$ is thrice the Angle of Refraction lek.

Which being Demonstrated, 'tis certain the Ray is refracted into eh, as if it came directly from k, and consequently k is the *Imaginary Focus* of the Ray ae. But this we shall thus Demonstrate.

In the Triangle lek ———————	14 $le = ld$ lk :: s∠lke s∠lek
But s∠lke = s∠ekf being Complements to 180°. ———————	15 $d : lk :: $ s∠$ekf : $ s∠lek
But ∠ekf = ∠mek therefore, the 15th is ———————	16 $ld . lk :: $ ∠$mek . lek$

And by Construction ld was put equal to 3 lk, therefore from this 6th step 'tis manifest, that the Angle mek is equal to Thrice the Angle lek. Which was to be Demonstrated.

Corollary.

Concerning *Convex-Glasses* exposed to Converging Rays.

Hitherto we have spoken of *Convex-Glasses* exposed either to *Parallel* or to *Diverging* Rays. Let us now consider their

T 15 F 2 Property exposed to Converging Rays *Tab.* 15. *Fig.* 2. Let be be a Ray of Light falling on the Convex-Glass ed, and converging

verging directly towards the point k; dk the distance of this Point of Convergence from the Glass, and sd the Focal length of the Glass being given, 'tis required to find da, the distance at which this Ray converges after passing the Glass.

We know that the Progress of a Ray is *reciprocal* (by *Exp.* 8.) and therefore, that if the Ray ae be refracted into eh, the Ray he shall be refracted into ea.

Wherefore it being by *Prop.* VIII ―― $ds — da = as : sd :: ad : dk$
Alternating we have it ―――― $sd : dk :: ds — da : ad$
And Compounding ―――― $sd + dk : dk :: ds : ad$

From which last Analogy this Rule arises, for solving the Problem in the Corollary.

As the Sum of the Focal Length of the Glass and the distance at which the strait Ray converges directly ―― $ds + dk$:
To the said *Distance at which the strait Ray converges* dk ::
So the *Focal Length of the Glass* ―― ds :
To the *Distance at which the refracted Ray converges* ―― ad :

Observation.

Dechales in his first Book of Dioptricks, *Prop.* 48. gives a Rule for solving this 8th Proposition. But therein he is the most egregiously mistaken as ever Man was, that pretended to Demonstration, and commits the most notorious Error that can be imagined. And yet herein he wants not his Followers, for *Zahn* in his *Telescopium Fundam.* 2. *Syntag.* 1. *Cap.* 4. *Prop.* 13 transcribes *Dechales*, and copies out even his *Errata Typographica*, besides the chief and great Error of the whole Solution. Which shews that *Zahn* was either very careless, or else that he understood nothing of the Matter, as indeed he seems to do very little, for he is a mere blind Transcriber from others.

[52]

Dechales Rule in his fore-cited Propofition is this. *As the Sum of the Diftance of the Object from the Glafs, and half the Glafs's Focus: Is to the Glafs's Focus :: fo the Diftance of the Object from the Glafs · to the Diftance of the Imaginary Focus beyond the Diftance of the Object:* That is, in *Tab.* 15. *F.*2. $af : sd :: ad : ak$. But how falfe this is, fhall appear not only from his miftaking one Angle for another in his Demonftration, but from the following Examples, which I have taken the pains to calculate for a more full Confutation of *Dechales,* and Illuftration of my own Rule.

Tab 15
Fig 2

1. *Example.*

Inch

Given in *T.*15. *F.*2. $\begin{cases} \text{Plan.-Conv. Gl. Foc } 144,00 = sd = 2\ ef \\ \text{Radi of the Convexit. } 72,00 = ef = fd \\ \text{Diftance of the Object } 48,00 = ad = az \\ \text{Breadth of the Glafs } 1,00 = ez \end{cases}$

By my Rule $\begin{cases} dk = 7200 \\ kl = 3600 \\ dl = 10800 = dk + kl \\ al = 6000 = dl - da \end{cases}$

By *Dechal. Prop.* 48. $\begin{cases} dk = 10560 \\ kl = 5280 \\ dl = 15840 = dk + kl \\ al = 11040 = dl - da \end{cases}$

Let us now try by Calculation, which of thefe is the Truth. *Tab.* 15. *Fig.* 2.

Tab 15
Fig 1

In the Right-angled Triangle efz, we have the Sides ef and ez, to find the Angle $efz = 0°\ 47'\ 40''$ and its Complement to $90°\ fez = 89°\ 12'\ 20''$.

Then in the Right-angled Triangle eaz, we have az, and ez to find the Angles and Side ae.

Thus

Thus $\angle eaz=$ 1° 11′ 40″
$\angle aez=$ 88 48 20
$ae=4801$

Then $aez+fez=aef=$ — — —178 0 40
And Compl. aef to 180° $=qea=$ Incl. $=$ 1 59 20
Then as 3 : 1 ∷ $s\angle qea : s\angle ieg=lea=$ 0° 39′ 50″ Ang. of Ref.
Moreover, $eal=180-eaz=$ — —178 48 20
And $ela=180-eal-lea=mel=ger=$ 0 31 50

Then in the Triangle eal, we have two Angles, lea and ela, and the Side ae, to find the Side al. Thus,

As $s\angle ela=$ 0° 31′ 50″ Log. C. Ar. 2.0333979726
To $ae=4801$ — — — — —3.6813317060
So $s\angle lea=$ 0° 39′ 50″ — — — —8.0639630497
To $al=6007$ — — — — — —3.7786927283

which is sufficiently agreeable to my $al=6000$, but differs vastly from *Dechales* $al=11040$.

I now proceed to find the Side dk, which by my Rule is 7200, but by *Dechales* is 10560.

$\angle qez=qea+aez=$ 1° 59′ 20″ $+$ 88° 48′ 20″ $=$ 90° 47′ 40″
$\angle qem=qez-90°=$ — — — — — — —0 47 40
$\angle mel=ale=ger=$ — — — — — — —0 31 50,

This is the Angle of Inclination or Incidence from Glass to Air, on the plane side of the Glass.

Then, As 2 : 3 ∷ $s\angle ger=$ 0° 31′ 50″ : $s\angle her=mek=ekd=$ 0° 47′ 40″.

And $kez=90-ekd=$ 89° 12′ 20″.

Then in the Triangle kez, all the Angles, and the Side ez are given, to find kd or kz (we supposing the Thickness of the Glass inconsiderable). Thus,

Rad. — — — — — — —
To $ez=100$ Log. 2.0000000000
So Tang $\angle kez=$ 89° 12′ 20″   11.8580312668
To $kd=7208$ 3.8580312668

Which

[54]

Which kd anſwers ſufficiently exact to what my Rule gives it 7200, the Eight Parts coming in for the Thickneſs of the Glaſs, and the Angles not being calculated more accurately than to 10" Seconds *Numero rotundo*. But this is much different from what *Dechales* Rule gives it 10560.

2. *Example.*

Given in *Tab.* 15. F. 2.
$$\begin{cases} \text{Glaſs's Focus} = & 14400 = sd = 2\,ef \\ \text{Rad. of the Conv.} = & 7200 = ef = fd \\ \text{Diſt. of the Object} = & 5763 = ad = az \\ \tfrac{1}{2}\text{Bread. of the Glaſs} = & 100 = ez \end{cases}$$

By my Rule
$$\begin{cases} dk = & 9608 \\ kl = & 4808 \\ dl = & 14412 = dk + kl \\ al = & 8549 = dl - ad \end{cases}$$

By *Dechales*, 48 Prop.
$$\begin{cases} dk = & 12165 \\ kl = & 6082 \\ dl = & 18247 = dk + kl \\ al = & 12484 = dl - ad \end{cases}$$

The Thickneſs of the Glaſs zd is but $\tfrac{1}{7200}$ and therefore inconſiderable, it being the Verſed Sine of the Angle efz. We ſuppoſe therefore kd and kz equal.

Then by Calculation, *ex Datis*, we find as follows,

1	$efz =$	0°	47'	40"
2	$fez =$	89	12	20
3	$eaz =$	0	59	40
4	$aez =$	89	00	20
5	ae	$= 5764$		
6	$aef =$	178	12	40

7 qea

$$\begin{array}{r|l}
7 & q\,e\,a = 1°\ 47'\ 20'' = \text{Inclination} \\
8 & l\,e\,a = 0\ 35\ 40 = \text{Refraction} \\
9 & e\,a\,l = 179\ 0\ 20 \\
10 & e\,l\,a = 0\ 24\ 0 \\
11 & a\,l = 8566
\end{array}$$

Which $a\,l = 8566$ is but 17 more than my Rule gives it, which (considering the Inaccuracy of the Calculation of the Angles, being only *Numero rotundo* to about 10" Seconds) proves my Rule sufficiently true, and shews *Dechales* as false, which makes $a\,l = 12484$.

Moreover, By my Rule $d\,k$ is $= 9608$, and by *Dechales* 12165. The Angles requisite to find $d\,k$ we have thus,

Before found—
$$\begin{array}{r|l}
1 & q\,e\,z = 90°\ 47'\ 40'' \\
2 & q\,e\,m = 0\ 47\ 40 \\
3 & a\,l\,e = 0\ 24\ 0 = g\,e\,r = m\,e\,l = \text{Inclin.} \\
4 & m\,e\,k = 0\ 36\ 0 = h\,e\,r = e\,k\,d. \\
5 & k\,e\,z = 89\ 24\ 0 \\
6 & k\,d = k\,z = 9550
\end{array}$$

Which $k\,d = 9550$ is but 58 less than my Rule gives it; and this small Discrepancy may easily arise from the Error of 10" Seconds in the Calculation of the Angles. But *Dechales* gives it 12165.

I have chosen a Plano-Convex Glass to demonstrate this Rule, which holds as true in double Convexes, but would in them be more difficult and intricate to demonstrate.

PROP.

Prop. IX.

In double Convex-Glasses of equal or unequal Convexities, the Rays proceeding from the Distance of a Diameter of one Convexity, are united at the Distance of a Diameter of t'other Convexity.

T.15 F.3. In *Tab.* 15. *Fig.* 3. Let us conceive the Glass *a b* divided by the Pointed Right Line *a b* into two Plano-Convex Glasses *a c b* and *a d b*. Let the Point *k* be distant from the Glass *a c b* the Diameter of the Convexity *a c b*. By what foregoes, *Prop*.II. The Rays *k a*, *k e*, *k c*, *k p*, &c. shall be sent parallel through the Glass *a c b*, so that they shall become *e g*, *c d*, *p q*. Then falling Parallel on the Plano-Convex Glass *a d b*, they are united thereby in *f*, at the distance of its Diameter: By the foregoing Doctrine. *Prop.* II.

Of Concave-Glasses.

Hitherto we have treated of *Spherical Convex Glasses* only. We now proceed to the Consideration of *Concave Glasses*.

Definition.

Virtual Focus, *or* Point of Divergence

T.15 F.5. In *Tab.* 15. *Fig.* 5. *a b c* is a Plano Concave Glass, whose Axis is *d e*, *f g* is a Ray falling thereon parallel to the Axis *d e*, *d* is the Centre of the Arch *a b c*. This Ray after it has passed the Glass at its Emersion at *g*, instead of proceeding directly to *h*, is refracted from the Perpendicular *d g*, and becomes *g k*. Draw *g k* directly to cross the Axis in *e*. I call the Point *e* the *Virtual Focus*, or *Point of Divergence*.

Concerning

Concerning Concaves, there is little to be said after our foregoing Method for Calculating the Progress of a Ray falling on a Spherical Convex, for this may easily be accommodated to Concaves.

I shall therefore slightly pass these over, and shall only lay down their Properties in brief, with their usual Demonstrations, referring to Calculation for a more accurate Scrutiny.

PROP. X.

A Ray falling parallel to the Axis from Air, on the Concave Surface of a Glass Medium, has its Virtual Focus by its first Refraction at the Distance of a Diameter and half of the Concavity.

Tab. 15. Fig. 4. $abkh$ is a Glass Medium terminated by the Concave Surface ab, de a Ray of Light falling parallel to the Axis gix. I say the Ray de, by its Refraction at the Point of Incidence e, is so refracted into eh, as if it proceeded directly from g the distance of a Diameter and half of the Convexity.

Let c be the Centre of the Concave-Arch aeb, draw ce directly to i, produce de directly to f, and he directly to g. The Angle $ced = fei$ is the Angle of Inclination, the Perpendicular is ei. By what foregoes, the Ray passing from Air a Rare Medium into Glass a Dense Medium, is refracted towards the Perpendicular by the Angle feh, which must be ⅓ of the Inclination fei. Therefore $feh = deg = egc$ is half $hei = gec$. Wherefore in the Triangle ceg, the Angle ceg being double the Angle egc, the Side cg that subtends ceg, shall be double the side ce that subtends egc. For we suppose these Angles to be so small, that Sines and Angles, or Sides and Angles are proportional. *Which was to be Demonstrated.*

I

PROP.

[58]

Prop. XI.

In Plano Concave Glasses, when the Rays fall parallel to the Axis, the Point of Divergence or Virtual Focus is distant from the Glass the Diameter of the Concavity.

T 15 F 5.   *Tab.* 15. *Fig* 5. *a b c* is a Plano-Convex Glass, whose Axis *e d*, *f g* is a Ray of Light falling on this Glass parallel to its Axis. This Ray after it has passed the Glass at *g*, is so refracted into *g k*, that *g k* being produced directly backwards, it shall intersect the Axis in *e*, so that *e b* shall be the Diameter of the Cavity *a b c*.

First, Let the plain Side be turned towards the Object, as in *Tab.* 15. *Fig.* 5. Because the Ray falls perpendicular on the plain Superficies, it is not at all refracted at its Immersion into the Glass. But at *g* it emerges from the Concave Side of the Glass into Air, and its Inclination is *g d b* (*d* being the Centre of the Cavity *a b c*) and 'tis now refracted from the Perpendicular *d g*, by the Angle *b g k*, which is half the Inclination *g d b*. But *b g k* is equal to *f g e* = *g e d*. Wherefore in the Triangle *g d e*, the Angle *g e d* is half the Angle *g d e*, and therefore the Side *g d* is half the Side *g e* = *e b* in Glasses of large Spheres.

F 16 F 1.   Secondly, *Tab.* 16. *Fig.* 1. Let the Concave Side *e c* be turned to the Ray *d e*. By the first Refraction the Ray suffers at its Immersion into Glass at *e*, 'tis refracted from *e* to *f*, and directed to the Point *k*, so that *c k* is thrice the Semidiameter *n c* (by the Xth hereof). Through the Point *f* draw *i h* perpendicular to the plain Side of the Glass, and continue *e f* directly to *l*. The Angle of Inclination of the Ray within the Glass is *h f e* = *i f l* = *d e k* = *e k c*. Now the Ray emerging from Glass to Air, the second refracted Ray

ought

Tab. 16. pag. 58

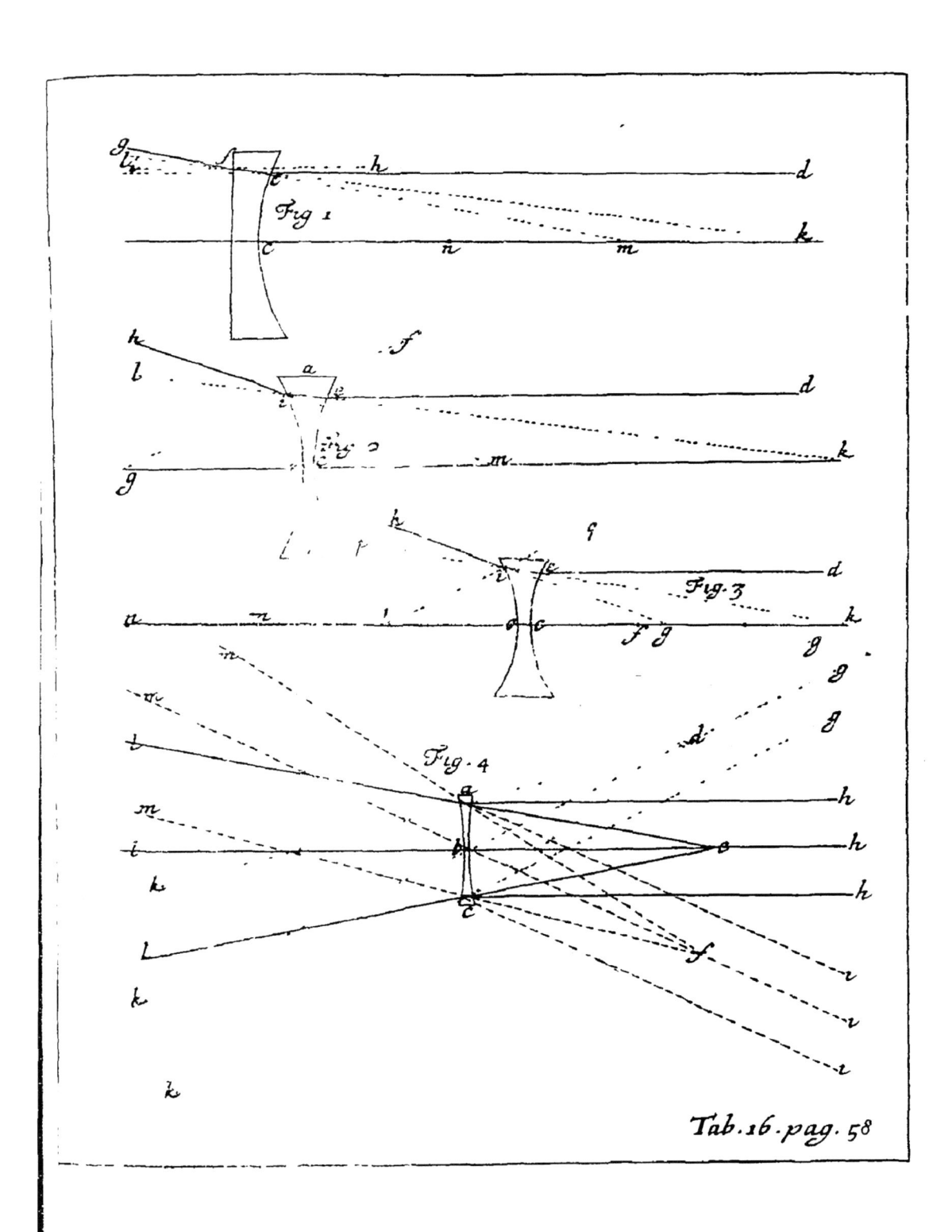

ought to recede from the Perpendicular if, so that the Angle gfi must be thrice the Angle gfl. Produce gf directly to m. Then gfi shall be equal to fmc. Wherefore in the Triangle kfm, As the Sine of the Angle kmf, or the Sine of the Angle fmc. To the Sine of the Angle fkm :: So fk · To fm, and (neglecting the Thickness of the Glass) So is kc · To mc. And Angles and Sines being proportional, kc shall be to mc as 3 to 2, but kc is Thrice the Semidiameter, therefore mc is the Diameter. *Which was to be Demonstrated.*

Corollary.

In Plano-Concave Glasses, as $300 - 193 = 107 : 193 ::$ So the Radius of the Concavity : To the Distance of the Virtual Focus.

Demonstration.

Tab. 15. F. 5. The Inclination is $hgd = gdb = fgz = 193$.
Refracted Angle is $zge = kgd = 300$.
Ang. of Refr. $kgh = kgd - hgd = 300 - 193 = 107 = fge = ged$.
In the Triang. gde. As $s\angle ged$: To $s\angle gde$ :: So Rad. $= gd$: To ge.
That is ———————— $107 : 193 :: gd : ge = eb$ in Glasses of large Spheres and small Segments.

PROP. XII.

In Double Concaves of equal Cavities, Parallel Rays have their Virtual Focus, or Point of Divergence at the Distance of the Radius of the Concavity.

Tab. 16. F. 2. ab is a Concave of equal Cavities, that is, mc the Radius of the Cavity ec, is equal to gn the Radius of the Cavity ni. Let the Ray de fall thereon parallel to the Axis λc. This Ray, after it has suffered a

double

double Refraction, shall proceed in ih, as if it came directly from m, the Centre of the Cavity.

Let ck be made three times cm, draw $keil$. By the first Refraction the Ray is propagated into ei, as if it proceeded from k (by *Prop.* X.). From the Centre g draw the Perpendicular gif. The Angle of Inclination of the Ray within the Glass is $eif = lig$. The Ray must therefore at its Egress at i be refracted, so that the Angle of Refraction $hil = kim$ must be half the Inclination lig. Wherefore in the Triangle kig, As the Sine of the Angle kig, or of the Complement to 180° viz. lig : To the Sine of the Angle at g ∷ So $kg = 4$. To ik or $nk = 3$. And as the Sines, so are the Angles, seeing they are supposed very acute: Therefore, As 4 : To 3 : So $\angle lig$: To the $\angle g$: Add $hil = 2$ to $lig = 4$, we have $big = 6$. Wherefore $\angle hig$: Is to the Angle g ∷ As 6 : To 3 :. or 2 : To 1. But the Sine of the Angle hig is equal to the Sine of the Angle gim, and consequently in the Triangle gim, As Sine of the Angle gim To the Sine of the Angle g ∷ So gm : To im Therefore gm : Is to im ∷ As 2 : To 1. So that neglecting the Thickness of the Glass, mi may be taken for the Radius of the Cavity, and gm is double thereto. Wherefore tis Demonstrated, that m is the Virtual Focus. *Which was to be Demonstrated.*

PROP. XIII.

In double Concaves of equal or unequal Concavities, the Virtual Focus or Point of Divergence of the Parallel Rays is determined by this Rule:

As the Sum of the Radii of both Concavities :
Is to the Radius of either Concavity ∷
So the Double Radius of t'other Concavity :
To the Distance of the Virtual Focus.

Tab.

[61]

Tab. 16. *Fig.* 3. fc is the Radius of the Concavity ec, make kc thrice fc, lo is the Radius of the Cavity oi; let lm be put equal to lo, and mn be put $=lm$, that is, on shall then be equal to thrice ol.

I say the Ray de, after a double Refraction, shall proceed in ih, as if it came directly from g, and that it shall be, As fl the Aggregate of the Semidiameters (neglecting the Thickness of the Glass) : To fc the Radius of one Concavity :: So om the Diameter of t'other Concavity : To gc the Distance of the Point of Divergence.

By the first Refraction the Ray proceeds in ei, as if it came directly from k, $keip$ being a Right Line (*Prop.* X.).

Then the Inclination within the Glass is $qie=pil$ And the second Angle of Refraction is $pih=gik$, which is to be half the Angle of Inclination pil.

Wherefore Sines and Angles being proportional, and the Thickness of the Glass neglected, we thus proceed in the Demonstration.

In the Triang. gik we have it ————————	1 | $gik=hip : gki :: kg : gi=gc$
Double the Antecedent on this side, and halve the Consequent on t'other —	2 | $2gik=pil : ikl :: kg : \frac{1}{2}gc$
Dividing the Second —	3 | $pil - ikl (=ilk\ 32.\ 1\ Eucl.)$: $ikl :. gk - \frac{1}{2}gc : \frac{1}{2}gc$
Then in the Trian. kli	4 | $lk : ikl :: ki=kc : il=lo$
From the Third and Fourth it follows ——	5 | $kc : ol .. kg - \frac{1}{2}gc : \frac{1}{2}gc$
Compounding the Fifth	6 | $kc + ol = kl \cdot ol :: kg : \frac{1}{2}gc$
Double the Consequents	7 | $kl : 2ol = om = ln \cdot\cdot kg : gc$
Compound. the Seventh	8 | $kl + ln = kn : om \cdot\cdot kg + gc = kc : gc$
Alternate the Eighth —	9 | $kn : kc :: om : gc$
But kn is equal to $3fl$,	

that

that is, thrice the Aggregate of the Semidiameters fc and lo. Also kc is equal to thrice the Semidiameter fc: and as the Triples are, so are their Thirds. Wherefore from the 9th. Step it follows —— $\tfrac{1}{3}ofl : fc :: om : gc$.

Which was to be Demonst.

Example.

Let fc be $= 8$ Feet or 96 Inches
$lo = 10$ Feet, or 120 Inches.
Then fl shall be $= $ to 216 Inches.
Say then $fl = 216 : fc = 96 :. 240 = 2 lo : 107 = gc$.
Or thus, $fl = 216 \cdot lo = 120 .. 192 = 2 fc : 107 = gc$.

Corollary.

It follows from the four last Propositions, that supposing a Ray falling on a Concave Glass, and tending towards the virtual Focus, after it has passed the Glass, it shall proceed Parallel to the Axis. Because the Progress of Light through Glasses is reciprocal. *Vid. Prop.* VI.

Scholium.

It is before Demonstrated in *Prop.* IV. that the Focus or Point of Convergence of a Convex-Glass, for the Parallel Rays that fall *obliquely* thereon is at the same Distance, as the Focus of the *direct* Parallel Rays. The same may be Demonstrated concerning the Virtual Focus or Point of Divergence in Concave Glasses, but 'tis sufficient only to illustrate this Matter by *Tab.* 16. *Fig.* 4. Let us imagine the uppermost Point of a distant Object

Object to send the Parallel Rays *g a, g b, g c*, on the Concave-Glass *a b c*, and its middle Point to send the Rays *h a, h b, h c*; and the lowermost Point to send the Rays *i a, i b, i c*. Here are therefore three Radious Cones, having their Vertices in their respective Points of the Object, and their Bases on the Surface of the Concave-Glass: the Axes of these Cones, are *g d b k*, *h e b l, i f b m*. These, by what foregoes preliminary to the *Prop.* IV. may be conceived to pass the Glass as it were unrefracted. But the other Rays of each Cone are refracted, that is, *g a* is so refracted at *a* into *a k*, as if it proceeded directly from *d* the Virtual Focus or Point of Divergence for this oblique Cone. And so *g c* is refracted at *c* into *c k*, as if it proceeded directly from *d*. And in like manner *h a, h b, h c*, are refracted into *a l, b l, c l*, as if they came from *e*. And the Rays *i a, i b, i c*, are propagated in *a m, b m, c m*, as if they proceeded directly from *f*. So that *d e f* is the Virtual Focus of the Glass exposed to the Object, that sends these direct and oblique Cones of Rays.

Converging Rays.

The Properties of Concaves exposed to *Converging* Rays are shewn in these two next following Propositions.

Prop. XIV.

In Concave Glasses, if the Point to which the incident Ray converges, be distant from the Glass farther than the Virtual Focus of Parallel Rays, the Rule for finding the Virtual Focus of this Ray, is this:

> *As the difference between the distance of this Point from the Glass, and the distance of the Virtual Focus from the Glass:*
> *Is to the distance of the Virtual Focus*
> *So the distance of this Point of Convergence from the Glass:*
> *To the distance of the Virtual Focus of this Converging Ray.*

Tab.

T 17 F 1.   *Tab.* 17. *Fig.* 1. *a b* is a Plano Concave Glass, *d* the Centre of the Concavity, *d a o* a right Line, *c f* the length of the Virtual Focus, which (by what foregoes, *Prop.* XI) is equal to 2 *a d* or 2 *d c*, so that *f d* is equal to 3 *d c* or 3 *a d*. Let *n a* be a Ray of Light converging directly towards the Point *g*. If it be made according to the Rule in the Proposition, *g f ⋅ f c ∷ g c ⋅ c h*. Then *h* shall be the Virtual Focus of the Ray *n a*, that is the Ray *n a* after the double Refraction it receives by the Glass shall proceed onwards in *a m*, as if it came directly from *h*, *m a h* being a Right Line.

The Proof hereof is after the same manner with the *Prop.* V. beforegoing; and we suppose (as in that) the Thickness of the Glass to be nothing in Comparison to the Focal Length, and likewise that the Angles of Incidence are so small, that they are as the Sines; also that the Breadth of the Glass is so little, that it makes the Angles *a g c*, *a d c*, *a h c*, *a p c*, &c. very small and Proportionable to their Sines.

Demonstration.

Let *p h* be made half *h c*, and consequently the third Part of *p c*. I say by virtue of the first Refraction which the Ray suffers at its entrance into Glass at *a*, 'tis refracted into *a k*, as if it proceeded directly from *p*, *p a k* being a Right Line.

To prove this we must observe that the Angle of Inclination or Incidence is *n a d = o a g*. If therefore it be proved, that the Angle of Refraction *g a k = n a p* is ⅓ of the Angle *n a d*, our first Position will be manifest, *viz.* That the Ray by the first Refraction is bent into *a k*.

First

Tab 17 pag 64

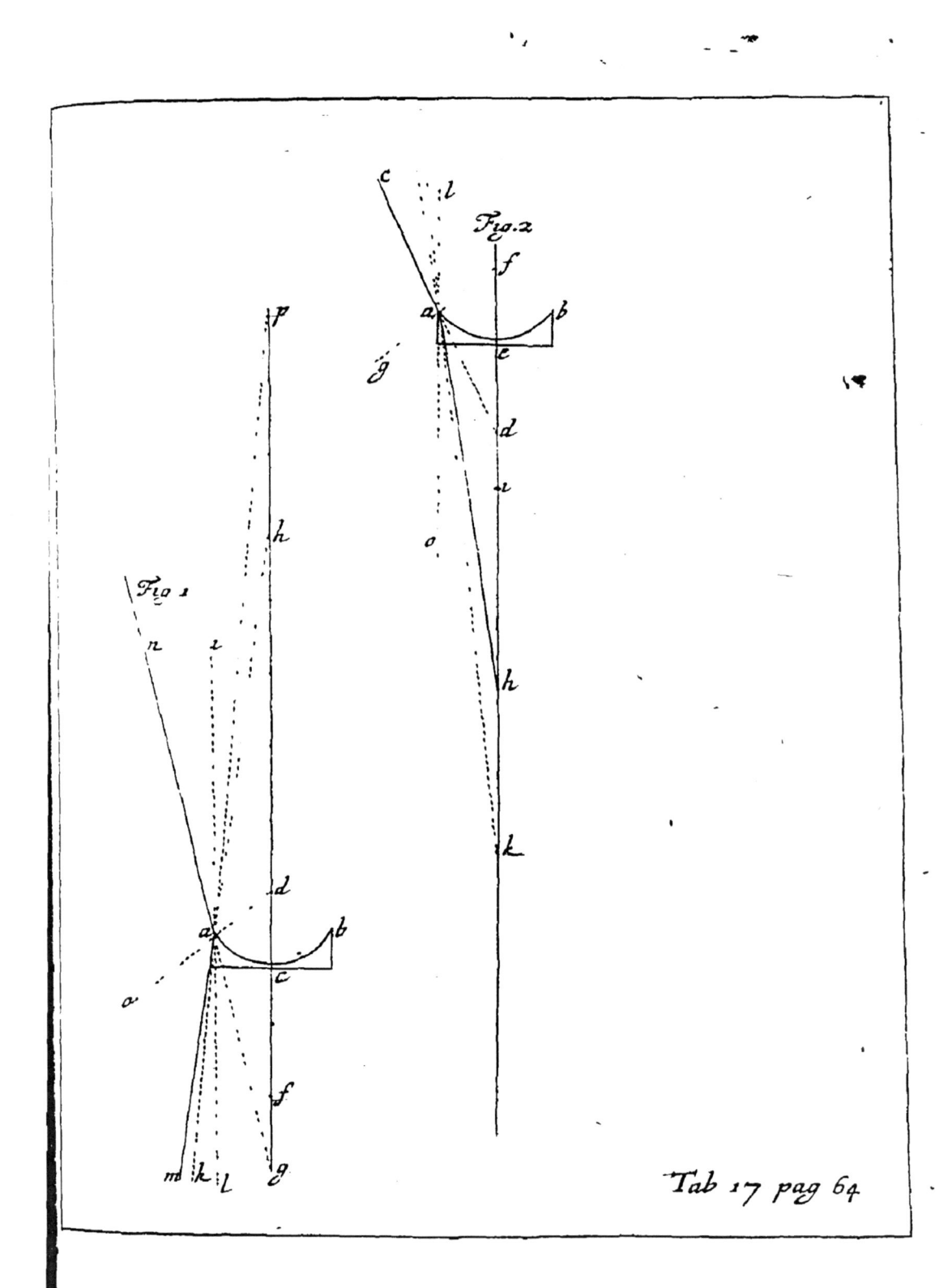

[65]

First therefore it is by Position	1	$gf : fc :: cg : ch$
Add to the Consequents their Halfs — — — — — — —	2	$gf : fd :: cg : cp = pa$
Compounding the second —	3	$gf + fd = gd : fd :: cg + cp = gp : pa$
Also in the Triangle gad —	4	$gd : da = dk :: s\angle dag = s\angle nad : s\angle g$
And Sines and Angles being proportional, it follows from the 4th. — — — — — —	5	$\frac{1}{3} nad \cdot \angle g :: gd : \frac{1}{3} ad = fd$
It then follows from the 5th. and 3d. — — — — — —	6	$\frac{1}{3} nad : \angle g :: gp : pa$
Moreover in the Triangle gap	7	$gp \cdot pa :: s\angle gap = s\angle nap \cdot s\angle g$
And Sines and Angles being proportional — — — — —	8	$gp \cdot pa :: \angle nap : \angle g$
From the 6th and 8th it follows	9	$\frac{1}{3} nad : \angle g :: \angle nap : \angle g$

From which 9th Step 'tis manifest that the first Angle of Refraction, nap, is equal to $\frac{1}{3}$ of the first Angle of Incidence nad. Which was first required to be Demonstrated.

We are secondly to Demonstrate, that by virtue of the second Refraction the Ray receives on the plane side of the Glass at its Egress into Air, 'tis refracted into ma, as if it came directly from h. Draw tal Parallel to the Axis hg, and Perpendicular to the plane side of the Glass; The Angle of Incidence is $lak = tap$; the Angle of Refraction is $mak = hap$; the refracted Angle $mal = hat$.

We are therefore to prove, that the refracted Angle mal is equal to triple the Angle of Refraction mak.

In the Triangle pah we have this Analogy $pa = pc : ph ::$ $s\angle ahp = s\angle ahc = s\angle hat = s\angle mal : s\angle hap = s\angle mak$. But pc is thrice ph, therefore (Sines and Angles being proporti-

K   onal

onal) the Angle *m a l* is thrice the Angle *m a k*. *Which was to be Demonstrated.*

Prop. XV.

Tab 17
Fig 2.

In Concave Glasses a b (T. 17. F. 2.) *if the Point* d *to which the Incident Ray* c a *converges, be nigher to the Glass than the Virtual Focus of Parallel Rays* i; *the Rule to find where it crosses the Axis at* h, *is this,*

> *As the Excess of the Virtual Focus more than this Point of Convergency* i d :
> *To the Virtual Focus* i e : :
> *So the distance of this Point of Convergency from the Glass* d e :
> *To the distance of the Point where this Ray crosses the Axis* h e

In the forementioned Figure *a b* is a Plano Concave Glass, *f* the Center of the Cavity *i e* the Length of the Virtual Focus of Parallel Rays, which we know is a Diameter of the Cavity, that is, $= 2 fe$. On this Glass there falls the Ray *c a* converging directly to the Point *d*. If it be made *i d . i e : : d e : h e*, I say *h* is the Point in the Axis, where the Ray *c a*, after its double Refraction, crosses it.

Demonstration.

For the Proof thereof we suppose all that we laid down as supposed in the last Proposition. Draw *f a* directly to *g*, and make *h k* equal to ½ *h e*. I shall first shew, that by virtue of the first Refraction, which the Ray suffers at *a*, 'tis refracted directly towards *k*. Here the first Angle of Incidence is *c a f*, $= g a d$. If therefore we prove that *k a d* is equal to ½ *c a f*, our first Position shall be manifest, that the Ray is refracted first towards *k*.

For

For by the Rule it is — — —	1	$id : ie :: ed : eh$
Add to the Consequents their Halfs — — — — — — — —	2	$id : if :: ed : ek$
Inverting and dividing the Second	3	$if - id = df : if :: ek - ed = dk : ek$
Moreover in the Triang. dfa	4	$df : af :: s\angle fad = s\angle caf : s\angle adf$
From the 4th Step it follows	5	$\frac{1}{3}\angle caf : \angle adf :: df : \frac{1}{3}af = if$
By the 3d and 4th it is — —	6	$\frac{1}{3}caf : adf :: dk : ek$
Also in the Triangle akd —	7	$kd : ka = ke :: s\angle kad . s\angle kda = s\angle adf$
Sines and Angles being prop.	8	$kd : ke :: \angle kad : \angle adf$
From the 6th and 8th it follows	9	$\frac{1}{3}caf : adf :: kad : adf$

Wherefore from this 9th Step 'tis manifest that kad is equal to $\frac{1}{3} caf$, which was first to be Demonstrated.

I shall next demonstrate, that by virtue of the second Refraction the Ray proceeds in ab.

Draw oal Parallel to the Axis fk, and therefore (by Supposition 2d) perpendicular to the plane side of the Glass. Here the Angle of Incidence from Glass to Air shall be oak. I am therefore to prove that the Angle of Refraction kab is equal to $\frac{1}{3} oab$ the refracted Angle. Thus,

In the Triangle kab it is $ka = ke$ $kb : s\angle abk = s\angle abe$, $= s\angle oab \cdot s\angle kab$

And Sines and Angl. being prop. $ke \cdot kb :: oab : kab$

But kb is $\frac{1}{3}$ of ke and therefore the Angle kab, is $\frac{1}{3}$ of the Angle oab. Which was to be Demonstrated.

K 2   *Diverging*

DIVERGING RAYS.

Corollary.

Concerning *Concave-Glasses* exposed to *Diverging Rays*.

The Virtual Focus of a Concave Glass exposed to *Parallel* Rays is found by *Prop.* X, XI, XII, XIII. And the Properties of a Concave exposed to *Converging* Rays are shewn in *Prop.* XIV. and XV.

T 17. F. 2. Let us now consider a Ray *Diverging* from the Axis, as suppose a nigh Object (*T.* 17. *F.* 2.) in *b*, whose Ray *b a* diverges from the Axis *b e*, and so falls on the Concave Glass *a b*. Let us conceive this nigh Object *b* either farther from, or nigher to the Glass, than the Glasses Virtual Focus. This Ray after passing the Glass diverges more, than before it entred it. And the Rule for determining the Point *d*, from which this Ray after passing the Glass does as it were directly *Diverge*, is this,

> *As the Sum of the distance of the Object from the Glass and the Glass's Virtual Focus*:
> *To the Distance of the Object from the Glass*:
> *So the Glasses Virtual Focus*:
> *To the distance of this Point of Divergency from the Glass*:

Demonstration.

By the foregoing XVth *Prop.* — $id \cdot ie :: de : eb$
And Alternating — — — — — $ie : eb :: id (= ie - de) \cdot de$
And Compounding — — — — $ie + eb \cdot eb :: ie \cdot de$

Which last Analogy gives the forementioned Rule in Words as is manifest by comparing it with the Scheme.

PROP.

Tab 18 pag 69

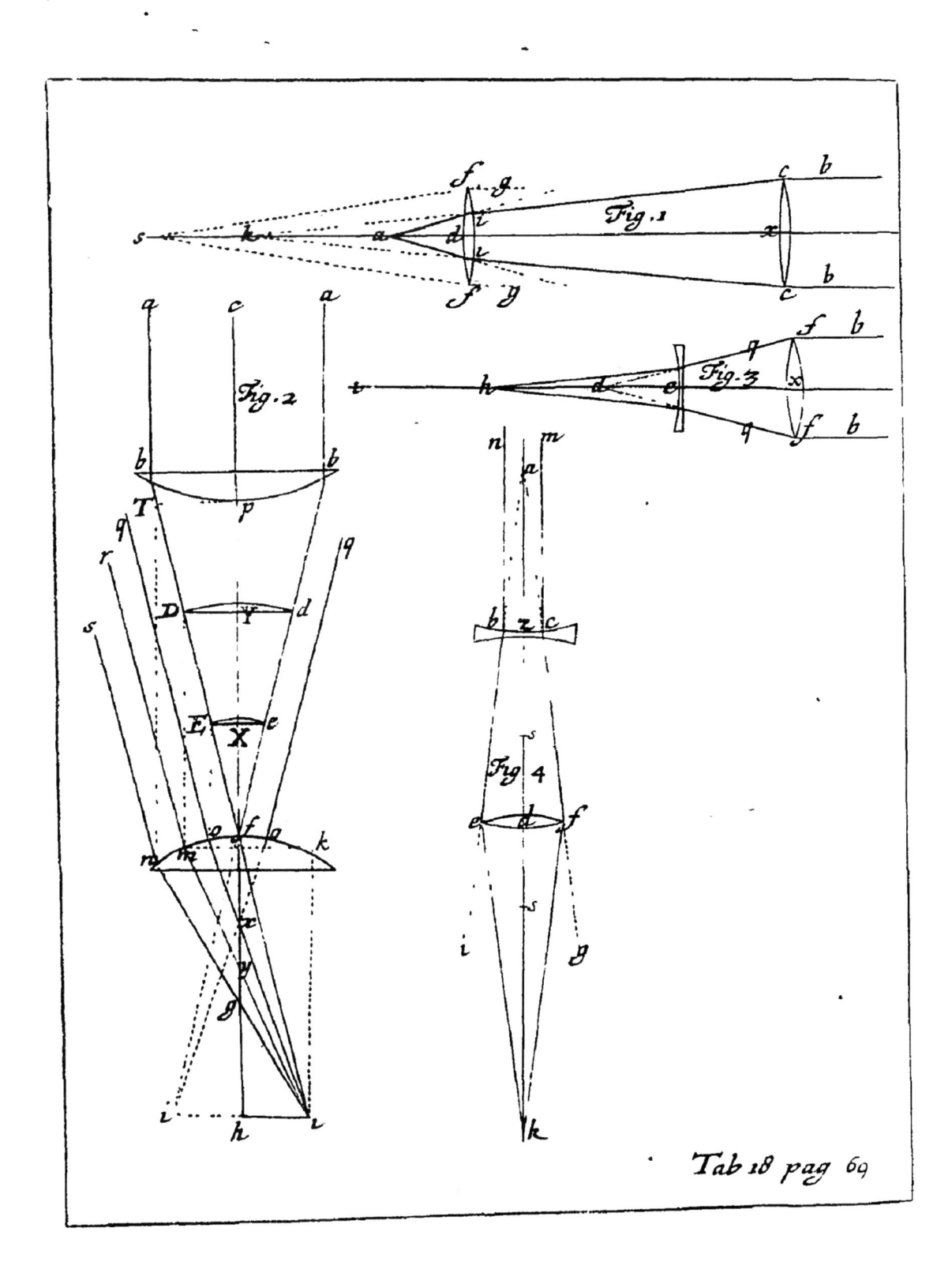

Prop. XVI. Probl.

The Focal Lengths of two Convex-Glasses being given, the longer being placed before the shorter at any given Distance less than the longer Focal Length; 'Tis required to determin the Distance of the Distinct Base from the shorter Glass.

This is solved from the VIII. *Proposition* hereof

Tab. 18. *Fig.* 1. cxc is a Convex Glass uniting the Parallel Rays bc, bc, in its Focus at k; fdf is a shorter Convex uniting the Parallel Rays gf, gf, in its Focus at s. In the Problem, kx the longer Focal Length, and sd the shorter Focal Length, and dx the Distance of the Glasses, are given; To find da, the Point wherein the Rays ci, ci, are united with the Axis by the Glass ff.

By the 8th. *Proposition* preceding, the Focal Length ds of the Convex Glass ff being given, and the Distance of an Object da being given less than the Focal Length ds, to find the Distance dk of the *Imaginary* Focus; the Rule is, As the Difference between the Distance of the Object da, and the Focal Length ds, that is, $ds - da = as$ To the Focal Length ds :: So the Distance of the Object from the Glass ad · To the Distance of the Imaginary Focus from the Glass dk.

Now whereas in the 8th. *Proposition* da is given, and dk sought, in this Problem da is sought, and dk is given; for dk is equal to the Difference between the Focal Length of the longer Glass kx, and the Glass's Distance xd.

Wherefore by the foresaid 8th. *Proposition*, and its Corollary, it being $ds - da = as \cdot ds :: ad \cdot dk$. It shall be also *alternando* $ds : dk :: ds - da : ad$. And Compounding $ds + dk : dk :: ds : ad$. But in this Problem the Three first Terms of this last Analogy are given, and the last ad required.

Where-

Wherefore by this Analogy, the laſt Term *a d* is found. And according to this Analogy we frame this Rule for ſolving this Problem.

As the Focal Length of the ſhorter Glaſs + the Difference between the Focal Length of the longer, and the Glaſſes Diſtance :
To the Difference between the Focal Length of the longer and the Glaſſes Diſtance : :
So the Focal Length of the ſhorter Glaſs :
To the Diſtance of the Diſtinct Baſe from the Glaſs.

Example.

Let the longer Focal Length be $xk = 20$, the ſhorter Focal Length $ds = 8$. The Diſtance of the Glaſſes $dx = 15$.

Then $xk - dx \; (= dk) \; + ds : dk :: ds : ad$

In Numb. $20 - 15 \; (= 5) + 8 = 13 : 5 :: 8 : 3,07692$.

Schol. 1. The ſame Solution holds, if the ſhorter Glaſs be placed before the longer, and the longer Glaſs at any Diſtance from the ſhorter leſs than the Focal Length of the ſhorter.

Let the ſhorter Focal Length be $= 8$, the longer $= 20$, and the Glaſſes Diſtance $= 6$; then $8 - 6 = 2$, and the Propoſition is $8 - 6 + 20 = 22 : 2 :: 20 : 1,8182 =$ to the Diſtance of the *Compound* Diſtinct Baſe (for ſo I'll call it) of theſe two Glaſſes from the laſt and longer Glaſs.

Corollary.

From hence is manifeſt the Rule which is before laid down after our 3d *Propoſition* for Determining the Focus of a double Convex-Glaſs. The Rule is this, *As the Sum of the Radii of both Convexities . To the Radius of either Convexity : So the double Radius of t'other Convexity : To the Diſtance of the Focus.*

For

For Example, Let the Radius of one Convexity be 20, and of t'other 8. Then 28 . 8 :: 40 : 11,4286. Or, 28 : 20 :: 16 : 11,4286 = Focus. Let us then conceive this double Convex-Glass to be divided into two Plano-Convex Glasses, formed on the same Spheres as the two Sides of the double Convex, *viz.* One on a Sphere whose Radius is 20; and t'other on a Sphere whose Radius is 8, and these two Glasses placed touching each other on their plain Sides, the larger Focal Length would be 40, and the shorter Focal Length would be 16, and the Distance of the Glasses would be *Nothing*. Then by the Rule of the XVI. *Prop.* 16 + 40 = 56 : 40 :: 16 : 11,4286 = To the Compound Focus.

Scholium 2.

By this Proposition, and by the Corollaries of *Prop.* XXVI. hereafter, the Eight first Propositions of *Dechales Second Book of Dioptricks* are manifestly solved.

Another Solution of the same Problem.

My esteemed Friend, the Learned and Ingenious Mr. JOHN FLAMSTEED, *Reg. Astron.* has very neatly solved this Problem, and communicated the Solution thereof to me, as follows.

Tab. 18 *Fig* 2. Let bpb represent a Convex-Glass, whose Focus is at f, let ab be two Rays falling upon it parallel to the Axis cf, which shall therefore be collected in f; let nfk be another Convex-Glass of any different Sphere, whose Focus is h, its Distinct Base ihi. 'Tis required to find, at what distance from the Point f, the Distinct Base shall be formed, the Glass nfk being placed any where nearer the Glass bb, as suppose in X, Y, or p.

Through

Through the Points X, Y, p, draw the Lines E X e, D Y d, T p, at Right Angles to the Axis. And from the Points E, D, T, wherein they cut the refracted Ray bf, draw the Lines E o, D m, T n, parallel to the Axis. And from the Points o, m, n, where they fall on the Glass nfk, draw the Lines oq, mr, ns, parallel to the refracted Ray bf, these represent this Ray fb falling upon the Glass nfk placed at X, Y, p.

Produce bf through the Glass to the Distinct Base, which it cuts in ι, we may now consider qo, rm, sn, as three parallel Rays proceeding from the same Point of an Object infinitely distant, which by the known Properties of Glasses, shall be collected into the same Point ι of the Distinct Base with the Ray bf. Draw therefore the Lines $o\iota, m\iota, n\iota$, intersecting the Axis in the Points x, y, g. Now, because the Focus is that Point, where the Ray falling upon the outward Glass is by the second Glass collected or made to converge with the Axis, the Points x, y, g, shall be the Foci sought, that is, fx shall be the Compound Focal Length for the Glass nfk placed in X, fy when 'tis placed in Y; and fg when 'tis placed in p, or when both the Glasses touch.

Now that we may find these Focal Lengths fx, fy, fg, draw mk parallel to the Distinct Base $\iota h \iota$, and ιk parallel to the Axis fh. We suppose the Thickness of the Glasses to be as little as possible, and therefore the Lines representing the Rays, passing *through* them, are *strait*, and not at all bent.

Wherefore the Triangles D Y f, $h \iota f$ are similar. Also the Triangles $mk\iota$, mfy are similar.

It shall therefore be ———	1	$fY : fb :: YD (=mf) : h\iota$
Converting and Compound.	2	$fY+fb . fY :: mf+h\iota : mf$
But by the Scheme ———	3	$mf+h\iota = mk$
Therefore the 2d is thus——	4	$fY+fb . fY :: mk : mf$
And by the sim. $\triangle$ $mk\iota$, mfy——	5	$mk . mf :: k\iota : fy$
From the 4th and 5th it foll.	6	$fY+fb : fY :: k\iota : fy$

Now

Now by Position $bf = pf$ is the longer Focal Length, and $fh = ki$ is the shorter Focal Length, and Yp the Distance of the Glasses; and therefore $fY = pf — pY$ is the longer Focus, — the Distance of the Glasses; and fy is the Distance of the Distinct Base from the inward Glass. From all which, the foregoing 6th Analogy, being resolved into Words, gives his Rule for solving the Problem,

>As the longer Focus — the Glasses Distance + the shorter Focus :
>To the longer Focus — the Glasses Distance ::
>So the shorter Focus :
>To the Distance of the Distinct Base from the inward Glass.

Or thus,

>As the Aggregate of the shorter Focus and the Difference between the longer and the Glasses Distance :
>To the Difference between the longer Focus and Glasses Distance ::
>So the shorter Focal Length :
>To the Distance of the Distinct Base from the inward Glass.

Which is the very same Canon with that I have given, deduced from the 8th Proposition hereof.

This Problem is of considerable Use in Dioptricks, being the Foundation of an excellent sort of Telescope much used in *England* for the Night. But it seems no Optick Writer has solved it. *Honoratus Faber* has clearly omitted it. And *Dechales*, though he offers at our foresaid VIII. Proposition, on which our Solution of this Problem is founded; yet missing so enormously as he has done in that, he could not pretend to the Solution of this. And had he rightly solved our VIII. Propsition, I question whether he would have pushed it on so far as to solve thereby this Problem; for in the two next succeeding Problems, he has rightly the Propositions on which their Solutions depend, but leaves the Problems themselves untouch'd.

[74]

PROP. XVII. PROB 4.

A Convex-Glass being given, with a Concave of a larger Sphere, the Concave being placed behind the Convex, at any Distance less than the Focal Length of the Convex; 'Tis required to find the Place of the Compound Focus, or Distinct Base of these two Glasses.

T 18 F 3   This Problem is solved by the XV. *Proposition* hereof. *Tab.* 18. *F.* 3. The Convex-Glass *x* is placed so before the Concave-Glass *e*, that this Convex would unite the Parallel Rays *b f*, *b f*, in its Focus at *d*, and the Rays *q d*, *q d*, would cross the Axis in *d*, unless the Concave *e* were interposed. Which Concave is supposed to have its Virtual Focus at *i* more distant than *d* the Distance of the Focus of the Convex *x*.

Wherefore here is a Ray *q* incident on the Concave *e*, and converges towards a Point *d*, nigher the Glass *e* than the Virtual Focus of parallel Rays *i* ; and 'tis required to determine the Point *h*, where it crosses the Axis. The Rule by the XV. *Proposition* is this,

> As the *Excess of the Focus of the Concave more than this Point of Convergency* i d :
> To *the Focus of the Concave* i e ::
> So *the Distance of this Point of Convergency from the Glass* d e :
> To *the Distance of the Point where this Ray crosses the Axis* h e :

Now in our present Problem, the three first Terms of this Analogy are given, and the last required. For the Problem gives *d x* the Focal Distance of the Convex, and *i e* the Focus of the Concave, and *e x* the Distance of the Glasses. Hence we have *d e* ($= d x - e x$) the Distance from the Concave of
the

the Point *d*, to which the Ray converges. And we have *i d* (= *ie* — *de*) the Excess of the Virtual Focus of the Concave beyond the Point of Convergency *d*.

Wherefore by the foresaid Analogy it being, As *i d* : *i e* :: *d e* : *b e*. The Rule for Solving this Problem is this,

From the Focal Length of the Convex subtract the Glasses distance. Mark the difference, then say,

  As the Focal Length of the Concave — this difference ·
  To the Focal Length of the Concave :
  So this difference :
  To the distance of the Distinct Base from the Concave.

1. *Example.*	2. *Example.*
Focus Convex = *d x* = 20	Focus Conv. = 12
Focus Concave = *i e* = 60	Focus Conc. = 15
Glasses Distance = *e x* = 10	Glasses Dist. = 2
Hence — — — = *d e* = 10 Diff.	Hence *d e* = 10 Difference
And — — — — = *i d* = 50	And *i d* = 5
Then *i d* = 50 : *i e* = 60 :: *d e* = 10 : *b e* = 12.	Then 5 : 15 :: 10 ; 30 = *b e*.

PROP. XVIII. PROBL.

The Focal Lengths of a Convex-Glass and a Concave-Glass being given, and the Concave placed towards the Object, distant from the Convex, so that the Sum of the Concaves Focal Length and Glasses distance may be greater than the Focal Length of the Convex, and this distance of the Glasses being given also; 'Tis required to determin the distance of the Distinct Base from the Convex.

This is performed by the V. *Proposition* hereof. *Tab.* 18.

T18.F4. *Fig.* 4. Let *b z c* be a Concave, on which there fall the parallel Rays *n b*, *m c*, which are so refracted by this Glass, that after passing it, they proceed on in *b e*, *c f*, as if they came directly from the Point *a* the Virtual Focus of the Concave, (by *Prop.* X. XI. XII. hereof) but in *e* and *f* meeting with the Convex-Glass, whose Focus is on each side it at *s*, *s*, the Rays diverge not to *i* and *g*, but are refracted, so that they cross the Axis in *k*.

We may therefore conceive these Rays, not as passing through the Concave *b c*, but as proceeding directly from the nigh Point *a*; and then to determine the Point *k*, where they cross the Axis, the Rule is in the *Prop.* V. thus,

As *s a* *the difference between the Focus* s d *of the Convex-Glass* e f, *and the distance* d a *of the Object from the Glass*:
To the Focus s d *of the Convex-Glass* ::
So *the distance* d a *of the Object from the Glass* :
To the distance of the respective Focus d k.

Now in this Problem, the three first Terms of this Analogy are given, and the fourth *d k* is required. For the Sum of the Concaves Focal Length and the distance of the Glasses, that is, $za + dz$ is equal to da; and $da - $ the Convex's Focal Length that is $da - sd$ is equal to sa.

Wherefore we solve the Problem by this Canon.

From the Sum of the Focus of the Concave and distance of the Glasses subtract the Focus *of the Convex, that is,* $za + dz - sd = sa$. *Keep this difference, then say,*

As this difference s a :
To the Focus of the Convex s d ::
So the Sum of the Concave's Focus and Glasses distance $za + dz = ad$:
To the distance of the Focus from the Convex d k.

Which is required by the Problem, and is the very Analogy of our *Prop.* V.

Tab 19 pag 77

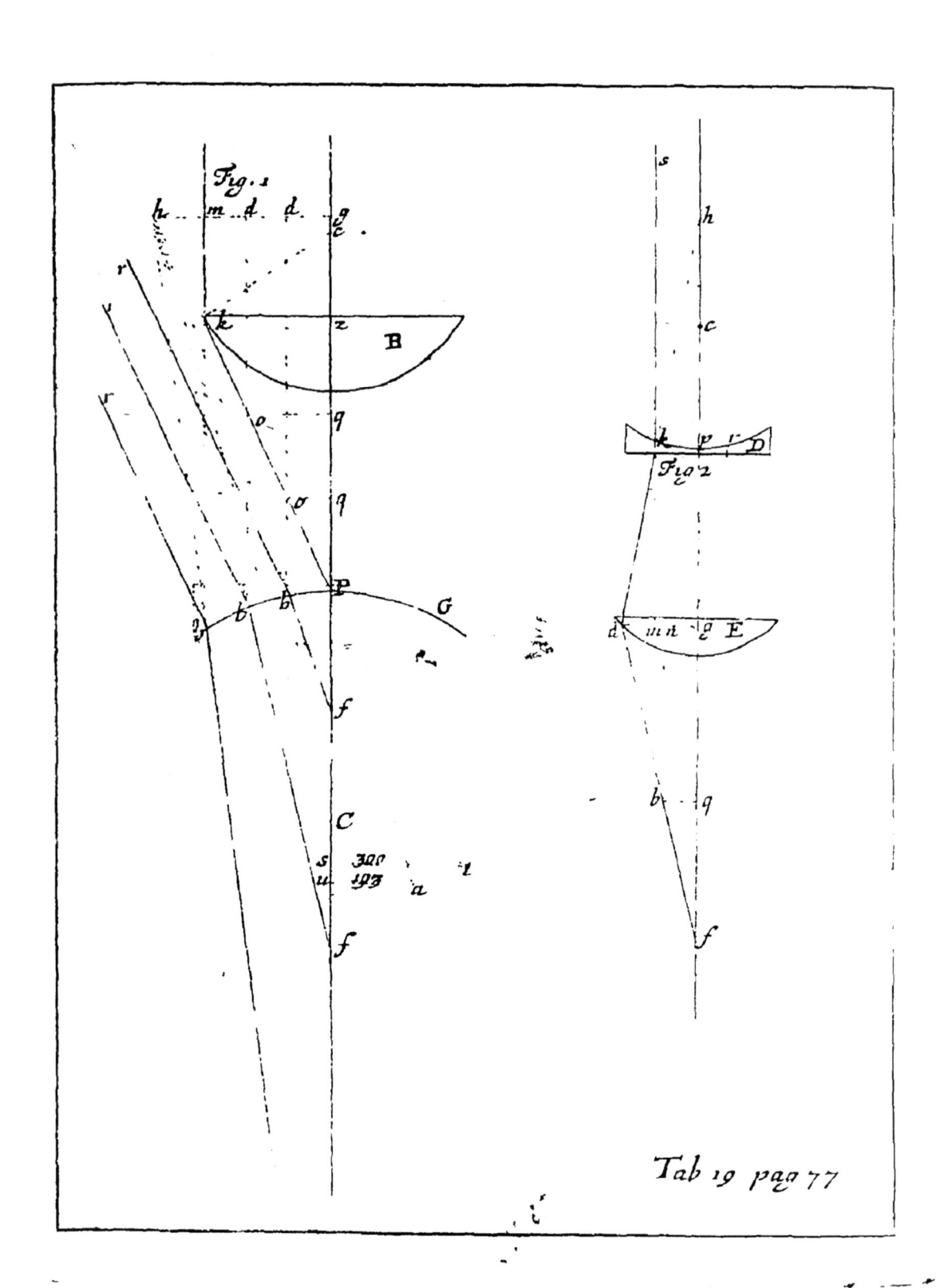

Another Solution of the Two last Problems in Prop. XVII. *and* XVIII.

These Two last Problems were likewise communicated to me, most ingeniously solved by my forementioned Honoured Friend Mr. J. Flamsteed. The Solutions I shall give in his own Words at large, as I have them in a Letter to me Dated from the *Greenwich Observatory, Jan.* 17. 168$\frac{4}{5}$. as follows.

The First Problem is this, *A Convex Glass being given, with a Concave of a larger Sphere; the Concave being placed at any distance less than the Focal Length of the Convex from it, and remoter from the Object; To find the Place of the Focus or Distinct Base.*

The Second Problem is, *From the same Data; the Concave being placed nigher the Object; To find the Distinct Base.*

For the First Problem, *Tab.* 19. *Fig.* 1. B is a Convex-Glass, T 19. F. 1. P its Focus, mk a Ray of Light falling upon it parallel to its Axis, which will therefore converge into its Focus at P. G is a Concave-Glass of a larger Sphere, placed upon the Focus of the Convex; C P the Radius of the Sphere whereon the Concave is formed. And we are always to conceive the Thickness of both these Glasses where the Rays of Light pierce them as small as possible.

Draw the Line k P, this shews the way of the Ray mk after its Emersion from the Convex B. Produce it both ways at pleasure to t and h. Then conceive the Concave G placed any where betwixt P and B, as in q, q; From which Places draw the Lines $q o, q o$, at Right Angles to the Axis. And from the Points o, o, k, wherein they intersect the refracted Ray k P; draw the Lines $o b, o b, k b$, falling on the Concave G in b, b, b. From these Points again draw the Lines br, br, br, parallel to the refracted Ray k P; these shall re-

present

present the Ray k P falling on the Concave G placed at q, q, and also when it touches the Convex B. Let these then be consider'd as so many parallel Rays, proceeding from the same distant Point. Wherever they shall intersect the Axis after they have passed the Concave, there shall be the true Focus for both Glasses, which I shall call the *Compound Focus*. To find which we are to remember;

That, as the Parallel Rays of Light falling on a Convex-Glass, are all collected very nearly in the same Point of the distinct Base; so also the Rays of Light falling Parallel to each other on a Concave, after they emerge from it, diverge and separate, as if they had all proceeded from the same Point, which I therefore call the *Point of Divergency* (*This, in my foregoing Propositions, I term with most Optick Writers, the* Virtual Focus) Which Point in a Concave Glass is just as far distant from it, as the Point of *Convergency*, or Focus of a Convex of the same Sphere or Spheres is distant from it. We know the Focal Point is some little nigher the Glass in the Parallel Rays that fall *widest* from the Axis, than in those that fall near it; so is the Point of *Divergency* for Concaves. But the difference is so small in Glasses of a large Sphere (such as in these Problems we suppose) that for all Rays falling on the Glass Parallel to each other, it may be taken as a *simple Point*. Such therefore we are to conceive it; and then to find this Point of Divergency, The Rule is (*Corol. Prop.* XI.) $300 - 193 = 107 : 193$ ∷ So C P the Radius of the Plano-Concave-Glass: To P h: Which in Glasses of a large Sphere, and where the Inclination of P h is small, will be insensibly different from P g; $h g$ being perpendicular to the Axis. Or we may determine this Point of Divergence Geometrically thus, On the Centre P with any Radius P t, on the void side of the Figure, strike the Arch $a t$; then make it $300 . 193 :: t s . a u$. Draw P a, and from C the Centre of the Concave draw C h Parallel to a P. The Point h, wherein it cuts the Line P k produced

duced upwards, shall be the Point of Divergency sought.

Lay a Ruler over the Point h, and the Points b, b, b; this, where it cuts the Axis $g\,p$ produced, as in f, f, shall give all the possible Compound Foci.

Then hg being perpendicular to the Axis, produce the Lines bo, till they cut it in d, d.

Then the Triangles hPg, oPq are similar: likewise the Triangles bfg, bfP are similar also.

It will then hold *ob similia Triangula* hPg, oPq	1. $hP : oP :: hg : dg$
Dividing the First ——	2. $hP - oP . oP :: hg - dg : dg$
That is, —— —— ——	3. $bo : oP :: hd : dg = oq$
Moreover by *Simil. Triang.* bfg, bfP —— ——	4. $hd : dg :: bb : bf$
From the 3d and 4th it follows —— —— ——	5. $bo : oP :: bb . bf$
And Compound the 5th —	6. $bo + oP : oP :: bb + bf : bf$
That is, —— —— ——	7. $hP : oP :: bf : bf$
And Dividing the 7th —	8. $hP - oP : oP :: bf - bf : bf$
That is, —— —— ——	9. $hP - oP : oP :: bb : bf$
But $hP = gP = bb$, and so likewise $oP = qP$, (the Inclination of kP, as is said before, being supposed very small, and the Glasses of small Segments of large Spheres.) Wherefore the 9th is thus —— ——	10. $gP - qP : qP :: gP : bf$

But by Position ⎰ Focus of the Concave 11. $= gP = hP$.
⎱ Focus of the Convex — 12. $= zP$.
⎰ Distance of the Glasses 13. $= zq$
⎱ Fo. Convex — Gl. dist. $= qP = zP - zq$.

Wherefore

[80]

Wherefore the 10th. Analogy, by the 11th, 12th, and 13th Steps, resolved into Words gives this Rule,

As the Focus of the Concave — Focus of the Convex + distance of the Glasses:
To the Focus of the Convex — distance of the Glasses ::
So the Focus of the Concave:
To bf = *to the distance of the Distinct Base from the Concave.*

And this Canon of Mr. Flamsteed is the very same with ours in the preceding 17th Proposition deduced from the 15th hereof.

But if the Concave be placed next the Object: Which is his Problem II, and our XVIIIth Proposition, my forementioned Learned Friend solves it thus.

T 19. F 2. *Tab.* 19. *F.* 2. D is a Concave, E a Convex, hp the Focal Length of the Concave, $gp = gq$ the Focal Length of the Convex. Let sk be a Ray of Light falling into the Concave at k. From the Point of Divergency h, through k draw the Line kd, this shall shew the refracted Path of the Ray sk after it has passed the Glass D. From q the Focus of the Convex E erect qb perpendicular to the Axis hf; and through g draw the Line igb Parallel to kd, intersecting the distinct Base of the Convex E in b, through which draw db, continuing it till it intersect the Axis in f: There shall be the compound Focus or distinct Base for these Glasses thus posited. Draw now the Line dg at Right Angles to the Axis; produce sk till it cut dg in m, and draw bn Parallel to qg.

Then the Triangles hdg, hkp, bgq, are similar. Also the Triangles bdn, fbq, are similar. And $hp + pg = hg$.

It shall therefore be — — —	1	$hg : gq :: dg : ng = bq$
And converting the First —	2	$hg : hg - gq :: dg : dg - ng$
Inverting the second — —	3	$hg - gq : hg :: dg - ng : dg.$
That is, by the Scheme —	4	$hg - gq . hg :: dn . dg.$

Then

Then by the similar Triangles dnb, dgf — — — — | 5 | $dn : dg :: nb = gq : gf$
From 4 and 5 it follows — | 6 | $hg - gq : hg :: gq : gf$
Then hg being = to $hp + pg$, the 6th is thus | 7 | $hp + pg - gq : hp + pg :: gq : gf.$

But by Position
- Focus of the Concave — | 8 | $= hp$
- Focus of the Convex — | 9 | $= gq$
- Distance of the Glasses — | 10 | $= pg$
- Focus of Concave + Glasses dist. — — — — | 11 | $= hg = hp + pg$
- Dist. of the distinct Base from Convex — — — | 12 | $= gf$

From all which the 7th Analogy may be thus expressed in words,

As the Focus of the Concave + the distance of the Glasses — the Focus of the Convex:

To the Focus of the Concave + the distance of the Glasses ::

So the Focus of the Convex:

To the Distance of the distinct Base from the Convex:

Which is the same Rule with that which I have before given in *Prop.* XVIII, deduced from the 5th hereof.

And these two last Propositions do naturally lead us to the Consideration of *Meniscus*-Glasses.

MENISCUS-GLASSES.

That is called a *Meniscus-Glass*, which is Convex on one side and Concave on t'other. 'Tis so named from its Resemblance to the New Moon or *Lunula*, in Greek μἡνίσκος.

In *Meniscus-Glasses* either the Semidiameter of the Convexity and Concavity are equal or unequal. If they are equal the Ray that falls thereon Parallel to the Axis, after Refraction proceeds

ceeds again Parallel If they are unequal, then either the Semidiameter of the Convexity is less than the Semidiameter of the Cavity, and then the Convexity prevails, and the Glass has a *Real Focus*: Or else the Semidiameter of the Cavity is less than the Semidiameter of the Convexity, and then the Cavity prevails, and the Glass has only a *Virtual Focus*. But of these more fully in the following Propositions, This *Observation* being premised, That the Focus of a *Meniscus*, the Semidiameter of whose Convexity is less than the Semidiameter of the Concavity, and these two Semidiameters being given, is easily determined by *Prop*. XVII preceding. For in that Proposition, two Glasses are given, one a Convex, and t'other a Concave, and the Focal Length of the Convex is shorter than that of the Concave. And whereas in that *Prop*. there is given a distance between the Glasses, let us conceive this Distance to be *nothing*, that is, let us imagine these Glasses to *touch*, and their Results a *Meniscus* whose Focus is determined by the same Rule in that *Prop*. Which is this,

Observ

> *As the Focal Length of the Concave — the Focal Length of the Convex + the Glasses Distance:*
> *To the Focal Length of the Concave:*
> *So the Focal Length of the Convex — the Glasses Distance:*
> *To the Distance of the Distinct Base from the Concave.*

But because we suppose, in the Case of a *Meniscus*, the two sides of the Glass to touch, that is, the distance of the two Glasses to be *nothing* (for every *Meniscus* may be conceived divided into two Glasses, a Plano-Convex, and a Plano Concave) or the Thickness of the Glass to be inconsiderable in Comparison of the Focal Length. The foresaide Rule applyed to a *Meniscus* shall be this,

As

Tab. 20 pag. 83

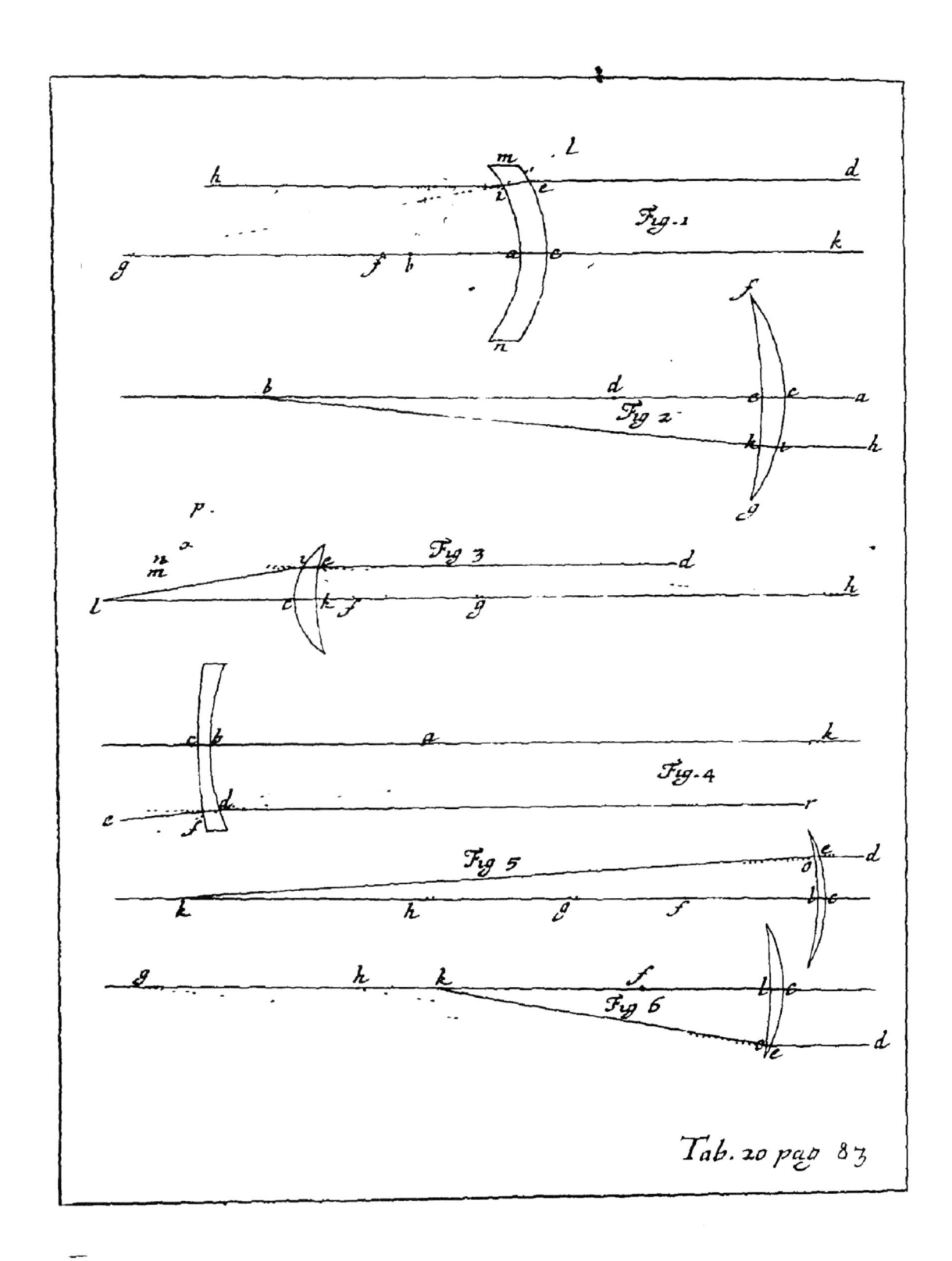

As the Focal Length of the Concave — the Focal Length of the Convex :
To the Focal Length of the Concave ∴
So the Focal Length of the Convex :
To the Distance of the Focus of the Meniscus.

Now if we have given the Semidiameters of the Convexity and Concavity of a *Meniscus*, we have given the Focal Lengths of the Plano-Convex and Plano-Concave of which this *Meniscus* is compounded. For these Focal Lengths may be assumed the Doubles of the Semidiameters, wherefore Halfs being as their Wholes, the foresaid Rule for finding the Focus of a *Meniscus* may be thus expressed,

As the Difference of the Semidiameters of the Convexity and Concavity :
To the Semidiameter of the Concavity ::
So the Diameter of the Convexity :
To the Focal Length.

Which is the Common Rule assigned by Optick Writers. But of this more fully hereafter *Prop.* XXIII. And tho this Rule in General were sufficient for determining the Foci of *Meniscus-Glasses*, yet I shall inlarge more fully thereon in the following Propositions.

PROP. XIX.

In a Meniscus, if both spherical Superficies have the same Diameter, the Ray that falls thereon Parallel to the Axis, after its second Refraction proceeds again Parallel.

Tab. 20. F. 1. mn is a *Meniscus*, bc the Semidiameter of the Convexity ec, fa the Semidiameter of the Concavity ia, de a Ray of Light Parallel to the Axis kg. I say this Ray after a double Refraction, one at e, and t'other at i, proceeds in ih Parallel to kg.

We here suppose the Thickness of the Glass inconsiderable in respect of the Semidiameter of the Sphere on which 'tis form'd; and therefore we wholly neglect it.

We suppose also that Sines and Angles and Sides in these small Angles are Proportional.

Let $gc = ga$ be made Triple $bc = fa$, the Ray de by its first Refraction at it's Entrance into the Glass at e is refracted towards g, eig being a Right Line; at i the Ray emerges from the Glass on the Concave Surface ia. Draw fil. Now the Angle of Inclination within the Glass is $lie = fig$, and if the Ray be refracted into ih, the Angle of Refraction is $hig = igf$, which ought therefore to be $\frac{1}{3}$ the Inclination fig, and, that it is so, I thus prove.

In the Triangle gif, As gf : To if :: So the Angle gif : To the Angle igf. But gf is double if, therefore $\angle gif$ is double $\angle igf$. Which was to be Demonstrated.

Prop. XX.

In a Meniscus, if the Semidiameter of the Concavity be triple the Semidiameter of the Convexity, the Focal Length is equal to the Semidiameter of the Concavity.

This is most evident, if the Convex side be turned to the Ray, as *Tab. 20. Fig. 2.* hi is a Ray parallel to the Axis ab, dc the Semidiameter of the Convexity $fcig$, $be = 3 dc$ the Semidiameter of the Concavity $fekg$. The Ray, by the first Refraction it suffers on the Convex Surface at i, is directed to concur with the Axis at a Diameter and an half of the Convexity, that is, in b. But b is the Centre of the Concavity; wherefore the Ray ik within the Glass falls perpendicularly on the Concave Surface fkg; and therefore is not at all refracted by its Emersion from the Glass, but proceeds onwards directly in ikb. Which was to be Demonstrated. But

[85]

But let the Concave-side be towards the Ray, as *Tab.* 20. *Fig.* 3. fc is the Semidiameter of the Convexity ic, $gk = 3fc$ the Semidiameter of the Concavity ek, de a Ray parallel to the Axis, produced directly to m. Let lc be made equal to gk, I say the Focus shall be at l, lc being equal to the Semidiameter of the Concavity. Draw geo. The Angle of the Rays Inclination on the Concave Surface is $deg = oem$ (Ang. ad *Verticem*) and the Ray by the first Refraction it receives on the Concave Surface at e is so refracted as if it came from the Point h distant a Diameter and half of the Concavity then draw $hein$ directly. Here $men = deh = ehg$ is the Angle of Refraction, which is therefore ½ of the Inclination $deg = egk = oem$. But we suppose, as the Angles so are the Sines, and so are the Sides. Wherefore in the Triangle egh, $s\angle egh = s\angle egk : s\angle ehk :: eh = kh : eg$, that is, $\angle egk : \angle ehk :: kh : eg$. But the Angle egk is equal to $3 \angle ehk$, and therefore kh is equal to $3 eg$, and consequently gh is double eg or gk. From f the Centre of the Convexity draw fip, this is perpendicular to the Convex Surface ic. Wherefore seeing gh is double gk, and gk is triple fc or fi, hf shall be octuple fi (by the Scheme). And the Second Angle of Inclination hif on the Convex Surface shall be octuple of the Angle at h, because their Correspondent subtending Sides are as 8 to 1. But hif is equal to pin (*Ang ad Vert.*) And because at the Rays Egress from Glass to Air, the Angle of Refraction nil ought to be half the Inclination pin, so let it be made; and then seeing the Angle pin is octuple the Angle at h, its half nil shall be quadruple the Angle at h, from the Angle nil subtract the Angle $nim = dih = \angle h$, there remains the Angle $mil = ilf = 3 \angle h$, wherefore the Angle at l and $egk = 3 ehk$ are equal. And then in the Triangle elg (neglecting the Thickness of the Glass) el and eg, or cl and kg the Semidiameter of the Concavity are equal. *Which was to be Demonstrated.*

Observation.

Observation.

This is the 28th. *Prop.* of *Dechales* First Book of *Dioptricks*, which he there huddles over in a most confused manner, omitting several Steps in the Demonstration. *Zahn* has the same in *Fund.* 2. *Syntag.* 1. *Cap.* 7. *Prop.* 32. and transcribes from *Dechales* not omitting his very Errors.

PROP. XXI.

In a Meniscus, the Semidiameter of whose Convexity is triple the Semidiameter of the Concavity, The Virtual Focus is distant the Semidiameter of the Convexity.

T 20 F 4. *Tab.* 20. *F.* 4. ab is the Semidiameter of the Concavity bd, $kc = 3\, ab$ is the Semidiameter of the Convexity cf, rd a Ray parallel to the Axis kc. This Ray by the first Refraction it receives on the Concave Surface at d, is refracted into de, as if it came directly from the Point k (by *Prop.* X.), wherefore de falls perpendicular on the Convex Surface (by *Def.* 10.) and consequently is not refracted at its egress from the Glass (by *Exp.* 3.) wherefore the Virtual Focus is at k. Which was to be Demonstrated.

PROP. XXII.

In whatever Meniscus wherein the Semidiameters of the Convexity and Concavity are unequal; The General Rule that assigns the Focus either Real or Virtual is this,

As the difference of the Semidiameters :
To either of the Semidiameters, whether of the Convexity or Concavity ::
So is the Diameter of the other Surface :
To the Focus Real or Virtual.

(Case

(*Case* 1.) I shall demonstrate this *Proposition* in Three several Cases, and the First shall be, Where the Semidiameter of the Concave is greater than the Semidiameter of the Convex, but less than triple the Semidiameter of the Convex.

(*Case* 2.) Wherein the Semidiameter of the Concave is greater than triple the Semidiameter of the Convex.

And in these Two Cases the Glass has a *Real Focus*.

(*Case* 3.) Wherein the Semidiameter of the Concave is less than the Semidiameter of the Convex, and then the Glass has only a *Virtual Focus*.

'Tis here supposed, that the Breadth of the Glass is so little, and the Angles so small, that Sines and Angles and Sides may be proportional. For an Angle, we often assume its Complement to 180°, as having the same Sine.

'Tis supposed likewise that the Thickness of the Glass is inconsiderable, and therefore 'tis wholly neglected.

First therefore for the First Case. *Tab.* 20. *Fig.* 5. Let de be a Ray parallel to the Axis ck, fc is the Semidiameter of the Convexity ec, gl is the Semidiameter of the Concavity ol. Make hc triple fc. Then by the first Refraction the Ray suffers at e, 'tis directed towards h (by *Prop* I.). Wherefore the Angle of Inclination upon its Emersion from the Glass is goh. Let the Angle of Refraction hok be made half goh. Then k is the Focus, and it being so made, I say, the difference of the Semidiameters $= fg$: Is to fc the one Semidiameter :: As $2gl$ the other Diameter : To ck the Focal Length.

Demonstration.

In the Triangle hog —— 1 | $\angle hog : \angle obg :: bg : go = gl$
And therefore —— — — 2 | $\frac{1}{2} hog = hok : obg :: bg : 2gl$
Moreover in the Triang. hok 3 | $hok : obg :: bk : ok = kl$
From 2 and 3 it follows — 4 | $bg : 2gl :: bk : kl$

By

[88]

By permuting the 4th.	5	$2gl \cdot kl :: hg : hk$
Compounding the 5th.	6	$2gl+kl : kl :: hg+hk = gk : hk$
But kl is equal to $kg + gl$, therefore	7	$2gl+kl = 2gl+kg+gl = 3gl+gk$
Wherefore the 6th. runs thus	8	$3gl+gk : kl :: gk : hk$
By permuting the 8th.	9	$3gl+gk : gk :: kl : hk$
Dividing the 9th.	10	$3gl : gk :: kl-hk = hl : hk$
And permuting the 10th.	11	$3gl : hl = 3fl :: gk : hk$
From 11 and 6 it follows	12	$3gl : 3fl :: 2gl+kl : kl$
And consequently from 12	13	$gl : fl :: 2gl+kl : kl$
Dividing the 13th.	14	$gl-fl=fg : fl=fc :: 2gl : kl=kc$

For the Thickness of the Glass is neglected, and therefore we assume $kl = kc$.

But this 14th. Analogy $fg : fc :: 2gl : kc$. Is the *Proposition* which was to be Demonstrated.

Note, *Zahn* does again in this *Proposition* transcribe from *Dechales*, and copies the very Mistakes of the Press. But in our foregoing Demonstration all is rectified.

Corollary

Because	$fg : fc :: 2gl : kc$
It shall also be	$fg : gl :: 2fc : kc$
For if it be	$fg : fc :: 2gl : kc$
Then Permuting	$fg : 2gl :: fc : kc$

Then halve the first Consequent and double the last Antecedent, and it shall be $fg : gl :: 2fc : kc$. *Which was to be Demonstrated.*

T 20. F. 6. In the 2. *Case*, Let fc, *Tab.* 20. *Fig.* 6. be the Semidiameter of the Convexity ec. Make ch equal to $3fc$. Let gl be the Semidiameter of the Concave lo, de a Ray parallel to to the Axis, which by the first Refraction tends towards h (by *Prop.* I.) Now the Angle of Inclination on the Concave Surface is hog; for go is the Perpendicular. Wherefore the Ray by the second Refraction from Glass to Air is bent from the Perpendicular by half the Angle of Inclination; Let koh be this Angle of Refraction $= \frac{1}{2} hog$. I say then, that As gf: To lf or fc (neglecting the Thickness of the Glass) :: So $2 gl$: To ch or lk.

Demonstration.

In the Triangle $g o b$ — —	1|$\angle ohg$ or $obl : \angle goh :: og = gl : gh$.
And therefore — — — —	2|$obl : \frac{1}{2} goh = hok :: 2gl : gh$
Moreover in the Triang. hok	3|$obl : hok :: ok = lk : kh$.
From 2 and 3 it follows —	4|$2gl : gh :: lk : kh$.
Permuting 4 — — —	5|$2gl : lk :: gh : kh$.
Compound the 4th. — —	6|$2gl+gh : gh :: lk+kh : kh$.
Permute the 6th. — — —	7|$2gl+gh : lk+kh :. gh : kh$.
From 5 and 7 it follows —	8|$2gl+gh : lk+kh = lh :: 2gl : lk$.
Compound the 8th.	9|$2gl+(gh+lh=)gl = 3gl : lh = 3 lf :: 2gl+lk : lk$.
And from the 9th. it follows	10|$gl : lf :: 2gl+lk : lk$.
And dividing the 10	11|$gl-lf = gf : lf :: 2gl : lk$.

Which was to be Demonstrated.

Corollary.

Because — — — $gf : lf :. 2gl : lk$.
It shall be also — — — $gf : gl :: 2lf : lk$, by the foregoing *Corollary.*

Lastly

Lastly in the third Case, *Tab.* 21. *f.* 1. fl is the Semidiameter of the Concavity il, nc the Semidiameter of the Convexity ec. Let cm be made Triple nc. de is a Ray Parallel to the Axis km. this Ray by its First Refraction proceeds in eim; at i it emerges into Air on the Concave Surface. Draw the Perpendicular fig. The Angle of Inclination on this Concave Surface is $eig = fim$, *ad Vert.* Let the Angle of Refraction him be made equal to $\frac{1}{2} fim$. as it ought to be. Then, I say, the Ray Proceeds after its Second Refraction in ih, as if it came directly from the Virtual Focus k, and that then it shall be, as $nf . nc :: 2fl : kc$.

Demonstration.

In the Trian. mif — —	1|$\angle mif : \angle m :: fm : fi = fl$.
Therefore — — — — —	2|$\frac{1}{2} mif = him : \angle m :: fm : 2fl$.
Also in Trian. mik — —	3|$\angle mik$ or its Compl. $\angle him :$ $\angle m :: mk : ik = kl$.
From 2 and 3 — — —	4|$fm : 2fl :: mk : kl = kc$ neglecting the Thickness.
Dividing 4 — — — —	5|$fm - 2fl : 2fl :: mk - kl =$ $ml = mc : kc$.
But by Position in the Scheme	6|$fm - 2fl = ml - 3fl$.
Wherefore the 5th Runs thus	7|$ml (= mc) - 3fl : 2fl :: ml$ $= mc : kc$.
And Permuting 7 — — —	8|$mc (= 3nc) - 3fl : mc ::$ $2fl : kc$.
And therefore — — — —	9|$nc - fl = nf : \frac{1}{3} mc = nc ::$ $2fl : kc$.

Which was to be Demonstrated.

Tab. 21. pag 90

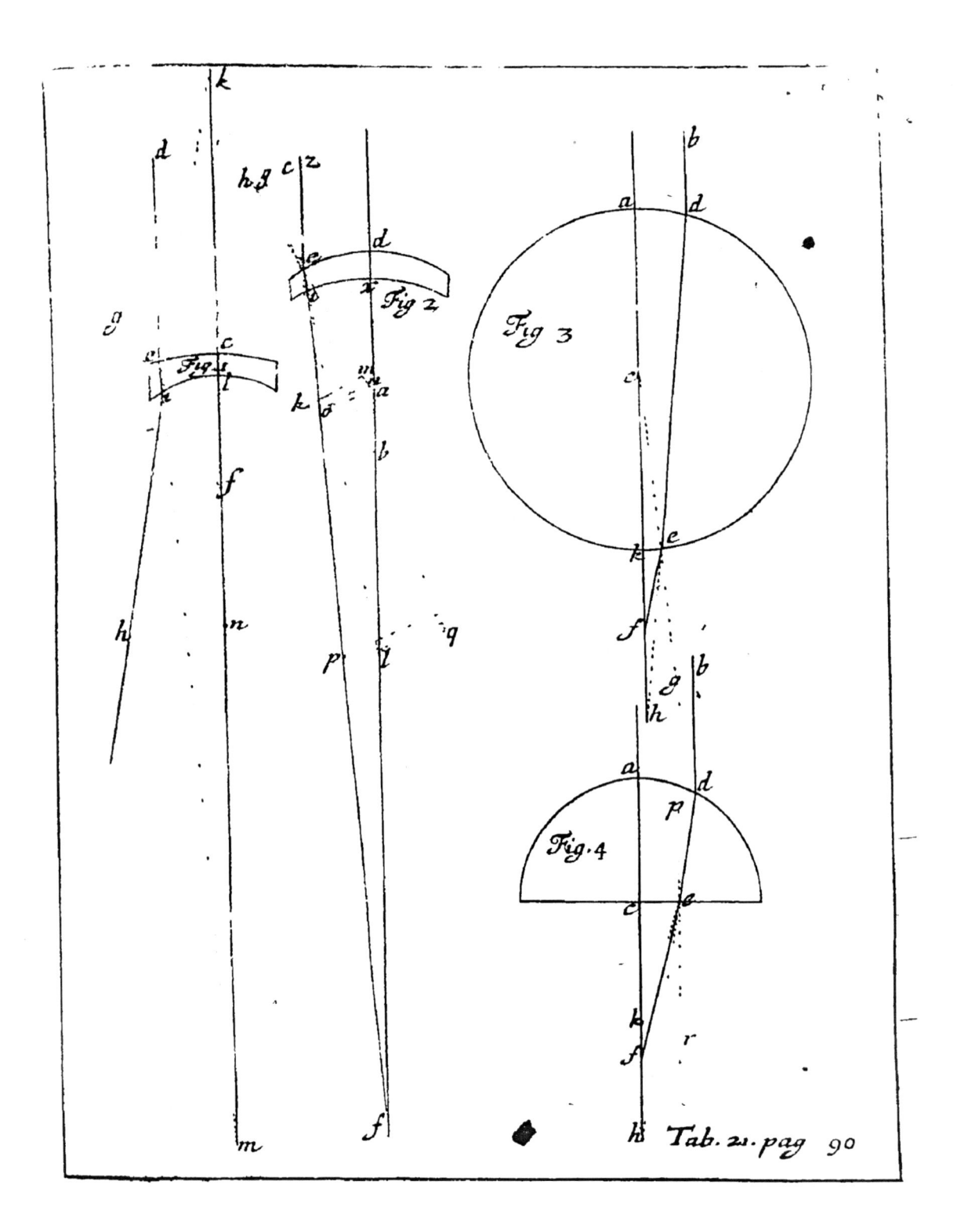

Corollary.

Seeing it is — — — $nf : nc :: 2fl : kc$.
It shall be also — — $nf : fl :: 2nc \cdot kc$.
Vid. Preceding Corollaries.

PROP. XXIII. PROBL.

The Semidiameter of the Convexity being given, 'tis required to find the Semidiameter of the Concavity, that a Meniscus formed with this Convexity and Concavity may unite the Parallel Rays at a given distance. Vid. Barrow Lect. Opt. 14. pag. 102. &c. Edit. Lond. 1672. 4to.

Tab. 21 F. 2. $ae = ad$ is the given Semidiameter of the Convexity, df is the given Distance, at which the Parallel Rays are to be united, ze produced to k is a Ray Parallel to the Axis df. Draw aeh on the Point of Incidence e as a Centre at any Interval, strike the Arch koa, and make the sine of the Angle of Incidence km, to the Sine of the first refracted Angle on, as 300 to 193, or as 14 to 9. Draw eol produced the other way to c. The Ray by the first Refraction is directed to l, in the Line le take any Point at Pleasure i, so that ei may be the Thickness of the Glass which is to be formed; which Thickness is here represented considerable, for Illustration sake, but it being really of no Moment in Glasses of small Segments of large Spheres, 'tis neglected altogether in Demonstration. Draw fi which we suppose equal to fd. And make the Angle liq. To the Angle lif :: As 193 : To 107. Draw qi which cuts the Axis in b. On b as a Centre strike the Arch of the Concavity ix. I say $bi = bx$ is the Semidiameter of the Concavity, which added on t'other side the Glass to the former given Convexity, shall unite the Parallel Rays at the given distance df.

Demonstration.

By the first Refraction the Course of the Ray is through eil, but at i it meets the Concave Surface, and emerges from thence into Air. Now the second Angle of Inclination is bil, for bi is perpendicular to the Concave Surface. But the Angle lif is (by Construction) To the Angle liq.: As 107 : To 193. Wherefore lif is the second Angle of Refraction agreable to the second Angle of Inclination bil (by *Exp.* 6.) Wherefore ipf is the refracted Ray. *Which was to be Demonstrated.*

Calculation of an Example.

Let the Semidiameter of the Convexity $ae = ad$ be given 10000. and the Focal Distance $df = fi$ 63000.

Let us suppose the first Angle of Inclination kea to be 5°. 0′. 0″.

Then as 300 : to 107 :: $s.\angle kea : s.\angle ila$, which is the first Angle of Refraction = 1°. 46′. 50″. Wherefore ilf = 178°. 13′. 10″.

Also (by *Prop.* 1.) As 107 : 300 : $ae = 10000$: To $el = il = ld = 28037$.

Then in the Triangle ifl, we have the three sides and the Angle ilf, to find the Angle, $ifl = 0°. 47′. 30″$ and $fil = 0°. 59′. 20″$.

Say then, As 107 : To 193 :: $s.\angle fil : s.\angle liq$ which we shall find to be 1°. 47′. 0″.

And $fil + liq = fib = 2°. 46′. 20″$. Also $180° - fib - ifl = ibf = 176°. 26′. 10″$.

Lastly in the Triangle fib

As $s.\angle ibf =$ 176°. 26′. 20″ Log. comp. ar. 1.2064785633
To $s.\angle ifb =$ 0 47 30 —————— 8.1404059077
So $if = 63000$ —————————— 4.7993405495
To $bi = 14000$ —————————— 4.1462250205

Where-

Wherefore I say that a *Meniscus*, whose Convexity hath the Semidiameter 10000, and the Concavity the Semidiameter 14000, has its Focal Length 63000.

Further Proof.

To Prove this by some of the foregoing Rules for finding the Focus of a *Meniscus*. Let us conceive such a *Meniscus* to consist of a Plano-Convex Glass, and a Plano-Concave Glass. And the Semidiameter of the Plano Convex to be 10000, and the Semidiameter of the Plano-Concave 14000. Then to find the Focal Lengths of these Glasses separately, say,

By *Corol. Prop.* II.   107 : 193 : : 10000 : 18037 = *Fo. Conv.*
And by *Corol. Pr.* XI. 107 : 193 : : 14000 : 25252 = *Fo. Conc.*
$$\text{Diff. } 7215$$

Then by the Observation Preliminary to *Prop.* XIX. 7215 : 25252 : : 18037 : 63128 = to the Focal length of such a *Meniscus*. Which comes sufficiently nigh 63000, considering the foregoing Angles are Calculated only in Round Numbers to every 10" seconds.

What is here performed by supposing the First Angle of Inclination $kea = 5°. 0'. 0''$, may be likewise done supposing it of an other Inclination, and as the Angle is smaller it will be the more exact.

Prop. XXIV.

An intire Glass-Sphere Unites the Parallel Rays at the Distance almost of half its Semidiameter behind it.

'Tis here supposed that the Incident Rays do not fall distant from the Axis more than 20 or 30 Degrees.

Tab.

Tab. 21. *f.* 3. *a k* is a Glass-Sphere. On the Point *d* there falls the Ray *b d* Parallel to the Axis *a k*. I say this Ray after a Double Refraction concurs with the Axis in the Point *f*, so that *f k* is almost half the Semidiameter of the Sphere.

c is the Centre of the Sphere, make *k h* equal to the Semidiameter *c k*, then *a h* is a Diameter and Half. And the Ray *b d* by the First Refraction proceeds in *d e* directly towards the Point *h*. But at *e* it emerges from Glass to Air. Draw the Perpendicular *c e g*, the Angle of this second Inclination is *c e d* = *g e h*. Now the Ray instead of proceeding directly to *h* is refracted from the Perpendicular *e g* by the Angle *f e h*, which is therefore to be half *c e d*. And that it is so, I thus prove. *c e d* is equal to *e c h* + *e h c* (32. 1. *Eucl.*) but *e c h* and *e h c* are to sense equal, their Subtenses *e h* and *e c* being very near equal: wherefore *e h c* is half *c e d*. But *e h c* is equal to *f e h* (their Subtenses *f e* and *f h* being as to sense equal; for *f k* by supposition is equal to *f h*, and *f e* is very near equal to *f k*, therefore *f e* is almost equal to *f h*) and consequently the Angle *f e h* is half *c e d* or *g e h*. Which was to be Demonstrated.

Prop. XXV.

A Glass Hemisphere Unites the Parallel Rays at the Distance of a Diameter and one third of a Semidiameter from the Pole of the Glass.

Tab. 21. *f.* 4. *a d c* is a Glass Hemisphere, *b d* a Ray of Light Parallel to the Axis *a h*. This Ray after a Double Refraction Crosses the Axis in the Point *f*, so that *f c* is a Semidiameter and one third of a Semidiameter. Make *c h* and

Tab. 22 pag. 95

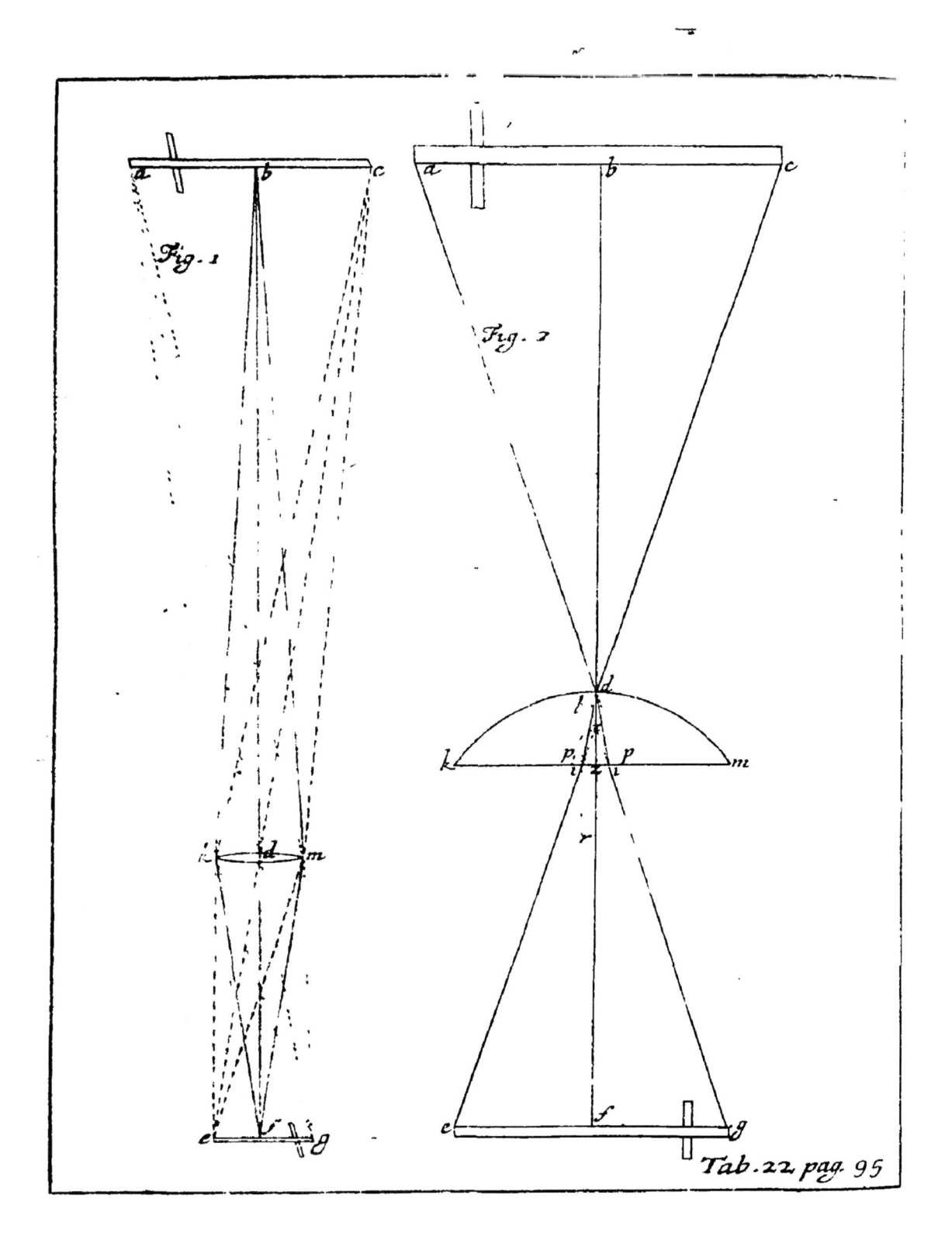

and kh each equal to ca. By the first Refraction at d, the Ray is directed towards h in deh. At e the Point where it emerges from the Glass, draw per Perpendicular to the Surface ce. Now the second Angle of Inclination is $dep = her$ (15.1.) $= khe$ (29.1) $= keh$. (For ke being nighly equal to kc, 'tis also nighly equal to kh, Then in the Equilateral Triangle keh, the Angle keh shall be nighly equal to the Angle khe) And the Angle of Refraction is feh. And this we are to prove equal to $\frac{1}{2}$ the Inclination her or ebf. Seeing kh is equal to ck, and kf is $\frac{1}{3}$ of kh by Construction, it follows that cf is double fh (for $ck + kf = cf = \frac{3}{3} + \frac{1}{3} = \frac{4}{3}$, and $fh = \frac{2}{3}$, but $\frac{4}{3}$ is $=$ to double $\frac{2}{3}$;) But ef is nighly equal to cf; therefore ef is nighly double fh. Then in the Triangle feh, as the Sides, so the Angles (by supposition) therefore the Angle ehf is nighly double the Angle feh. Which was to be Demonstrated.

Definition.

The Projection of an Object in the Distinct Base of a Convex Glass, I call the *Image*.

Prop. XXVI.

As the Distance of the Object from the Glass:
To the Distance of the Image from the Glass ::
So the Diameter of the Objects Magnitude :
To the Diameter of the Image.

Tab. 22. f 1. abc is an Object, kdm a Convex Glass in the Hole of a Dark Chamber, efg the Image formed by this Glass on a White Paper in the Distinct Base. I say,

As

As *c d* the Distance of the Object from the Glass: To *e d* the Distance of the Image from the Glass ∷ So *a c* the Objects Magnitude: To *g e* the Magnitude of the Image.

To shew this, we are to remember the Premises to the IV Proposition. For by them we shall find, that the Axes *a d*, and *c d* of the Luminous Cones *k a m*, *k c m*, may be consider'd as passing the Glass unrefracted. Because that after they have passed the Glass and become *d g*, *d e*, they proceed Parallel to their Course before they entred the Glass. So that in Glasses of large Spheres, and small Segments, the thickness of the Glass being inconsiderable in respect of the Focal Distance, we may neglect it. And then we have here two Similar Triangles *a d c*, *g d e*; For ∠*a d c* is equal to ∠*e d g* (15. 1. *Eucl.*) and the Side *e g* is Parallel to the Side *a c* (by supposition) and consequently the Angle *c a d* is equal to the Angle *e g d* (29. 1.) and *a c d* is equal to the Angle *g e d*. Wherefore it shall be *c d* : *e d* ∷ *a c* : *g e*. *Which was to be Demonstrated.*

Note. From hence appears the Mistake committed by Monsieur *Comiers* in *DeBlegny's Zodiacus Medico-Gallicus. An. 3tio. pag* 117. Who says, *Diameter Imaginis Solis in Distinctâ Basi obtinebit ad minimum in sua Diametro Funem seu Chordam Dimidii Gradus magni Circuli Sphæræ, cujus Vitrum est segmentum.* Whereas it should be, *Magni Circuli Sphæræ, cujus Radius est Distantia Focalis Vitri.*

What is here Demonstrated concerning the Real Image of a Convex Glass may be accommodated to the Virtual Image of a Concave.

Scholium.

But if we are yet more scrupulous, and will consider also the thickness of the Glass; Then the Point within the Glass

Glaſs from whence the Diſtance of the Diſtinct Baſe is to be counted, may be thus determin'd in a Plano-Convex Glaſs. *Tab. 22. f. 2, k d m* is a Plano-Convex Glaſs with its Convex Side towards the Object *a b c*; *a d, c d*, the Axes of Radious Cones falling Obliquely on the Glaſs in its Pole *d*, Which (if the Glaſs were not interpoſed) would proceed directly on to *p, p*, but by the Glaſs are now refracted into *d ı, d ı*; But at *ı ı* meeting with the Second ſurface of the Glaſs, inſtead of going ſtrait onwards, they are again Refracted into *ı e, ı g*, Parallel to *a d, c d*. Let *e i, g ı* be produced backwards till they Interſect the Axis *b f* in *x*, I ſay *x* is the Point in the Glaſſes Axis, from whence the Diſtance of the Diſtinct Baſe is to be reckon'd. *And as the Thickneſs of the Glaſs* d z : *To the Diſtance of this Point* x *from the Inner ſurface* z x :: *So is the Co-tangent of the Angle of Incidence from Glaſs to Air* : *To the Co-tangent of the Refracted Angle.*

Tab. 22. F. 2.

For to the Point of Incidence *ı* draw *l i r* Perpendicular to *k m*. Here the Angle of Incidence from Glaſs to Air is *l ı d = ı d z* and the Complement of *ı d z* is *d ı z*, whoſe Tangent is *d z* (making *ı z* Radius) and the Refracted Angle is *r ı e = ı x z* whoſe Complement is *x ı z*, and the Tangent hereof is *x z*.

In Double Convexes the Caſe is ſomething different, but 'tis needleſs to inlarge any farther thereon.

Wherefore we ſee, that if we uſe a Plano-Convex Glaſs with its Convex-ſide towards the Object, and if we allow for its Thickneſs, we are to compute the Diſtance of the Object from the Pole of the Glaſs *d*, and the Diſtance of the Diſtinct Baſe from the Point *x*. But ſuppoſing the Plane Side towards the Object *e f g*, then we are to reckon the Diſtance of the Object *e f g* from the Point *x*, and the Diſtance of the Diſtinct Baſe *a b c* from *d* the Pole of the Glaſs. *Vid. Prop.* XXVII.

Corollary 1.

It follows from this *Prop.* XXVI. That the Diameter of the Sun subtending an Arch of 32 Minutes in a Great Circle of the Heavens, the Diameter of the Sun's Image, Represented in the Distinct Base of a Convex-glass, subtends an Arch of 32 Minutes in a Circle, whose Radius is the Distance of the Distinct Base from the Glass.

T 23 F 1   But *Tab.* 23. *Fig.* 1. *b* is a Convex-Glass, *a b* a Ray of Light proceeding from the Sun's Eastern Limb, *d b* a Ray from its Centre, *c b* a Ray from its Western Limb. Let the single Glass *b* Represent the Image of the Sun in the Distinct Base *h q i*, and let us suppose the Sun's Diameter to be 32' Minutes. Draw *b h*, *b q*, *b i*. Let *e x z f* be another Plano-Convex-Glass, so placed behind the Glass *b* that both these Glasses together (according to *Prop.* XVI.) may Represent the Sun's Image in the Distinct Base *k p o*: 'Tis required to find the Breadth or Diameter *k o* of this Image, from these Data, *h b q* the Angle of the Sun's Semidiameter 16' Minutes, *b q* the Focal Length of the Glass *b*, *b f* the Distance of the Glasses, *p f* the Distance of the Distinct Base from the Glass *f x*, *e g* the Radius of the Convexity *e x z*, or instead thereof, the Focal Length of the Plano Convex Glass *e x z f*, for having one we may easily obtain the other.

We suppose that the Central Ray *d b x q* is Co-incident with the Axis of the Glasses.

First therefore in the Right Angled Triangle *h b q*, we have the Angle *h b q* (and consequently *b h q = b e f*) and *b q* to find *b q*.

(2) Then $bf + fp = bp$. And $bq : hq :: bp . pn :: bf : ef$.

(3) In the Right-Angled Triangle *e f g*, *e f* and *e g* are known to find the Angle *f e g*.

(4) 180

Tab. 23. pag. 98

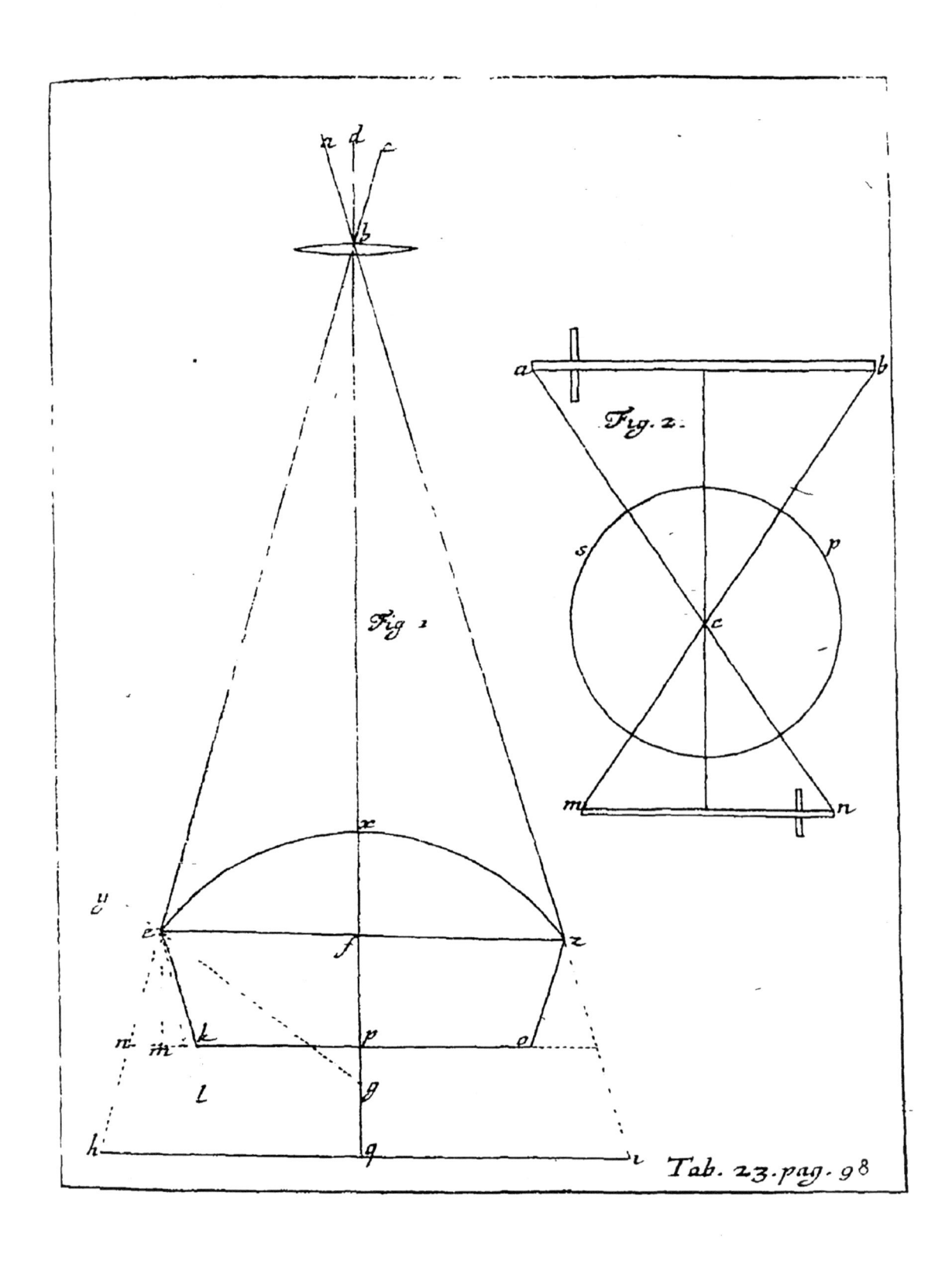

(4) $180 - bef - feg = yeb = geh$, Which is the Angle of the Inclination of the Ray be on the Convex furface ex.

(5) $300 : 193 :: s. \angle heg : s. \angle hel$, Wherefore the Ray by its firſt Refraction would proceed in el.

(6) Draw me Perpendicular to the Plane Surface ef, then $ef = mp$. And $me = pf$. And $np - mp = nm$; And the Angle nem is $=$ to qbh, And $hel - nem$ is $=$ to mel; Which is the Inclination of the Ray on the Plane Surface ef.

(7) Then $193 : 300 :: s. \angle mel : s. \angle mek$.

(8) In the Right-angled Triangle mek, me and the Angles are known to find mk.

(9) Laſtly $nm + mk = nk$, and $pn - nk = pk = \frac{1}{2} ko$; Which was required to be found.

Corollary 2.

The foregoing Trigonometrical Calculation in the firſt Corollary I had from my Eſteem'd Friend Mr. *John Flamſteed Aſtr. Reg.* But Inſtead thereof, or as an Additament thereto, I ſhall ſubſtitute this Problem.

To Determine the Breadth of the Diſtinct Baſe Reſulting from the Combinations of Glaſſes expreſſed in Prop. XVI, XVII, XVIII. There being given (together with the Data in thoſe Propoſitions) the Breadth of the Object, or the Angle it ſubtends before the outermoſt Glaſs, And if it be a nigh Object, its Diſtance from the outermoſt Glaſs.

We here ſuppoſe our Glaſſes of the leaſt Thickneſs Imaginable, or that all the Refractions are performed in the Right Line, that paſſes through the Glaſſes Breadth at Right Angles to the Glaſſes Axis, for avoiding Confuſion in the Schemes.

[100]

T.24. F.1, 2,3,4,5.   Wherefore in *Tab.* 24. *Fig.* 1, 2, 3, 4, 5. *b* is the Glaſs next the Object, whether Convex (as in *Prop.* 16, 17.) or Concave (as in *Prop.* 18.) We ſhall take the Sun for our Object, and ſuppoſe *a b* a Ray proceeding from its Eaſtern Limb, *d b* a Ray from its Centre, *c b* a Ray from its Weſtern Limb. Let the ſingle Glaſs *b*, in the firſt and ſecond *Figures*, Repreſent the Image of the Sun in the Diſtinct Baſe *h q i*. The Breadth of the Baſe *h q i* is eaſily obtain'd from the Data. Let *e f z* be another Glaſs, ſo placed behind the Glaſs *b*, that both theſe Glaſſes together may Repreſent the Suns Image in the Diſtinct Baſe *k p o*, 'Tis required to find the Breadth or Diameter *k o* of this Image from theſe Data ; *b q* the Focal Length of the Glaſs *b* ; The Breadth of the Image *h i*, or the Angle *a b c* = *e b z* ; The Focal Length of the Glaſs *e z* ; The Diſtance of the Glaſſes *f b* and *p f* the Diſtance of the Diſtinct Baſe from the Glaſs *e z*.

Through *p* at Right-angles to the Axis *d s b f p* of the Glaſſes draw *k p o* infinitely. Firſt from theſe Data, let us obtain the Breadth of the Glaſs *e z*, where the Rays *b e*, *b z*, meet it, or its half breadth *e f*, which is eaſily had in the Right-angled Triangle *e f b*, the Angle *e b f*, and the Side *f b* being given.

Let us then conſider *b* as a radiating Point, either farther from or nigher to the Glaſs *e z* than its Focus ; And by *Prop.* V. and VIII. for Convexes, and by *Corol.* XV. for Concaves, let us determine the Reſpective, Imaginary, or Virtual Focus *s*, whereby we obtain *f s*. From *s* draw *s e*, *s z*, directly ; Where theſe Lines *s e*, *s z*, meet the Diſtinct Baſe in *k* and *o*, there the Breadth of the Diſtinct Baſe is determin'd, To obtain the Meaſure whereof, ſay as *s f* : *f e* :: *s p* : *p k* = *p o* = ½ *k o*.

And note that in *Fig.* 1 and 3. *s p* = *s f* − *p f*. But in *Fig.* 2, 4, 5. *s p* = *s f* + *f p*.

Corol-

Tab. 24 pag. 100

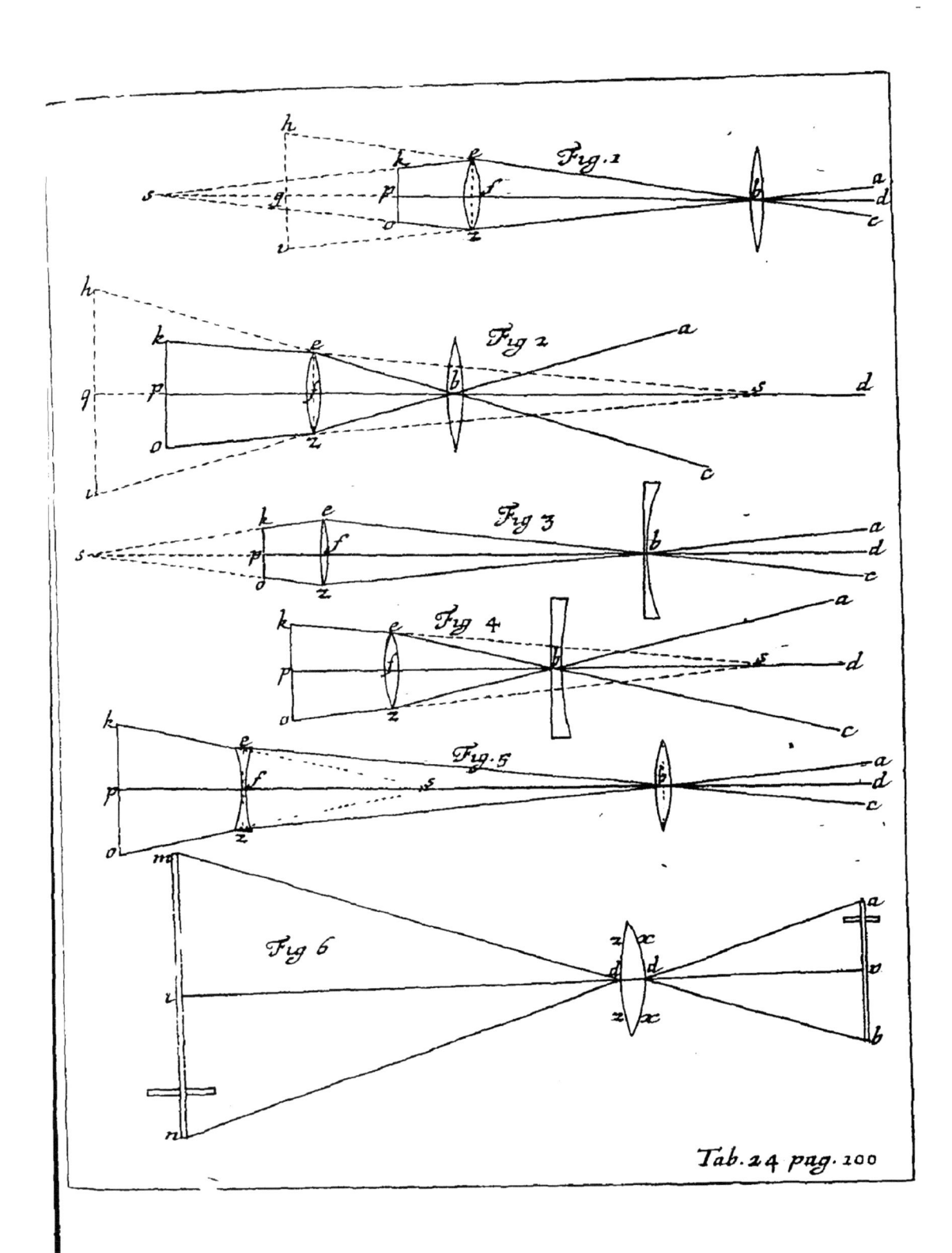

Corollary 3.

If the Glaſs be a Compleat Sphere; Then, as the Diſtance of the Object from the Centre of the Glaſs : To the Breadth of the Object :. So the Diſtance of the Image from the ſame Centre of the Sphere : To the Breadth of the Image.

This is Manifeſt from *Tab.* 23. *Fig.* 2. Whereby it appears, T23.F2. that a Glaſs Sphere *s p c* expoſed to an Object *a b*; From each point *a, b*, of the Object there proceeds one certain Ray *a c n*, *b c m*, which paſſes Unrefracted, And theſe Rays Croſs in the Centre *c* of the Sphere, by which means they are Perpendicular to both Sides of the Sphere, at their Ingreſs and Egreſs, and ſo paſs Unrefracted.

Corollary 4. PROBL.

The Diſtance of an Object, and its Diameter being given, 'tis required to Repreſent its Image in the Diſtinct Baſe under a given Meaſure, The Thickneſs of the Glaſs being given alſo.

This is the 52 Problematical Propoſition of *Gregorii Opt. Promot.* And is thus ſolved by our Doctrine.

Tab. 24. *Fig.* 6. *a v b* is an Object, whoſe Diameter *a b* T24.F6. is given, and its Diſtance from the Glaſs *v d* is given alſo: 'Tis required to Project this Object under a Given Meaſure *m n*; The Thickneſs of the Glaſs *d d* being alſo given. Let it be made, As *a b : v d :: m n : d ı*. Then ſtrike the Arch *x d x* with ſuch a Radius, that the Rays flowing from the Point *v* may thereby be tranſmitted Parallel within the Body of the Glaſs (which ſhall be by the foregoing Doctrine, by making $\frac{1}{2}$ *v d* the Radius) Afterwards ſtrike the Arch *z d z* with ſuch

a

a Radius, that it may Unite the Parallel Rays at ι, which shall be by making ½ $d\iota$ the Radius: I say the Glass $z\,x$ shall project the Image of $a\,b$ under the given Measure $m\,n$. This is so manifest from *Prop.* IX. together with the foregoing Doctrine, that it wants no farther Explication.

Note. I have here consider'd the whole Thickness $d\,d$ of the Glass in Conformity to *Gregory*'s Proposition. But what foregoes concerning the Consideration of the Glasses Thickness may be apply'd here.

Prop. XXVII.

The Object and its Image in the Distinct Base are Reciprocal. vid. Prop. VI.

T.22.F 1.   *Tab.* 22. *Fig.* 1. $a\,b\,c$ being an Object, and the Convex Glass $k\,m$ Representing the Image thereof in the Distinct Base $e\,f\,g$. Let us now conceive $e\,f\,g$ an Object, I say the same Glass $k\,m$ the same way posited shall project the Image thereof in the Distinct Base at $a\,b\,c$.

This does necessarily follow from the precedent Proposition, and from *Exp.* 8. And therefore needs no farther Demonstration.

Corollary.

Hence it follows that the Image in the Distinct Base may be sometimes larger than the Object. On which depends the Doctrine of the double *Microscope*, as hereafter shall appear more fully.

Let us imagine the Image of the Sun projected in the Focus of a Convex-glass, And let us now conceive the *Converse, viz.* That this Image were now the Real Sun, the Distinct Base

Tab 25. pag 103

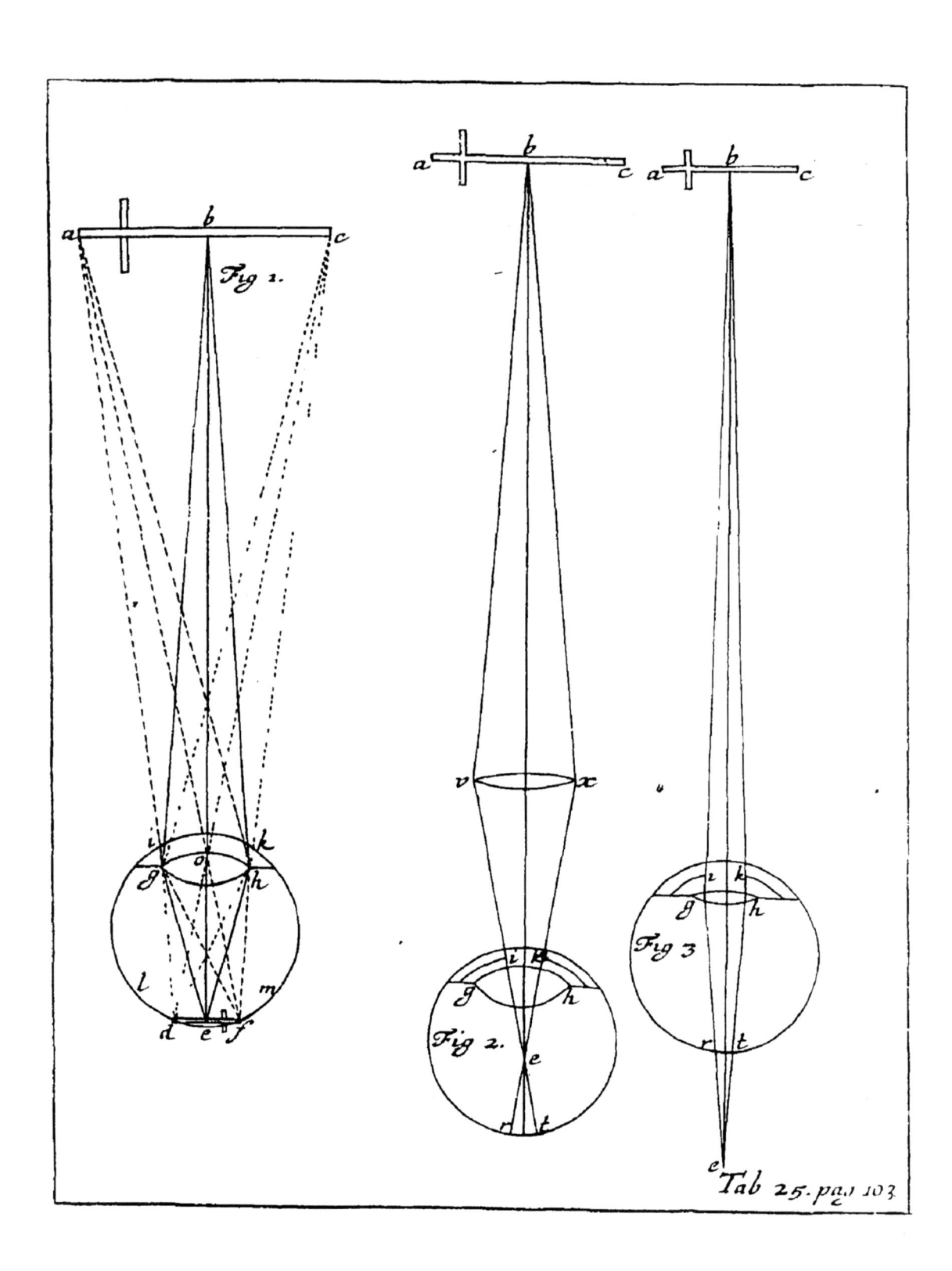

[103]

of this would be as Large and as Remote as is now the Sun. So that every Convex-glass may be conceived to two Foci, or Distinct Bases; one at the Object, t'other at the Image.

PROP. XXVIII.

The manner of Plain Vision with the naked Eye is expounded.

Tab. 25. F. 1. *a b c* is an Object, *i k l e m* is the Globe of the Eye, furnish'd with all its Coats and Humors; But in this Figure we have only expressed the Crystalline Humour *g o h*, as being Principally concern'd in Forming the Image on the Fund of the Eye.

(1) From each Point in the Object we may Conceive Rays flowing on the Pupil of the Eye *i k*; as here from the middle Point *b*, there proceed the Rays *b g*, *b o*, *b h*; These by means of the Coats and Humours of the Eye, and especially by the Chrystalline Humour *g h*, are refracted and brought together on the *Retina* or Fund of the Eye in the Point *e*, and there the Point *b* is represented. For we may conceive the Crystalline Humour *g h* as it were a Convex-glass, in the Hole of a Dark Chamber *i l m k*, and that *d e f* is the Distinct Base of this Glass. What is here said of the Point *b*, and its Representation at *e*, may be understood of all the other Points in the Object, as of *a* and *c* and their Representations at *f* and *d*.

(2) And as in a dark Chamber, that has a Hole furnish'd with a Convex-glass, if the Paper, that is to receive the Image in the Distinct Base, be either nigher to, or farther from the Glass, than its due distance, the Representation thereon is confused; For then the Radious Pencils do not exactly determine with their Apices on the Paper; But those from one Point are mixt and confused with those from the Adjacent Points: so in the

the Case of Plain Vision, 'tis requisite that the Pencils should exactly determine their Apices at *d, e, f,* on the Retina, or else Vision is not Distinct.

'Tis therefore contrived by the *Most Wise and Omnipotent Framer of the Eye,* That it should have a Power of adapting it self in some Measure to *Nigh* and *Distant* Objects. For they require different Conformations of the Eye; Because the Rays proceeding from the Luminous Points of *Nigh* Objects do more Diverge, than those from more Remote Objects.

But whether this variety of Conformation consist in the Crystallines approaching nigher to, or removing farther from the Retina; Or in the Crystallines assuming a different Convexity, sometimes greater, sometimes less, according as is requisite, I leave to the scrutiny of others, and particularly of the curious Anatomist. This only I can say, that either of these Methods will serve to explain the various Phænomena of the Eye; And I am apt to believe, that both these may attend each other, *viz.* a Less Convex Crystalline requires an Elongation of the Eye, and a more Convex Crystalline requires a shortning thereof; As a more Flat Convex Object-glass or of a Larger Sphere requires a Longer Tube, and one more Protuberant, bulging or of a smaller Sphere requires a shorter Tube.

(3) By the forementioned Scheme we perceive, the Rays from each Point of the Object are all confused together on the Pupil in *g h,* so that the Eye is placed in the Point of the Greatest Confusion. But by means of the Humors and Coats thereof each Cone of Rays is separated, and brought by it self to determine in its proper Point on the *Retina,* there Painting distinctly the Vivid Representation of the Object, Which Representation is there perceived by the *sensitive Soul* (whatever it be) the manner of whose Actions and Passions, He only knows who Created and Preserves it, *Whose Ways are*

Past

Past finding out, and by us unsearchable. But of this Moral truth we may be assured, *That He that made the Eye shall see.*

(4) We are likewise to observe, that the Representation of the Object *a b c* on the Fund of the Eye *f e d* is Inverted. For so likewise it is on the Paper in a dark Room; there being no other way for the Radious Cones to enter the Eye or the dark Chamber, but by their Axes *a o, b o, c o,* crossing in the Pole *o* of the Crystalline or Glass. And here it may be enquired; How then comes it to pass that the Eye sees the Object *Erect*? But this Quæry seems to encroach too nigh the enquiry into the manner of the Visive Faculties *Perception*; For 'tis not properly the Eye that *sees*, it is only the Organ or Instrument, 'tis the *Soul* that *sees* by means of the Eye. To enquire then, how it comes to pass, that the Soul perceives the Object *Erect* by means of an *Inverted* Image, is to enquire into the Souls Faculties; which is not the proper subject of this Discourse. But yet that in this Matter we may offer at something, I say, *Erect* and *Inverted* are only Terms of Relation to *Up* and *Down*, or *Farther from* and *Nigher to* the Centre of the Earth, in parts of the same thing: And that that is an *Erect* Object, makes an *Inverted* Image in the Eye, and an *Inverted* Object makes an *Erect* Image; That is, that part of the Object which is *farthest from* the Centre of the Earth is Painted on a Part of the Eye *Nigher* the Centre of the Earth, than the other parts of the Image. But the Eye or Visive Faculty takes no Notice of the Internal Posture of its own Parts, but uses them as an Instrument only, contrived by Nature for the Exercise of such a Faculty.

But to come yet a little nigher this difficulty; This enquiry results briefly to no more than this, How comes it to pass, that the Eye receiving the Representation of a Part of an Object on that part of its Fund which is *Lowermost* or nighest the Centre of the Earth, perceives that part of the Object as *Uppermost*

most or fartheft from the Centre of the Earth? And in anfwer to this, let us imagine, that the Eye in the Point f receives an Impulfe or Stroke by the Protrufion forwards of the Luminous Axis aof, from the Point of the Object a; Muft not the Vifive Faculty be necefſarily directed hereby to confider this ftroke, as coming from the Top a, rather than from the bottom c, and confequently fhould be directed to conclude f the Reprefentation of the Top?

Hereof we may be fatisfy'd by fuppofing a Man ftanding on his Head: For here, tho the Upper Parts of Objects are painted on the Upper Parts of the Eye, yet the Objects are judged to be *Erect*. And from this Pofture of a Man, the Reafon appears, why we have ufed the Words *Fartheft from*, and *Nigheft to the Centre of the Earth*, rather than *Upper* and *Lower*. For in this Pofture, becaufe the *Upper* Parts of the Object are painted on that part of the Eye nigheft the Earth, (though really the upper Part of the Eye) they are judged to be fartheft removed from the Earth.

What is faid of *Erect* and *Reverfe* may be underftood of *Siniſter* and *Dexter*. But of thefe Phyfical Conjectures enough.

(5) The Image of an *Erect* Object being Reprefented on the Fund of the Eye *Inverted*, and yet the fenfitive Faculty judging the Object *Erect*; it follows that when the Image of an *Erect* Object is Painted on the Fund of the Eye *Erect*, the fenfe Judges that Object to be *Inverted*.

This is a neceffary Conclufion, and is of confequence for explaining fome Particulars that follow.

(6) The *Magnitude* of an Object is Eftimated by the Angle the Object fubtends before the Eye. Thus in the fame foremention'd *Tab.* 25. *Fig.* 1. the Length of the Object ac is eftimated by the Angle $aoc = fod$, this we call *The Optick Angle*.

From

From hence, & from *Prop.* XXVI, XXVII. it follows, that if the Eye were placed inſtead of the Glaſs at *d* (*T.*22.*F.*1.) and *a b c* or *e f g* were Objects, the Eye would perceive them of Equal Bigneſs. *T* 22. *F* 1

I know very well the Point *o*, which is the Vertex of the Optick Angle, is variouſly aſſigned by various Authors; ſome placing it in the Centre of the Eye; Others in the Vertex of the Cryſtalline; Others in the Vertex of the outward Coat or Cornea of the Eye: But 'tis a Matter of no great conſequence, where-ever we place it, for according to the Bigneſs of this Angle *a o c*, the Image on the Fund of the Eye is Bigger or Leſs. *Vid. Tacquet Optica. Lib.* 1. *Def* 4. and *Prop.* 3.

I know likewiſe, that by a curious Experiment in Opticks diſcover'd by an Ingenious *French-Man* Monſieur *Mariotte*, 'tis controverted, whether the *Retina* or *Choroide* be the Seat of Viſion, or the Place on which the Pictures of outward Objects are expreſſed (*vid. Philoſoph. Tranſact.* Num. 35. and 59.) But to our buſineſs it matters not which of them we pitch on; and therefore I chuſe to ſpeak as commonly 'tis preſumed; and mention the *Retina*, or rather the *Fund of the Eye*, as the Place that receives this Picture.

(7) In the ſame (*Tab.* 25. *Fig.* 1.) We perceive the Rays that flow from the Point *b* do proceed to the Eye *Diverging*, as *b g*, *b o*, *b h*, And if the Object *a c* were infinitely diſtant from the Eye, or ſo diſtant from the Eye, that the Breadth of the Pupil *i k* were inſenſible in Compariſon to this Diſtance, then the Rays *b g*, *b o*, *b h*, would proceed as it were Parallel, and ſo fall on the Eye. In both which Caſes, by means of the Refractions in the Eye, they are brought together, and paint the Image of the Point *b* on the Fund of the Eye at *e*. *Vid. Gregorii Opt. Prom Pr.* 30. *T* 25. *F* 1.

But in *Tab* 25. *Fig.* 2 If the Diverging Rays *b v*, *b x*, that flow from the Point *b*, meet the Convex Glaſs *v x*, and are thereby made to converge as *v i*, *x k*, and ſo fall on the Eye, *T* 25. *F* 2.

P 2 and

and there paffing through the Cryftalline *g h*, are made to Converge yet more as *i e*, *k e*; Here they crofs in the Point *e*, before they reach the Retina *r t*, and confequently do paint thereon the Image of the Point *b* confufedly, for 'tis Painted on the fpace *r t*; whereas to caufe diftinct Vifion, it fhould only be painted on a correfpondent *Point* on the Retina.

And this is the Fault of their Eyes, who are called *Myopes*, *Purblind*, or *Short fighted*. For in them the Cryftalline is too Convex (as in this *Tab.* 25. *Fig.* 2. both the Convex Glafs and Cryftalline joyn'd together make too great a Convexity) uniting the Rays before they arrive at the Retina. And therefore they are helped by Concave glaffes, which take off from the too great Convexity of their Cryftalline fome part of its Refractive Power. Or rather thefe Concaves make the Rays *Diverge* fo, that their Cryftalline fhall be fufficient only to bring them again together, fo that they be not united, till they arrive at the Fund of the Eye.

Myopes are alfo helped by holding the Object very near; for then the Rays that fall on their Eye from any fingle Point do more Diverge, than when the Eye is farther from the Point, and confequently their too Convex Cryftalline does but fuffice to bring them together on the Retina

(8) On the contrary, the Eyes of Old Men have their Cryftalline too Flat (as *Tab.* 25. *Fig.* 3.) and cannot correct the Divergence of the Rays *b i*, *b k*, to make them meet on the Retina *r t*, but beyond the Eye at *e*. Wherefore for their Help 'tis requifite they add the Adventitious Convexity of a Glafs, that both it and the Cryftalline together, may be fufficient to unite the Rays juft at the Retina: And from hence it appears, that Spectacles help Old Men, not by magnifying an Object, but by making its Appearance Diftinct; for Old Men cannot read the largeft Print without Spectacles, and yet with Spectacles, they read the fmalleft, though thefe with Spectacles

cles do not appear so large, as those without Spectacles.

(9) What is said of the *Confused* or *Distinct* Representation of a *Point* in the Object, may be understood of the *Confused* or *Distinct* Representation of the whole Object; at least for those Parts that lye pretty nigh adjacent to that Point that is looked at. For here we do not take a *Point* in the strict sense of the Mathematicians, but in a Physical Sense, for the smallest Part imaginable; or as we have assumed it in the first supposition. And the whole Object consisting of such Points, what is shewn of one Point may be understood of every Point in the Object, that is, of the whole Object.

(10) 'Tis Requisite also (before I proceed farther) to explain, what I mean by *Clear* Vision, and *Faint* Vision; *Distinct* Vision, and *Confused* Vision.

By what foregoes, I suppose these two latter Terms are pretty well understood, *viz*. *Distinct* Vision is then caused, when the Pencils of Rays from each Point of an Object do accurately determine in Correspondent Points of the Image on the *Retina*. *Confused* Vision on the contrary, when these Pencils do intermix one with another.

But *Clear* Vision is only caused by a Great Quantity of Rays in the same Pencil, illuminating the Correspondent Points of the Image *strongly* and *vigorously*.

Faint Vision is then when a Few Rays make up one Pencil; And tho this may be *Distinct*, yet 'tis *Dark* and *Obscure*, at least not so *Bright* and *Strong*, as if more Rays concurr'd.

Of Single Glasses apply'd to the Eye.

Hitherto I have spoken of Glasses by themselves; And of the Eye by it self: I come now to consider them both together.

But

But first 'tis to be Noted, that when we speak of the *Distinct* or *Confused* Appearance of an Object, 'tis needful only to explain my self concerning some one single Point in the Object; and for this we chuse the middle Point; for if we shew that single Point in the Object to be *Distinctly* or *Confusedly* Represented on the *Retina* (according to the XXVIII. *Prop.*) the same may be understood of the Adjacent Points in the Object.

But when we discourse of the *Erect* or *Inverted* Appearance of an Object: Or of the *Magnify'd* or *Diminish'd* Appearance of an Object; 'tis requisite we consider the whole Object. For a single Point, though Physical, cannot properly be consider'd as *Erect* or *Inverted*, or *Magnify'd* or *Diminish'd*.

So that we perceive *Distinct* or *Confused* Vision to depend on the Formation of Rays proceeding from each single Point. But *Erect* and *Inverted*, or *Magnify'd* and *Diminish'd* Appearances depend on the Consideration of Rays proceeding from different Points of the Object. I shall always consider those, that proceed from the extremities of the Object.

Prop. XXIX.

An Object seen through a Plain Glass whose Surfaces are Parallel is Magnify'd thereby.

This Proposition being directly contradictory to what Honoratus Faber asserts in the XLIII. *Prop. Sec.* 2. of his *Synopsis Optica*, I shall mark my *Tab.* 26. *Fig.* 1. with the same Letters wherewith he marks his 89th Fig. He acknowledges that the *Apparent Place* of an Object is changed by a Plain Glass, but not that the Visual Angle is alter'd thereby. But I shall shew that the Optick Angle is Magnify'd thus; Let *m l* be a Plain Glass, *a b* an Object, *a f* a Ray produced

Tab. 26 pag. 110

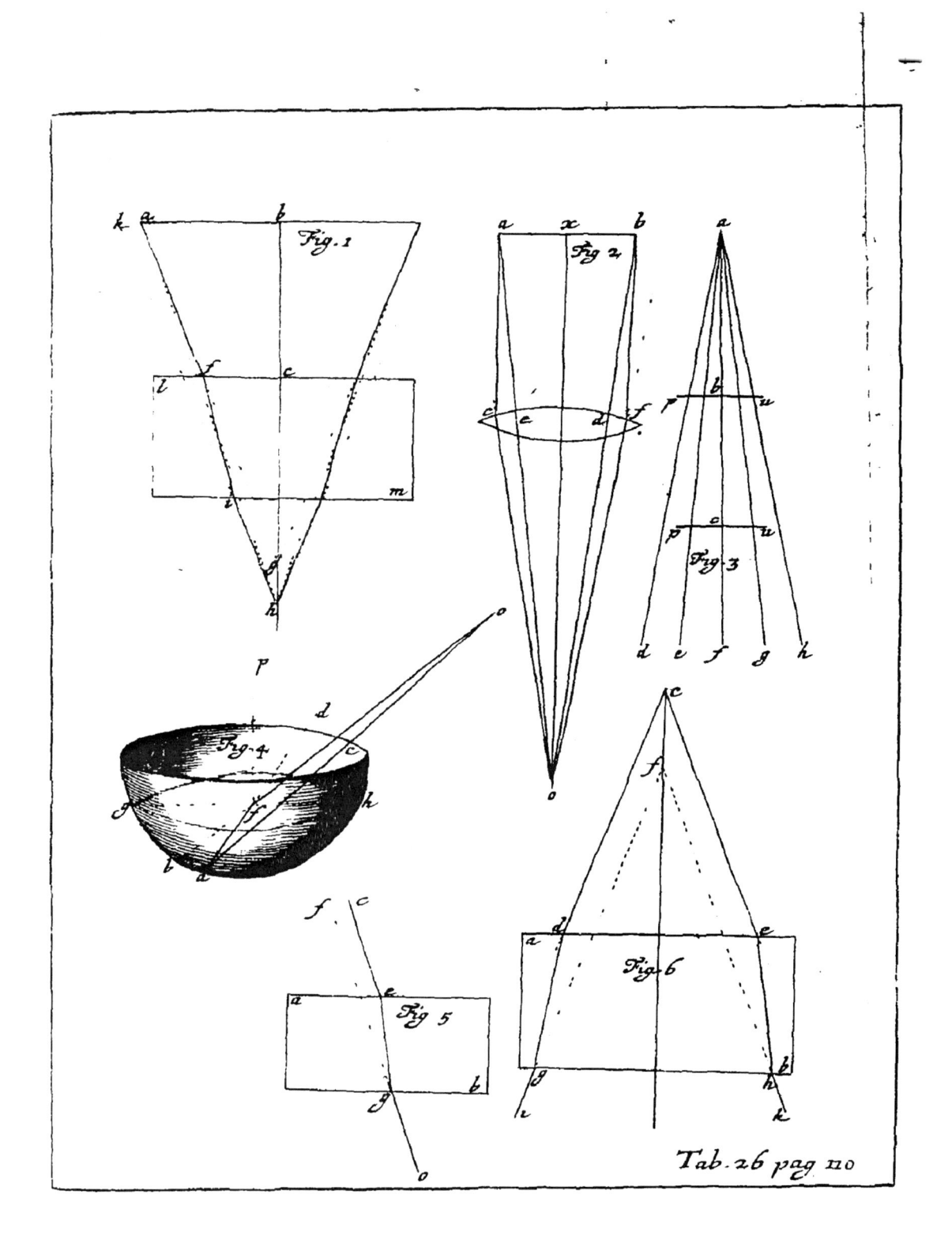

duced directly to *g*, but Refracted into *f i*; And at its Emersion from the Glass at *i*, Refracted again into *i h*, parallel to *a f g*. (by *Experim.* 1, 2.) Produce *i h* directly towards *k*; let the Eye be at *h*, draw *h a*. The Angle, under which the Object *a b* appears through the Glass *m l* to the Eye at *h*, is *i h b*, or *k h b*, which is certainly greater than *a h b*, which is the natural Optick Angle. Wherefore the Eye at *h* through the Glass sees the Object *a b*, under a greater Angle than it would do without the Glass, and consequently the Object is magnify'd by the Glass. *Which was to be Demonstrated.*

But that which deceived FABER is, that because the Angle *a g b* is equal to the Angle *k h b*, therefore (says he) the Optick Angle *with* and *without* the Glass are the same; or (as he has it) the Eye at *g* without the Glass would see the Object *a b* under the Angle *a g b*, and through the Glass the Object is seen under the Angle *k h b* equal to *a g b*. Which is granted him. But this does only prove, that the naked Eye at *g*, and the Eye through the Glass at *h*, sees the Object under the same Angle. Whereas he should have proved (if it were possible), that the naked Eye at *h*, and the Eye through the Glass at *h*, sees the Objects under the same Angle; And then indeed he had rightly proved what he proposed, *viz*. that the Optick Angle is not magnify'd by the Interposition of the Glass: For 'tis not Mathematical, first to place the Eye at *g without* the Glass, and then at *h with* the Glass, and proving the Optick Angles the same, to conclude that therefore the Plain Glass does not magnifie. For at that rate one may shew that even a Convex Glass does not magnifie; For at *one* Station an Object shall appear under as great an Angle *without it*, as at *another* Station *through* the Glass.

The Reason, why the Common Window Glass, &c through which we look, causes no sensible Alteration of Objects, is because 'tis too Thin. *Vid. Barrow Lect. Opt.* 15.

Con-

Concerning the *Apparent Place* of an Object through a Plain Glass, more hereafter.

PROP. XXX.

All Objects seen Erect through Convex Glasses are Magnify'd thereby.

T26 F2   *Tab.* 26. *Fig.* 2. Let *a x b* be an Object, *o* the Eye, draw *a e o*, *b d o*, directly strait from the extremities of the Object to the Eye. The Angle comprised by the Direct Rays *a e o*, *b d o*, that is the Angle *a o b*, is the *Natural* Optick Angle. Let now the Glass *c f* be interposed, here because the Rays *a e*, *b d*, would *naturally* and by their *Direct* course concur at *o*, now the Glass is interposed, their Concourse shall be accelerated before they arrive at *o*. Wherefore the Eye at *o* shall not perceive the extremities of the Object through the Glass by the Rays *a e*, *b d*, but by some *other Rays*. And these *other Rays* must fall either *without* (that is, farther from the Axis *o x*, than) *a e*, *b d*, or they must fall *within a e*, *b d*: But they cannot fall *within a e*, *b d*, for if *a e*, *b d* themselves be made by the Glass to concur *before* they arrive at *o*, much more shall any other Rays that fall *within a e*, *b d*, be made to concur *before* they arrive there: And consequently they cannot convey the Appearance of the Extreme Points *a*, *b*, to the Eye at *o*. Wherefore it remains, that the Rays that do this must fall *without a e*, *b d*. Let these Rays be *a c*, *b f*, which by the Refractive Power of the Glass are bent from their Direct Course and are made to proceed in *c o*, *f o*, crossing at the Eye in *o*; Here the Optick Angle through the Glass is *c o f*, which is greater than the Natural Optick Angle *a o b*, and consequently the Object is Magnify'd. *Which was to be Demonstrated.*

Prop.

[113]

Prop. XXXI.

Concerning the Apparent Place of Objects seen through Convex-glasses.

(1) In Plain Vision the Estimate we make of the *Distance* of Objects (especially when so far removed, that the Interval between our two Eyes, bears no sensible Proportion thereto; or when look'd upon with one Eye only) is rather the Act of our *Judgment*, than of *Sense*; and acquired by *Exercise* and a Faculty of *comparing*, rather than *Natural*. For *Distance* of it self, is not to be perceived; for 'tis a Line (or a Length) presented to our Eye with its End towards us, which must therefore be only a *Point*, and that is *Invisible*. Wherefore Distance is *chiefly* perceived by means of Interjacent Bodies, as by the Earth, Mountains, Hills, Fields, Trees, Houses, *&c.* Or by the *Estimate* we make of the *Comparative Magnitude* of Bodies, or of their *Faint Colours, &c.* These I say are the *Chief Means* of apprehending the Distance of Objects, that are considerably *Remote*. But as to *nigh* Objects, to whose Distance the Interval of the Eyes bears a sensible Proportion, their Distance is perceived by the turn of the Eyes, or by the Angle of the Optick Axes. (*Gregorii Opt. Promot. Prop.* XXVIII.) This was the Opinion of the Antients, *Alhazen, Vitellio,* &c. And tho the Ingenious Jesuit *Tacquet* (*Opt. Lib.* I. *Prop.* II.) disapprove thereof, and Objects against it a New Notion of *Gassendus* (of a Man's seeing only with one Eye at a Time one and the same Object) yet this Notion of *Gassendus* being absolutely False (as I could Demonstrate, were it not beside my Present Purpose, but I refer to the 7th Chap. of the 2d Part.) it makes nothing against this Opinion.

(2) Wherefore Distance being only a *Line*, and not of it self perceivable; if an Object were convey'd to the Eye by

Q one

[114]

one single Ray only, there were no other means of judging of its Distance, but by some of those hinted before. Therefore when we estimate the Distance of *nigh* Objects, either we take the help of both Eyes, or else we consider the Pupil of one Eye as having *Breadth*, and receiving a *Parcel* of Rays from each Radiating Point. And according to the various Inclination of the Rays from one Point, on the various Parts of the Pupil, we make our Estimate of the Distance of the Object: And therefore (as is said before) by one single Eye we can only Judge of the Distance of such Objects, to whose Distance the Breadth of the Pupil has a sensible Proportion. To illustrate all this by *Tab.* 26. *Fig.* 3. Let *a* be a Radiating Point, sending forth the Rays *a d*, *a e*, *a f*, *a g*, *a h*, with all the intermediate Rays. Let *p u* be the Breadth of the Pupil, and first placed at *c*, there receiving only *a e*, *a f*, *a g*: Let *p u* be translated to *b*, where it receives all the Rays, and 'tis manifest that the Rays from *a* are differently inclined on the Pupil in one and t'other Posture, for the Rays, which fall on the Pupil when placed at *b*, diverge very much more than those that fall upon it, when placed at *c*: And therefore the Eye, or Visual Faculty will apprehend the Distance of *a* from *b* and *c* to be *Different*. For it is observed before (*Prop.* 29. *Sect.* 2. see also, *Gregorii Opt. Promot. Prop.* XXIX.) that for viewing Objects *Remote* and *Nigh*, there are Requisite Various Conformations of the Eye: The Rays from *Nigh* Objects, that fall on the Eye, Diverging more than those from more *Remote* Objects.

(4) If therefore by Refraction through Glasses, that parcel of Rays which falls on the Pupil from each Point in *Nigh* Objects be made to flow as close together as those from *Distant* Objects; or the Rays from *Distant* Objects be made to Diverge, as much as if they flow'd from *Nigh* Objects, the Eye through such Glasses shall perceive the *Place of the Object changed.*

(5) But

(5) But first for a sensible and common Experiment, to shew the *Change* of an Objects *Place* by Refraction. *Tab.* 26. *F.* 4. represents a Vessel, on whose Bottom at *a* there is laid a piece of Mony, or any other remarkable Object, so that the Eye at *o* may just perceive the Mony over the Edge *c* of the Vessel. The Mony now appears to the Eye *o* by the direct Line *a c o*. Let now the Vessel be fill'd with Water up to *g f h*; let the Ray *a f* proceed from the Mony, and draw *p f* perpendicular to *g h*, the Ray *a f*, instead of going onwards directly to *d*, emerging from Water, a dense Medium to Air, deflects from the perpendicular *p f*; and becomes (suppose) *f o*. Wherefore the Eye *o*, now the Vessel has Water in it, sees the Silver, not by the direct Ray *a c o* (for that is bent from it, and escapes it) but by the refracted Ray *a f o*. Produce *o f* directly to *b*, the Mony shall appear as if it were at *b*. For the Eye is not sensible of the bending of the Ray, but is affected by it, as if it were directly strait.

(6) In like manner *Tab.* 26. *F.* 5. if the Point *c* send its Ray *c e* obliquely on the plain Glass *a b*; and after a double Refraction it arrive at the Eye *o*; This Point *c* is not now seen in its own proper Place, but somewhere in the Ray *o g* produced, as at *f*. For the Eye is not sensible of the outward accidental Refraction, that attends the Ray at its passage through the Glass, but is directed by the next immediate Ray *o g* that falls upon it, and considers it as *strait*, and coming directly from the Point *f*.

I say moreover, that by a plain Glass, the place of an Object is changed, and brought nigher the Eye. *Tab.* 26. *F.* 6. *c* is an Object sending its Rays *c d*, *c e*, upon the plain Glass *a b*, these after a double Refraction proceed (by supposition) in *g i*, *h k*. Produce these directly towards *f*; and suppose the Pupil of the Eye large enough to receive the Rays *g i*, *h k*; the Point *c* shall appear to the Eye as at *f*.

Q 2

(7)

(7) *To determine the Locus Apparens of an Object placed nigher a Convex-glass than its Focus.*

To perform this, we are to have, the Power of the Glass, the Distance of the Object from the Glass, and the Length of the Object given. *Tab.* 27. *Fig.* 1. *a b c* is an Object, whose Distance from the Glass *b z* is given. Let us suppose the Glass of the least thickness imaginable, that we may not be at the trouble of considering the Optick Angle, both at the Immersion and Emersion. Let the middle Point *b* Radiate upon the Glass, and after the Rays have passed the Glass, let them be so Refracted, as if they came directly from the Point *e*. From the forementioned *Data*, this Point *e*, being the *Imaginary Focus*, is easily determin'd by *Prop.* VIII. hereof: Through *e* draw the Infinite Right Line *d e f* Parallel to *a b c*. Wherefore as the *Locus Apparens* of the Point *b* is at *e*, so the *Loci* of the Collateral Points *a, c*, shall be somewhere in the Line *d e f* (unless perhaps Convexes on very small Spheres, will Represent the Object Crooked or Bowed, but of this we shall take no notice) to determine which, from the Vertex of the Glass *z* draw the Lines *z a d, z c f* (or if the Glass have any Thickness, as in *Tab.* 27. *Fig* 2. from the Vertex of Immersion, or outward Vertex, draw *z a, z c*; And from the Vertex of Emersion or Inward Vertex, draw *z d, z f,* Parallel to *z a, z c*, and then the Thickness of the Glass must be one of the *Data. Vid. Prop.* 47. *Gregorii Opt. Promot.*) the Points *d* and *f* are the *Loci Apparentes* of the Points *a* and *c*. For certainly were the Eye behind the Glass just at *z*, the Object *a b c* would appear under the Angle *a z c*, and the Point *b* would appear as at *e*, and therefore the Points *a* and *c* would appear somewhere, so as to make the Object keep the same Angle, But that can only be by the Points *a* and *c* appearing at *d* and *f* (supposing the Object to appear in its own Natural strait shape) Wherefore *d* and *f*

Tab. 27. pag. 116

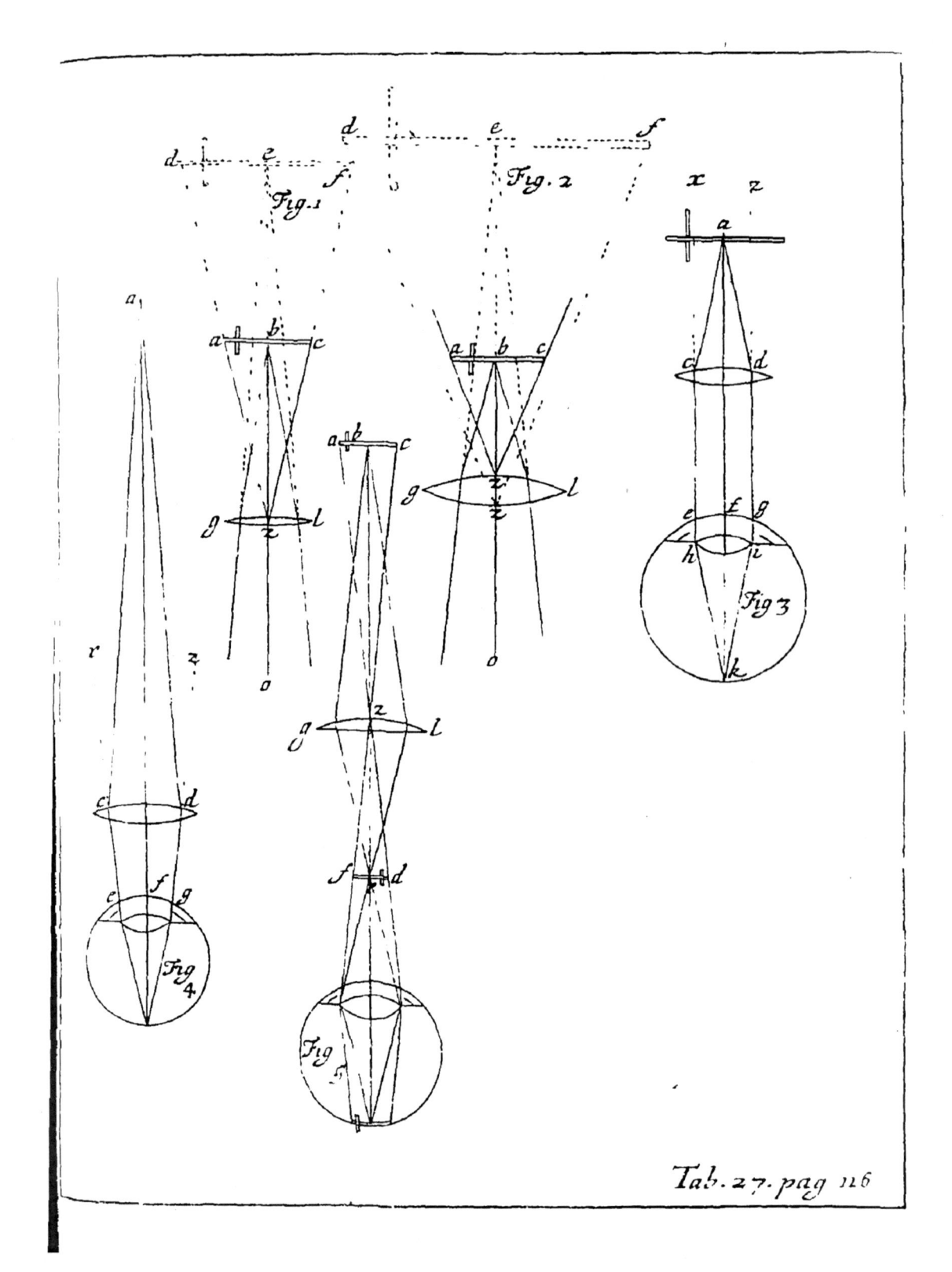

are the *Loci* of the Points *a* and *c*, and *d e f* is the *Locus* of the Object *a b c*.

Hence it appears, that a Convex-Glass Represents Objects as farther off than really they are: And this is the Reason, why Pieces of Perspective (as of Churches and Long Porticoes) appear very Natural and strong through Convex-Glasses duly apply'd. For these Glasses making Objects appear further off than really they are, must consequently make the Parts of the Perspective seem really *Hollow'd* or sunk in, the *French* term it *Renfoncé*.

Hence also tis Manifest, why Convex Glasses help the Eyes of those, that see only *Distant* Objects, as *Old Men*, for these make *Nigh* Objects appear as *Distant*. *Vid. Prop.* XXVIII. *Sec.* 8.

We may perceive also that the Distance between the Object and Glass continuing the same, the *Locus Apparens* is never alter'd, though the Eye be removed to and from the Glass *Gregorii Opt. Promot. Corol. Prop.* XLVII. For the Distance between the Object and Glass continuing the same, the Imaginary *Focus e* shall always be the same.

(8) *The Locus of an Object expos'd to a Convex-Glass in its Focus is not to be determin'd.*

When the Radiating Point *a*. Tab. 27. Fig. 3. is placed in the *Focus* of the Convex-Glass *c d*, the Rays *c e*, *d g*, after passing the Glass, run Parallel, and being produced to *c x*, *d z*, they never Intersect. Wherefore in this Case there is no Rule whereby to determine the *Locus* of the Object. And *Barrow* tells us only, *Quod Remotissime Positum Æstimatur*. Lect. 18. *ad Finem.* T27 F3

(9) *The Locus of an Object, beyond the Focus of a Convex-Glass, to the Eye between the Glass and Distinct Base, cannot be determined.*

Tab.

T 27 F 4. *Tab.* 27. *Fig.* 4. Let *a* be a Radiating Point placed more diſtant from the Glaſs *c d* than its Focus, the Rays *c e*, *d g*, after paſſing the Glaſs, do *Converge* towards the Diſtinct Baſe, let the Eye *e f g* be placed between the Glaſs and Diſtinct Baſe, it ſhall then receive the Rays *c e*, *d g*, Converging, and they being produced towards *x* and *z* ſeparate the further.

In this and the laſt Section lies the great Difficulty, which the *Incomparable* and *moſt profoundly Learned* B A R R O W (*Lect. Opt.* 18. *Sect.* 13.) confeſſedly paſſes over as inſuperable, and not to be explained by whatever Theories we have yet of Viſion. For ſeeing that the Object which applies to the Eye by *Leſs-diverging* Rays, is judged the *more remote*; And that which applies to the Eye by *Parallel Rays*, is reputed *moſt remote*; it ſhould ſeem reaſonably to follow, that what is ſeen by *Converging Rays*, ſhould appear yet *moſt remote* of all. And yet Experience contradicts this, and teſtifies, that the Point *a, Tab,* 27. *Fig.* 4. appears variouſly *diſtant*, according to the various Situations of the Eye between the Glaſs and Diſtinct Baſe; and that it does almoſt never (if ever) appear *more diſtant* than the Point *a* it ſelf to the naked Sight, and ſometimes it appears *much nigher*: Or rather, by how much the Rays, which fall through the Glaſs on the Eye, do *more Converge*, by ſo much the *nigher* does the Object appear to approach, inſomuch, that if the Eye approach the Glaſs *very nigh*, the Object *a* appears in its *natural Place* The Eye being a little farther removed from the Glaſs towards the Diſtinct Baſe, the Point *a* ſeems yet to approach. The Eye being yet farther, the Point ſeems yet *nigher*, and ſo by degrees, till at laſt the Eye being placed at a certain ſtation, as at the *Diſtinct Baſe*, the Point *a* appears *very nigh*, ſo that it begins to vaniſh away in mere *Confuſion*. All which (continues the candid B A R R O W) ſeems repugnant, or at leaſt not ſo well to agree to what we have laid down. And ſo he

leaves

leaves this Difficulty to the solution of others, which I (after so great an Example) shall do likewise, but with the resolution of the same admirable Author, of not quitting the *evident* Doctrine, which we have before laid down, for determining the *Locus Objecti*, on the account of being pressed by *one Difficulty*, which seems inexplicable, till a more intimate Knowledg of the *Visive Faculty* be obtained by Mortals. In the mean time, I propose it to the consideration of the ingenious, whether the *Locus Apparens* of an Object placed as in this 9th. Section, be not as much *before* the Eye, as the Distinct Base is *behind* the Eye. Vid. Corol. 1. Prop. LVII.

(10) *If an Object be more distant from a Convex Glass than its Focus, and the Eye beyond the Distinct Base, the* Locus Apparens *of the Object is in the Distinct Base.* Vid. Prop. XXXIX. Sect 5. item Schol. Prop. L.

Tab. 27. Fig 5. The Object *a b c* is projected by the Glass *g z l* in the Distinct Base *d e f*. The *Locus* of each Point in the *Object* is in the correspondent Point of the *Image* in the *Distinct Base*: Thus *a* appears at *d*, *b* at *e*, *c* at *f*. *Gregorii Opt. Prom. Prop.* XLVI.

Dechales (*Dioptr. Lib.* II. *Prop.* XI.) remarks a Matter of some moment in this Business of the *Locus Objecti*. The reason (says he) that the Appearances through Glasses of the Change of the Objects Place, do not so strongly strike the Sense, as the Doctrine here laid down seems to intimate, proceeds from hence; that Optick-Glasses are seldom or never made so large, as to be look'd through by both Eyes at once, for if they were, he asserts, That the *Locus apparens Objecti* would be much more plainly and sensibly determin'd to the sight. In this particular certainly he is much in the right; for we see at all times, that two Eyes make a more exact estimate of the Position of an Object, than one single Eye. And we have a sensible Experiment hereof in *Catoptricks,*

tricks, by the large concave Miroirs, where an Hand and Dagger presented beyond the Focus, seem to strike far without the *Speculum*, at him that presents it: But not so strongly if the *Speculum* be but small, so that the Image can be seen but by one Eye at once.

Scholium.

To this Property of the Change of the *Apparent Place* of an Object, may we attribute that common Effect of Objects seeming to *Dance* and *Move*, being seen through Spherick-Glasses, whether Convex or Concave, nimbly shaken between the Eye and the Object. 'Tis a noted Experiment, that to know, whether a Glass be Plain or Spherical (which is not to be found by Inspection of the Glass it self, or by Touch, if the Glasses be formed on large Spheres, and be but small portions thereof), the common Tryal is, to shake them something nimbly between the Eye and an Object; and if the Object seem to move by the motion of the Glass, the Glass is *not Plain*: The reason hereof is this; That toward the *Extremities* of a Glass, the Glass refracts *more* than towards the middle (for the very middle Ray, that is perpendicular, is not refracted at all) and consequently the *Apparent Place* of an Object is more changed by the Refraction in the *Extreme* parts of the Glass, than in the *middle* of the Glass: So that the Object, by the Motion of the Glass, appearing sometimes through the middle of the Glass, sometimes through the extremities of the Glass, the *Apparent Place* thereof is *varied* likewise, and the Object seems therefore to *change its Place*, or to *move*. But in a plain Glass the Case is otherwise, for the Refraction thereof is equally prevalent throughout the whole Glass, and neither *stronger* nor *weaker* in the *middle*, than in the *extremities*, so that the shaking of it between the Eye and

and Object, makes no other difference in the *Apparent Place*, than if the Glass were look'd through fixt and immoveable; and therefore the Object seems not through it to shake and move. And tho the *Locus* be changed by a Spherick Glass's being removed *to and from* the Eye, yet in Glasses of large Spheres, the *Locus* is not so *sensibly* changed, as by being shaken *before* the Eye. The same Reason holds for the apparent Dancing of Objects seen through rising Smoaks or Vapors.

Prop. XXXII.

An Object being placed in the Focus of a Convex-Glass, and the Eye on t'other side the Glass, sees this Object distinctly and erect.

That an Object so posited, is seen distinctly, is evident, because the Rays from each particular Point, after passing the Glass, become parallel (by *Prop.* VI.) and so fall on the Eye. And therefore (by *Prop.* XXVIII. *Sec.* 7.) they are fit to cause Distinct Vision. *Tab.* 27. *Fig* 3. The Point *a* sendeth forth its Diverging Rays *a c*, *a d*, on the Convex-Glass *c d*; these are transmitted by the Glass parallel in *c e*, *d g*, and so fall on the Eye; by whose Coats and Humors, especially by the Crystalline *h i*, they are refracted and brought together in the Point *k* on the *Retina*, there representing distinctly the Point *a* of the Object. T 27. F 3.

Or thus, *Tab.* 28. *Fig.* 1. The Eye *o p*, being in the place where some of the Rays from every Point in the Object are mixt together, is in the place of the greatest *Confusion*; and therefore by *Prop.* XXVIII. *Sec.* 3. the Vision is distinct. T 28. F 1.

I say also the Object is seen *erect*. In the same Figure *g k* is a Convex-Glass, *a b c* an Object; we may imagin that each Point of this Object sends from it a Cone of Rays, fall-

R

ing on the whole Surface of the Glafs; but for avoiding Confufion in the Scheme, I only exprefs and confider the Rays *c g*, *c h*, from the Point *c*; and *a k*, *a i* from the Point *a*. *o p* is the Cryftalline of the Eye. The Rays *c g*, *c h*, after paffing the Glafs become parallel as *g o*, *h p*, and fall fo on the Cryftalline, by whofe Refractions they are again brought together in the Point *d* on the Retina, there painting the lively Reprefentation of the Point *c*, and the fame may be fhewn of the Reprefentation of the Point *a* at *f* on the Retina. Wherefore the *finifter* Point *c* is reprefented on the *dexter* part of the Fund of the Eye *d*; and the *dexter* part of the Object *a* is painted on the *finifter* part of the Eye *f*. And confequently the Image on the Retina being *inverted*, the Object is feen erect (by Prop. XXVIII. Sec. 4, 5.). *Which was to be Demonftrated.*

Prop. XXXIII.

An Object being placed in the Focus of a Convex Glafs, and the Eye being placed in the Focus, on t'other fide the Glafs, fees this Object under the fame Angle, as were the naked Eye placed at the ftation of the Glafs

T.28.F 2.   *Tab.* 28. *Fig.* 2. *a x b* is an Object placed in the Focus of the Glafs *e f* (which we fuppofe of the leaft thicknefs imaginable). Let the Rays *a e*, *b f*, run parallel to the Axis *x c o*, thefe Rays are united in the Focus at *o*, at which Point we fuppofe the Eye. Produce *o e* and *o f* directly to *g* and *h*, and draw *e c f* (which by fuppofition is parallel to *a x b*, and then draw *a c*, *b c*. The Optick-Angle through the Glafs is *e o f*, which we are to prove equal to *a c b*. Thus, *a x* and *e c* being parallel, and *a e*, *x c*, being fo likewife, *a x* is equal to *e c*, and *a e* to *x c*, being the oppofite Sides of a Parallelogram. But *x c* is equal to *c o* (the Focal Length on one
fide

Tab. 28 pag. 121

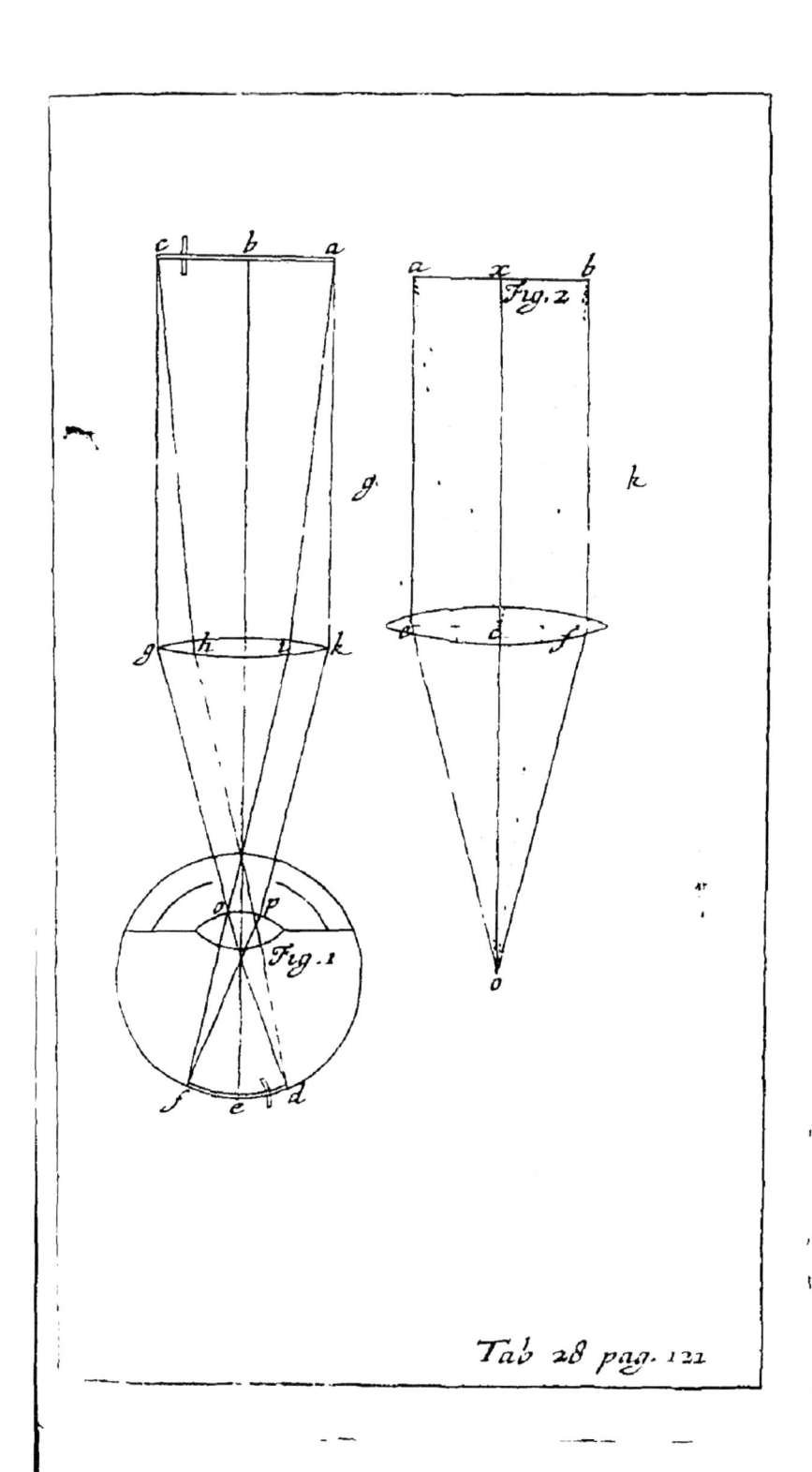

side and t'other). Wherefore the Right-angled Triangle *e c o* is equal and similar to the Right-angled Triangle *a x c*. Wherefore the Angle *e o c* is equal to the Angle *a c x*, or *e o f* is equal to *a c b*. And consequently the Eye at *o* sees the Object through the Glass under the same Angle, as the naked Eye being placed at *c*, would see it. *Which was to be proved.* Vid. *Gregorii Opt. Prom. Prop.* XLIV.

Scholium.

This is the Posture of both Eye and Object for causing the most perfect Vision possible through a single Convex Glass; unless perhaps we say, That seeing all Objects, which we perceive most distinctly are pretty nigh our Eyes; therefore we may conceive the Rays flowing from each Point of them, as falling on the Pupil *Diverging*. And consequently, that to see an Object most perfectly through a Convex Glass, 'tis best that the Object be placed a very little nigher the Glass than its Focus. For then the Rays, after passing the Glass, do something *Diverge*, and fall so on the Pupil; and this being the most natural and usual occurrence of Objects, it suits best, and is best adapted and most agreeable to the Eye; which by its refractive Coats and Humors easily collects each Cone of these *Diverging* Rays, and brings them together in a Point on the Fund of the Eye.

Corollary 1.

The Eye and Object being so placed as above; the Eye sees this Object *magnify'd* under an Angle almost *double* to that under which the Object would appear to the Eye, were the Glass removed; that is, the Angle *e o c* or *a c x* is almost double the Angle *a o c* (*a o* and *b o* being drawn directly) for the Angle *a c x* is equal to *a o c* + *c a o* (32. 1.) but *c a o* is almoſt equal to *a o c*. Therefore the Angle *a c x* is almoſt double *a o c*. *Which was to be Demonſtrated.* That *c a o* is almoſt equal to *a o c*, is manifeſt; for the Triangle *o c a* is almoſt Iſoſceles, *o c* (= *c x*) being almoſt equal to *c a*.

If now we ſuppoſe the Eye to continue in the Focus at *o*, and the Object *a x b* to be brought nigher the Glaſs *e f*, ſtill the Optick Angle through the Glaſs ſhall be *e o f*. By which (tho it continue the ſame, yet) the Object would not be magnifi'd by the Glaſs in this ſecond Poſture, as much as in the former. For the Angle *e o f* in this latter Poſture would not ſo much exceed the natural Optick Angle *a o b*. For at laſt *a x b* being brought ſo near *e c f*, as to be *coincident* therewith, the Angles *e o f* and *a o b* would be *coincident* alſo.

The ſame may be ſhewn, if we ſuppoſe the Object to continue in the Focus, and the Eye *o* to approach the Point *c*. For at laſt the Eye arriving at *c*, perceives the Object through the Glaſs under its own natural Angle *a c b*.

Corollary 2.

Hence it appears, that the Eye being in the Focus of a Convex-Glaſs, and the Object in the Focus alſo, the Eye can perceive no greater an *Area* or Space of the Object, than the Breadth of the Glaſs, or the Breadth of that Portion thereof, which the Eye makes uſe of; for *a b* is equal to *e f*. And the reaſon is, becauſe thoſe Rays *a e*, *b f*, that come from the Extremities of the Object *a* and *b*, and concurr at the Eye in the Focus *o*, muſt neceſſarily fall on the Glaſs parallel to the Axis *x c*.

PROP.

Tab. 29 pag. 129

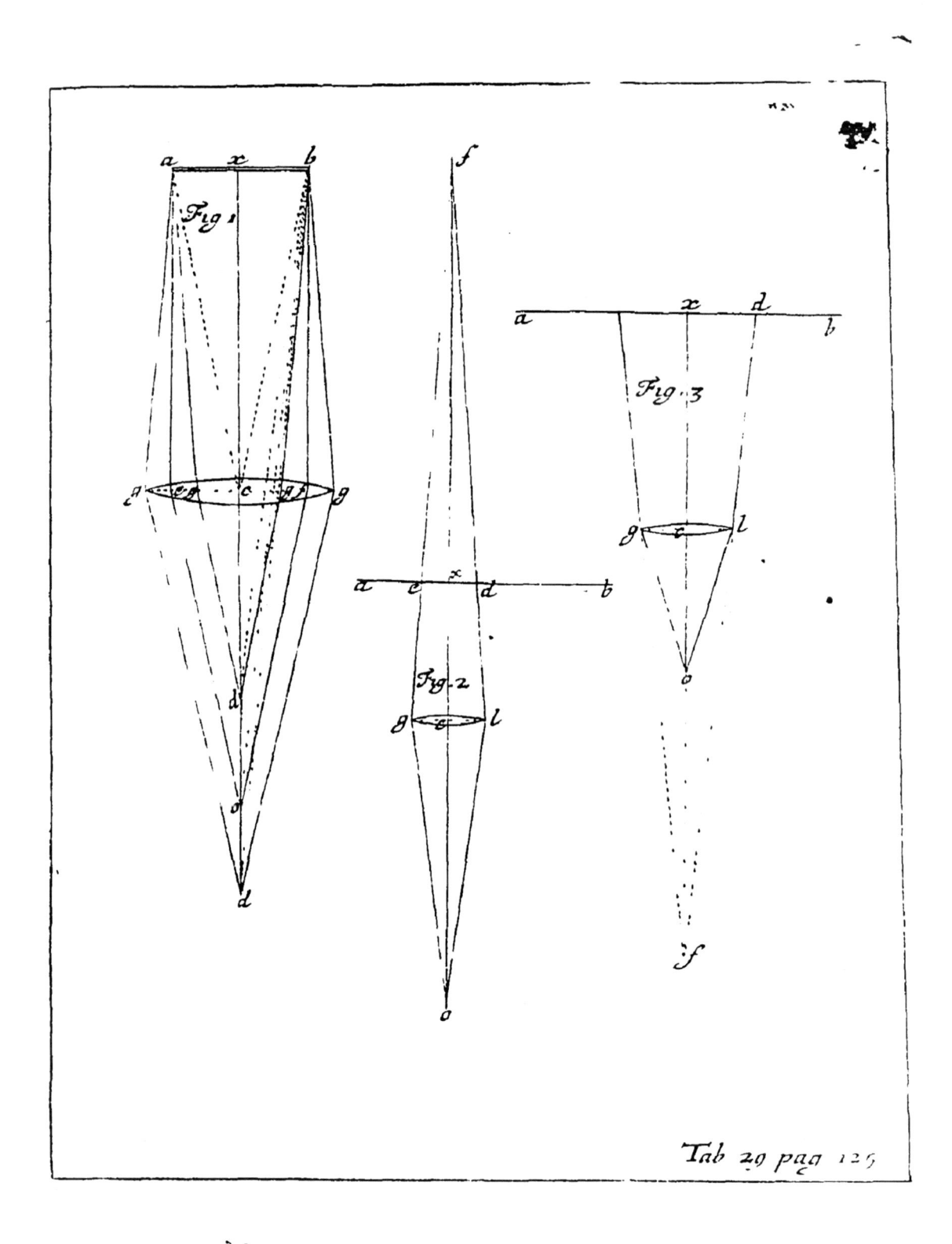

PROP. XXXIV. PROB.

To determine the Optick Angle, or apparent Magnitude of an Object in the Focus of a Convex-Glass, to the Eye at any other station, from these Data, the Glasses Focal Length, or the Distance of the Object from the Glass x c, Tab. 29. F. 1. *The Distance of the Eye from the Glass* c d, *and the Breadth of the Object* a b.

T.29. F1.1

The Thickness of the Glass I take no notice of, because I would not perplex the Scheme. And therefore the Glass is supposed of the least Thickness imaginable; or all the Refractions are supposed performed at the Line in the middle of the Glass g e c f g.

Wherefore let a x b be an Object, and let the Rays a e, b f, fall parallel to the Axis x c o; these are united in the other Focus at o, where if the Eye be placed, it sees the Object under the Angle e o f = a c b, by the preceding Prop. Wherefore having b x the half Object, and x c; in the Right-angled Triangle b x c, we may find the Semi-optick Angle b c x. Draw the prickt Line b o directly; the Angle b o x is the natural Optick Angle of the Object b x, which is easily obtained, in the Right-angled Triangle b o x, having b x and x o.

Let now the Eye be out of the Focus at d; the Rays a g, after passing the Glass, become parallel to e o (Prop. VI.) And therefore the Angle g d x is equal to e o x or a c x, which we have found before. Draw the prickt Line b d directly; the Angle b d x is the natural Optick Angle of the Object b x, were the Glass removed, and is easily had in the Right-angled Triangle b x d, having b x and x d ($=xc+cd$). So the Problem is satisfied.

PROP.

Prop. XXXV. Probl.

To determine the Visible Area of an Object in the Focus of a Convex Glass; from these Data, the distance of the Object from the Glass or the Glasses Focal Length, the distance of the Eye from the Glass, and the Breadth of the Glass.

It is shewn before in the 2d. *Corollary* to *Prop.* XXXIII. That the Visible Area of an Object in the Focus of a Convex Glass, to the Eye placed in t'other Focus, is equal to the Breadth of the Glass. Wherefore I shall only here consider the two other Cases.

T 29. F 2. And first, Let the Eye at o, *Tab.* 29. *Fig.* 2. be placed *further* from the Glass $g\,l$ than its Focus, the Object $a\,x\,b$ is in the Focus, $g\,l$ the Glasses Breadth, $x\,c$ the Glasses Focus or distance of the Object, and $c\,o$ the distance of the Eye from the Glass are given. Draw $g\,o$, $l\,o$, and produce the Axis $o\,c\,f$ infinitely. Let us now imagin the Point o a nigh Radiating Point or Object, sending its Rays $o\,g$, $o\,c$, $o\,l$, on the Glass. By *Prop.* V. Let us determin the Distinct Base or Respective Focus of this Point projected by this Glass, which by the foregoing *Data* is easily performed. Suppose this respective Focus to be $c\,f$. Draw $g\,f$, $l\,f$, where these Lines intersect the Object in e and d, the Visible Area of the Object is determined by $e\,d$.

Demonstration. For by Exper. 8. the Progress of a Ray through different Mediums is *Reciprocal*. Wherefore if the Rays $o\,g$, $o\,l$, be refracted into $g\,e$, $l\,d$; it will necessarily follow, that $e\,g$, $d\,l$, being consider'd as two Rays flowing from the Points e and d, they shall be refracted into $g\,o$, $l\,o$; wherefore this Analogy will hold, $f\,c : c\,l \;.\; f\,x \;(=f\,c-x\,c) : x\,d$. Which $x\,d$ is half the Visible Area to the Eye at o.

Secondly,

Secondly, Tab. 29. F. 3. Let the Eye at *o* be placed *nigher* T 29. F 3. the Glass than its Focus. Draw *g o*, *l o*. And produce the Axis *o c* infinitely backwards towards *f*. Then (as before) supposing the Point *o* a Radiating Point or Object; by the *Data*, and by *Prop.* VIII. we may easily determin the *Imaginary* Focus thereof, which let be *c f*. From *f* draw *f g* directly to *e*, and *f l* to *d*. *e d*, by the foregoing Demonstration, is the Visible Area of the Object *a b*. And *c f* : *c l* :: *f x* ($= f c + c x$) : *x d*. Which is half the Visible Area to the Eye at *o*.

Scholium.

The same Rules may be used, when the Object is *nigher* to or *further from* the Glass than its Focus. So that this Proposition is universal to all Cases in *Erect Vision* through Convex Glasses. But whether this Area be *distinctly* visible or not, depends on other Considerations; and will be obvious enough to those that consider what *has been before*, and what *shall* be hereafter laid down concerning the *distinct* and *confused* appearance of Objects.

Prop. XXXVI.

An Object being placed more distant from a Convex Glass than its Focus, and the Eye placed on t'other side this Glass nigher to the Glass than the Distinct Base to the Glass, sees this Object erect and confused.

I have shewn before (*Prop.* V. XXVI, XXVII.) that if an Object be placed more distant from a Glass than its Focus, this Object is projected in a distinct Base somewhere on t'other side the Glass. And that this Distinct Base, may be sometimes *Less*, sometimes *equal to*, and sometimes *Greater* than the Object it self

Tab.

Tab. 30. *Fig.* 1. *a b c* is an Object expofed to the Glafs *g l*, and projected in the Diftinct Bafe *f e d*. Each Cone of Rays from the Object is made to *converge*, as *b l g* is formed into *g e l*. Let the Eye be placed at *k*. I fay, firft the Object appears *erect*. For the Rays from *a* the upper part of the Object tend to, and determin in the lower part of the Fund of the Eye. And the Rays from *c* the lower part of the Object tend towards the upper part of the *Retina*; and therefore the Appearance is *erect*, (by *Prop.* XXVIII. *Sec.* 4, 5.)

Moreover, the Eye being placed any where between the Glafs *g l*, and the Diftinct Bafe *f e d*, does not receive the Species of the Object *inverted*; for that only happens juft in the Diftinct Bafe it felf. And on this account, 'tis manifeft, that the Appearance to the Eye in this pofture shall be *Erect*.

I fay likewife, that the Apearance of the Object is *confufed*. Let us conceive the Pupil of the Eye at *m n*; here it receives the Rays from the Point *b converging*; and therefore by *Prop.* XXVIII. the Reprefentation of the Point *b* on the Fund of the Eye shall be *confufed*. And fo of the other Points in the Object, that is, of the whole Object. And if the Eye recede from the Glafs, as to *h i*, the Vifion is *more confufed*, becaufe the Rays are *nigher* converged.

PROP. XXXVII. PROBL.

To determin the Optick Angle, or Apparent Magnitude, and the Vifible Area of an Object placed as in the laft; from thefe Data, The Breadth of the Object a b c *(Tab.* 30. *Fig.* 2.), *Its Diftance from the Glafs* z b, *The Glaffes Power, The Glaffes Breadth* g l, *And the Diftance of the Eye from the Glafs* k z.

(1.) From

(1.) From these *Data* by the foregoing Doctrine of Convex Glasses, 'tis easie to determine the Breadth of the Distinct Base. For by *Prop. XXVI, XXVII. As the Distance of the Object from a Convex Glass : To the Breadth of the Object :: So the Distance of the Image in the Distinct Base :* (which is easily obtained from the foregoing *Data*) *To the Breadth of the said Image.* That is (in the foresaid Figure) $bz : ac :: ez : df$. And As $ab : bz :: de : ez$. And consequently the Angle ezd is equal to the Angle azb; the Triangles ezd and azb being similar. And in the Right-angled Triangle abz, we have ab and bz, to find the Angle $azb = ezd$; which is the Angle, under which the Object would appear to the Eye placed just touching the Glass at z; supposing the Glass to be there of the least Thickness imaginable.

(2.) Let us now suppose the Eye at k. I say if the Rays from the single Points a, c, in an Object be converged by the Convex Glass gl to any other Points d, f; the Object shall appear under the Optick Angle xkm, as do the *Apices* of the Pencils from the Extreme Points of the Object, which is $dkf = xkm$. Vid. *Gregorii Opt. Promot. Prop. XLV.*

(3.) Wherefore in the Right-angled Triangle ekd, we have ek and ed, To find the Angle $ekd = zkx$, which is the Semi-Optick Angle to the Eye at k. In like manner may we find the Optick Angle at any other given Station of the Eye, as at n, $end = gnz$ being equal to half fnd.

(4.) As to the *Visible Area* of the Object, 'tis determin'd as before, *Prop. XXXV.* and *Schol.* I shall only add, That if the Eye be at q, and the Line dq being drawn, and produced towards h, it does not fall upon the Glass gl; then the Eye at q shall not see through the Glass the Point a, the *Apex* of whose Pencil is in the Point d. And from hence we may perceive, that at k, we may see through the Glass a *greater* space than the Area of the Object abc. At n we can but *just* see the *whole* Object *a b c*; and at *q* we cannot see the extreme Point *a c*. By which the 81 and 82 *Prop.* of *Kepler*'s *Dioptricks* are manifest.

(5.) If the Glass have any Thickness considerable, see *Prop.* XXXI. concerning the *Locus Objecti*, Sec. 7.

Scholium.

If we first determine the *Visible Area* by *Prop.* XXXV. the Breadth of the Object need not be one of the *Data* for determining the *Optick-Angle*. For the Breadth of the Object is found by obtaining the *Visible Area*.

Prop. XXXVIII.

An Object being more distant from a Glass than its Focus, and the Eye placed in the Distinct Base, the Object appears most confused.

By *Prop.* XXXVI. 'tis manifest, that the nigher the Eye approaches the Distinct Base, the more *confused* the Object appears; because the Rays from each particular Point, do fall on the Eye *closer Converged*, and more orderly separated by the Glass from the Rays of adjacent Points. But in the Distinct Base, the Rays are most of all Converged, and most orderly united in their proper Points, each with the Rays flowing from the same Point in the Object. Wherefore the Eye is there in the greatest Confusion.

Moreover (by *Prop.* XXVIII. *Sec.* 3.) 'tis requisite to Distinct Vision, that the Rays from the several Points in the Object, fall on the Eye altogether *confused* thereon (as they do on the Glass in the Hole of a dark Room), that the Coats and Humors of the Eye may refract them, and bring them together,

ther, diftinctly painting the Image on the *Retina*. But when the Eye is in the Diftinct Bafe, all this is fruftrated.

Prop. XXXIX.

The Object being more Diftant from the Glafs than the Focus; and the Eye further from the Glafs than the Diftinct Bafe, begins to perceive the Object inverted; and, at a proper diftance, Diftinct.

(1.) This is manifeft by *Tab.* 30. *Fig.* 3. wherein *a b c* is an Object, *g s l* the Glafs projecting the Diftinct Bafe *f e d, o* is the Eye. And becaufe half the Pencils of Rays that flow from each of the extreme Points of the Object *a* and *c*, proceeding forwards from the Points *d* and *f* in the Diftinct Bafe, after they crofs in the aforefaid Points *d* and *f*, by reafon of their too great Divergence, do efcape the Eye. Therefore, for avoiding Perplexity in the Scheme, I have only expreffed the Half Cones *s a l, s d l,* and *s c g, s f g,* which incurr the Eye.

(2.) Wherefore we may obferve, that the Diverging Rays *p f o* and *o d q*, falling diverging and confufed on the Cryftalline *p q*, are thereby collected, and made to concurr on the *Retina* in the Points *n* and *r*; and there paint the *upper* Point *a* of the Object on the upper part *r* of the Eyes Fund; and the *lower* Point *c* of the Object on the lower part *n* of the *Retina*. Therefore by *Prop.* XXVIII. *Sect.* 4, and 5. the Object appears *inverted*, becaufe the Image reprefented on the *Retina* is *Erect*.

(3.) Or more plainly thus, We may now conceive the Diftinct Bafe it felf *f d* to be as it were an *inverted* Object (as here the Crofs turned with its head downwards). Therefore the appearance thereof to the Eye, fhall feem *inverted*. For if the Eye perceive an *erect* Object, *erect*, it muft needs perceive the Diftinct Bafe, being an *inverted* Object, *inverted*.

S 2 And

And this may be laid down as a General Rule, That where an Object, or the Image, or Representation of an Object, which is next the Eye, is *inverted*, there the Object shall appear *inverted*. And where the Object, or Image next before the Eye, is *erect*, the Object appears *erect*.

(4.) I say also, *At a proper distance the Inverted Appearance is Distinct*. For when the Eye is so far removed from the Distinct Base, as to be able to correct the Divergence of the Rays, that come to it from each Point in the Distinct Base, and to form them into correspondent Cones determining their *Apices* on the *Retina*, the Vision is Distinct, otherwise not.

Moreover there are two other *Phænomena* of this Posture of Object, Glass, and Eye; which I shall here explain as follows.

(5.) If the Eye be moved *upwards* towards z, the Object shall appear to move *downwards*. If the Eye be moved downwards towards x, the Object seems to move *upwards*. To explain this, let us consider the Point c, and how the appearance thereof is brought *to* and formed *in* the Eye. And we shall find, that in the Posture of the Scheme, the Point c is expressed in the Eye, only by that parcel of its Rays that fall on the half Glass sg, for these are brought together in sfg, and flowing forward, become pfo: But the other parcel of Rays scl, that fall on the half Glass sl, and are brought together in sfl, proceeding forwards, escape the Eye; for they go on in pfz. Wherefore the Point c is now represented through the half Glass sg, or seen somewhere between g and s. But the Eye moving upwards towards z, so that it miss the Rays pfo, and receive only the Rays pfz; the Point c shall then be represented through the half Glass sl, or seen somewhere between s and l, and consequently shall seem to move *downwards* What is shewn of the Point c, may be conceived of the other Points in the Object, that is, of the whole Object.

And

And this *Phænomenon* is the strongest Confirmation imaginable, that the *Locus Apparens Objecti*, in this Case, is in the *Distinct Base* (as is said before, *Prop.* XXXI. *Sec.* 10). For by raising the Eye, we depress the Point f; and by depressing the Eye, we raise the Point f. Wherefore the appearance of the Point c is at f. For the Point c in the Object seems to move contrary to the motion of the Eye.

From the foregoing Explication it follows, that if the Glass be moved *upwards*, the Object appears to move *upwards*. And if the Glass be moved *downwards*, the Object appears to move *downwards*; for the moving of the Glass *upwards* is the same as moving the Eye *downwards*; but moving the Eye *downwards*, makes the Object appear to move *upwards*; therefore the moving of the Glass *upwards* makes the Objects appear to move *upwards*.

Or thus, Because moving the Glass *upwards*, the Distinct Base is moved *upwards* (for it follows the Glass), and the Distinct Base is in this case as it were the Object. (*Prop.* XXXI. *Sec.* 10.) Therefore by the Glasses motion *upwards*, the Eye shall perceive the Object moved *upwards*.

(6.) If with both Eyes we look at the inverted Appearance of an Object through a Convex-Glass, we shall perceive the Object double. Supposing the Eyes not very far removed from the Distinct Base. *Tab.* 30. *Fig.* 4. abc is an Object projected by the Glass gl in the Distinct Base fed, the Point e being correspondent to the Point b. Let the Cone of Rays gel flow forwards from e, and become zey. Let the two Eyes n, m, meet the Cone of Rays zey. I say the Eye n perceives the Point e (the Representation of the Point b) by the Rays zeq, which flow forward from sel; and consequently the Eye n perceives the Point b or e, as it were, somewhere between s and l. In like manner, the Eye m perceives the Point b or e somewhere between s and g: Wherefore the two Eyes seeing the Point b or e, as it were, *in two places*, see it *Double*.

Double. What is said of the Point *b*, may be understood of any other Point in the Object, and consequently of the whole Object. And if we shut the *Right* Eye *m*, the *Left* Appearance of *b* vanishes; if the *Left* Eye *n*, then the *Right* Appearance of the Object vanishes.

But if the Eyes be removed very far from the Distinct Base *f e d*, their Interval continues the same; and the Rays *e k*, *e p*, Diverging continually, *they* shall at last fall on the Eyes, that is, *e k* on the Eye *n*, and *e p* on the Eye *m*. By which the Eye *n* shall perceive *e* as it were at *u* (*k e u* being one Right Line), and the Eye *m* shall perceive the same *e* as it were at *r* (*p e r* being one Right Line), whereby the Difference of the Places *r* and *u* becomes less than before, till at last the Eye be got at such a Distance from the Distinct Base, that this Difference of the Apparent Places becomes so small, that 'tis insensible to the sight.

Quære. How Dr. *Briggs* would explain this *Phænomenon* of *Double Vision* by his Theory of sight. *Philosoph. Collect.* Numb. 6.

Prop. XL.

T.30 F.5.

To determine the Optick-Angle or Apparent Magnitude, and the Visible Area of an Object, placed as in the last, from these Data; The Breadth of the Object a b c, *(Tab. 30. F. 5.) Its Distance from the Glass* s b, *The Glasses Power or Focal Length, The Glasses Breadth* g l, *And the Distance of the Eye from the Glass* o s.

(1.) It is shewn before (*Prop.* XXXVII) how we may from these *Data* obtain the Breadth of the Distinct Base *f e d*, and its Distance from the Glass *e s*. Wherefore *o s — e s = o e*. Then in the Right-angled Triangle *o e f*, we have *o e* and *e f* to find the Angle *f o e*, which is the Semi-Optick Angle, under

der

der which the Eye perceives the Inverted Appearance of the Object. In like manner may we find the Optick Angle to any other station as at *n*.

(2.) The Learned GREGORY in his *Opt. Promot. Prop.* 46. has a curious Theorem to this purpose, 'tis this, *The Rays from each single Point in an Object* a b c, *being formed by the Glass* g s l *into the Distinct Base* f e d ; *and the Eye* o *being placed behind the Points of Concourse* f e d ; *the Image of each Point in the Object shall appear in the* Apex *of its Pencil* (That is, The Image of the Point *a* shall appear in the *Apex* of its Pencil at *d, &c.*), *And the Object shall appear Inverted, And under that Optick-Angle, as the* Apices *of the Pencils of the Extreme Points of the Object*; That is, under the Angle *f o d*.

(3) The *Visible Area* is thus determined, *Tab.* 30. *Fig.* 6. The Object *a b c* is projected by the Glass *g s l* in the Distinct Base *f e d*. Let the Eye be at *o*; draw *o g, o l*; the Eye at *o* shall see no more of the Object, than what is represented between *z* and *r*, where the Lines *o g, o l*, intersect the Distinct Base. To determine the Points in the Object, that answer the Points *z, r*, in the Distinct Base. From the Centre of the Glass *s* (for I suppose it of no Thickness), draw *z s x, r s k*, the Point *k* answers *r*, and *x* answers *z*. Lastly, from the foregoing *Data* to determine the Measure of *z r* say, As *s o : s g :: e o : e z = ½ z r*; but the three first are known, therefore the fourth is known also. *Which was to be found.*

(4) If the Line *o y* produced, do not fall on the Glass, then that Point in the Object, whose *Apex* of its Pencil is at *y*, or which is projected in the Distinct Base at *y*, shall not be seen through the Glass by the Eye at *o*. Vid. *Schol. Prop.* XLVI. *Gregorii Opt. Promot.*

Corollary.

Corollary.

Hence it follows, That the *further* the Eye is removed from the Distinct Base, it perceives the *greater* Area of the Object; but can never see more than what is projected in the Breadth of the Glass; that is, *z r* can never be *greater* than *g l*, nor ever equal thereto, unless the Eye *o* be at an infinite Distance.

PROP. XLI.

An Object being placed nigher a Convex Glass than its Focus, and the Eye on t'other side the Glass, at any Distance within the Eyes power, sees this Object Distinct and Erect.

I say, *Within the Eye's Power*; for 'tis shewn before in *Prop.* VII. and VIII. That when an Object is placed nigher a Convex Glass than its Focus, the Rays from each Point thereof, after passing the Glass, do Diverge, but not so much as if the Glass were away. Wherefore, tho the Eye looking at an Object within the Focus of this Glass, may be *nigher* the Object, than if the Glass were away, and yet see it *distinctly*; yet there is a *mean* to be observed; for even with the Glass it self the Eye may be *too nigh* the Object, and not able to correct the Divergence of the Rays it receives.

But that an Object thus posited appears *Distinct* to the Eye at a convenient Distance, is manifest; for the Rays from each Point proceed *moderately Diverging*, and so fall on the Eye. *Prop.* XXVIII. *Sec.* 7.

That an Object thus posited is seen *Erect*, is evident from *Prop.* XXXII. and XXXIX.

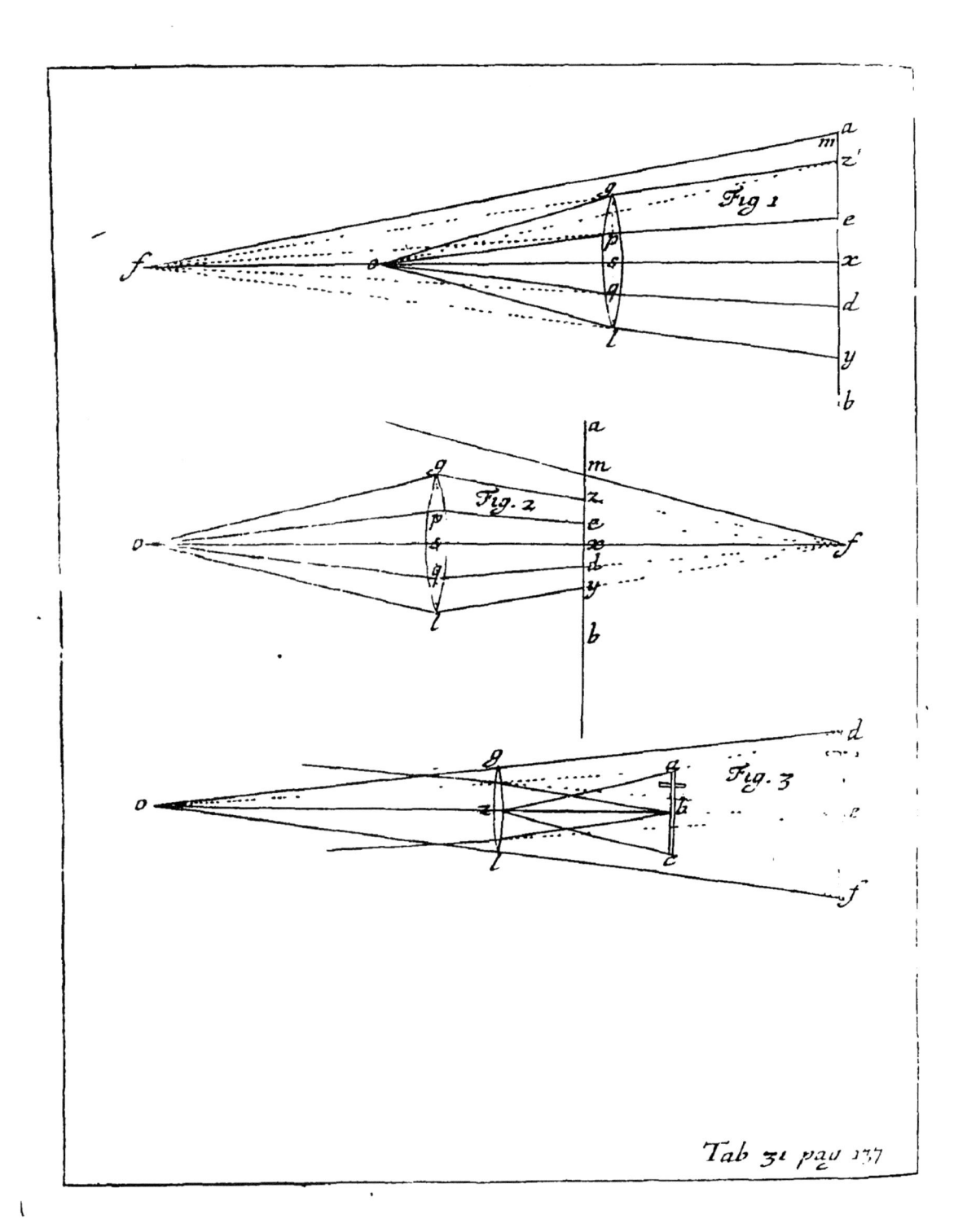

Fig. 1

Fig. 2

Fig. 3

Tab 31 pag 137

PROP. XLII.

To determine the Visible Area, and the Optick-Angle or Apparent Magnitude of an Object placed as in the last, from these Data, The Power or Focal Length of the Glass, The Distance of the Object from the Glass, The Distance of the Eye from the Glass, and the Breadth of the Glass.

Tab. 31. *Fig.* 1. and 2. *a b* is an Object exposed to the Glass *g l*, nigher to it than its Focus. *o* is the Eye, which in *Fig.* 1. is supposed *nigher* the Glass than its Focus; and this is the First Case. But in *Fig.* 2. the Eye *o* is supposed *further* from the Glass than its Focus; and this is the Second Case. 'Tis shewn before (*Prop.* V. VIII.), how the *Respective* and *Imaginary* Foci *f* are determined in one and t'other Case.

First let the given Breadth of the Glass be *g l*. By *Prop.* XXXV. we determine the Visible Area *z y*. Let us then suppose the given Breadth of the Glass to be *p q*. By the same *Prop.* XXXV. we determine the Visible Area *e d*.

As to the Optick-Angles *g o l* (supposing the Object *z y*) or *p o q* (supposing the Object *e d*) they are determined from the *Data*, by Plain Trigonometry of Right-angled Triangles, as before in *Prop.* XXXIV.

And we shall find by Calculation (as indeed 'tis evident by the very Inspection and Consideration of the Schemes), that the Collateral Parts *z e*, *d y*, of the Object *z y*, are much more magnifid (in respect of their Natural Appearance) by Broad Glasses formed on small Spheres, than the Middle Parts *e x*, *d x*, for the Angle *g o p* is the Optick-Angle, through the Glass, of the Part *z e*, and the Angle *p o s* is the Optick-Angle, through the Glass, of the Part *e x*, but the former exceeds the Natural Optick-Angle much more than the latter.

[138]

As to the Natural Optick-Angle of the Object zx, were the Glass away; draw zo directly (*Fig.* 1.), then in the Right-angled Triangle zxo, we have zx and xo to find the Angle zox, which is the Natural Optick-Angle of the Object zx.

From hence it is, that by Broad Glasses formed on small Spheres, the Extreme Parts of *strait* Objects, seem to be *incurved* and *bent*, as is manifest in the Case of the *Micrometer*, or Lattice of fine Hairs, strained before the Eye Glass in a Telescope, for Measuring the Diameters of Objects. As *Pere Cherubin* complains in his *Dioptrique Oculair. Part.* III. *Sec.* 7. *Chap.* 1. *pag.* 239. but understood not the reason. Of this we may make Experiment, by looking with a very Convex Glass at two Parallel Lines drawn pretty close on a Paper.

Schol. 1.

If instead of the Glasses Breadth, we have the Breadth of the Object ed given, we may easily determine the Breadth of the Glass, through which this Portion of the Object is seen: For from the Point f, draw fe, fd, these intersect the Glass in p, q. I say this is the Portion of the Glass, through which ed is visible. And if the Line fm, being produced, do not fall on the Glass, the Point m in the Object is not visible through the Glass gl to the Eye at o.

Schol. 2.

This XLII. *Proposition*, as it relates to the Optick-Angle, may be solved another way by Determining the *Locus Objecti*. But then, to the former *Data* in that *Proposition*, instead of the *Glasses Breadth*, we must add the *Breadth of the Object*. Wherefore, *Tab.* 31. *Fig.* 3. Let the *Locus* of the Object abc be determin'd def, by *Prop.* XXXI. *Sec.* 7. Let the Eye

[139]

Eye be at o, draw do, fo directly; if the Right Line do do not fall on the Glass, the Eye at o cannot perceive through the Glass the Point of the Object a (Vid. *Prop.* XXXVII. *Sec.* 4. *Prop.* XL. *Sec.* 4. *& Schol. Prop.* XLVI. *Gregorii Opt. Promot.*). But if do, fo, fall on the Glass; I say, the Angle dof is the Angle under which the Object abc appears to the Eye at o through the Glass. For the Object abc is seen through the Glass under the same Angle, as the Image def would be seen without the Glass (by *Prop.* XXXI. *Sec.* 7.). Now because we have ab and bz given, and ez found, we may find also ed; for $bz : ba :: ez : ed$. Then in the Right-angled Triangle doe, we have de and eo ($= ez + zo$) to find the Angle $doe = \frac{1}{2} dof$. Draw then ao directly; the Angle aob is the Natural Optick-Angle, under which the Object ab would appear to the Eye without the Glass. Now having ab and bo ($= bz + zo$) we may find the Angle aob; the Difference between which and the Angle doe (that is doa) shews how much the Object is magnified by the Glass.

I. *Example of the First Case computed by the Method in* Prop. XLII. *Tab.* 31. *Fig.* 1. T 31 F.1.

Glasses Focus = — — — — — — — 4637
Dist. of the Eye from the Glass = so = 2500
Dist. of the Obj. from the Glass = sx = 2721 } *Data.*
½ Breadth of the Glass = ½ gl = sg = 145

½ Visible Area = — — — — — zx = ?
½ Optick-Angle = — — — ∠ gos = ? } *Quæsita.*

First supposing the Point o a Radiating Point,
By *Prop.* VIII. As Focus Glass — so : to Foc. Glass :: so : fs
That is in Numbers — — — 2137 · 4637 :: 2500 : 5425

T 2 Then

[140]

Then — — — — $fs : sg :: fx (=fs+sx) : zx$

That is $5425 : 145 :: 8146 : 217 = xz$ the Visible *Area* in this Case according to the *Data*.

Secondly, To find the Optick-Angle gos, under which this $zx = 217$, appears; say,

so : Rad. :: sg : Tang. $\angle gos = 3° \ 19' \ 10''$.

The foregoing *Example* calculated according to *Schol.* 2. *Prop.* XLII. But the Letters refer to *Tab.* 31. *Fig.* 3.

T.31.F.3.

$$\left.\begin{array}{l}\text{Glasses Focus} = \text{———————} 4637\\ \text{Dist. of the Eye from the Gl.} = zo = 2500\\ \text{Dist. of the Obj. from the Gl} = zb = 2721\\ \frac{1}{2} \text{ Breadth of the Object} = \text{——} ab = 217\end{array}\right\} Data.$$

$$\left.\begin{array}{l}\text{Distance of the Imaginary Focus } ze = ?\\ \text{Breadth of the Imaginary Focus} = de = ?\\ \text{Optick-Angle ————} \angle doe = ?\end{array}\right\} Quæsita.$$

First, Supposing the Point b a Radiating Point, to determine the Imaginary Focus at e, by *Prop.* VIII. we must say,

As Focus Glass — zb : Focus Glass :: zb : ze
That is in Numbers 1916 : 4637 :: 2721 : 6585
Then by *Pr.* 2. 6. *Eucl.* zb : ba :: ze : ed
That is in Numb. 2721 : 217 :: 6585 : 525

Lastly, As $eo (= ze + zo)$: Rad. :: de : Tang. $\angle doe = 3° \ 18' \ 30''$, which wants only 40" Seconds of the former Calculation, by reason of the neglect of the Fractions.

II. Ex-

II. *Example of the Second Case calculated according to* Prop. XLII. *Tab.* 31. *Fig.* 2. T 31 F 2

Glasses Focus = — — — — — — 4637
Dist. of the Eye from the Glass = *s o* = 5000
Dist. of the Obj. from the Glass = *s x* = 2721
½ Breadth of the Glass = ½ *g l* = *s g* = 145
⎬ *Data.*

½ Visible Area = — — — — — *z x* = ?
½ Optick-Angle = — — — ∠ *g o s* = ?
⎬ *Quæsita.*

First, Supposing the point *o* a Radiating Point, Then by *Prop.* V.
As *s o* — Foc. of the Gl. : Foc. of the Gl. :: *s o* : *f s*
That is in Numbers 363 . 4637 :: 5000 : 63870
Then — — — *f s* : *s g* : *f x* (= *f s* — *s x*) : *z x*
That is in Numbers 63870 : 145 :: 61149 . 138, being the Visible *Area* in this Case, according to the *Data*.

Secondly, To find the Optick-Angle *g o s*, under which this *z x* = 138 appears, say,
As *s o* : Rad. :: *s g* : Tang. ∠ *g o s* = 1° 39′ 40″

The foregoing II. *Example* calculated according to the Solution in *Schol.* 2. *Pr.* XLII. The Letters relate to *Tab.* 31. F. 3. T 31 F 3

Glasses Focus = — — — — — — — 4637
Dist. of the Eye from the Glass = *z o* = 5000
Dist. of the Obj. from the Glass = *z b* = 2721
½ Breadth of the Object = — — *a b* = 138
⎬ *Data.*

Distance of the Imaginary Focus = *z e*
½ Breadth of the Imaginary Focus = *d e*
Optick-Angle through the Glass = ∠ *d o e*
⎬ *Quæsita.*

Let

Let us suppose the Point b a Radiating Point. To determine the Imaginary Focus at e, by *Prop.* VIII. say,

As Foc. of the Glass $- z\,b$. Foc. of the Gl. :: $z\,b$: $z\,e$

That is in Numbers 1916   4637 :: 2721 : 6585

Then — — — — — $z\,b$: $b\,a$ :: $z\,e$: $e\,d$

That is in Numbers 2721 : 138 :: 6585 : 334

Lastly, As $e\,o$ ($= z\,e + z\,o$) : Rad. :: $d\,e$: Tang. $\angle d\,o\,e =$ = 1° 39′ 0″, which by reason of the neglect of Fractions wants 40″ Seconds of the foregoing Calculation.

Of CONCAVES.

I Now proceed to the Consideration of Vision through *Concave* Glasses.

PROP. XLIII.

All Objects seen through Concave Glasses appear Erect and Diminish'd.

That the Object shall appear *Erect* is manifest; for 'tis before (*Prop.* XXXIX. *Sec.* 3.) laid down as a General Rule, *That where the Object, or Image that is next before the Eye, is Erect, the Eye shall perceive the Object Erect; and where Inverted, the Eye sees it Inverted.* But Concaves have no *Distinct Base* (as Convexes have) wherein they represent the *Image* of the Object *Inverted*, and consequently, wherever the Eye is placed behind a Concave Glass, it shall perceive the Object through it, in its Natural Posture. That Concaves have no *Real Distinct Base*, is most plain from the Doctrine that foregoes relating to them: For a Distinct Base is caused by the Collection

Tab. 32 pag. 143

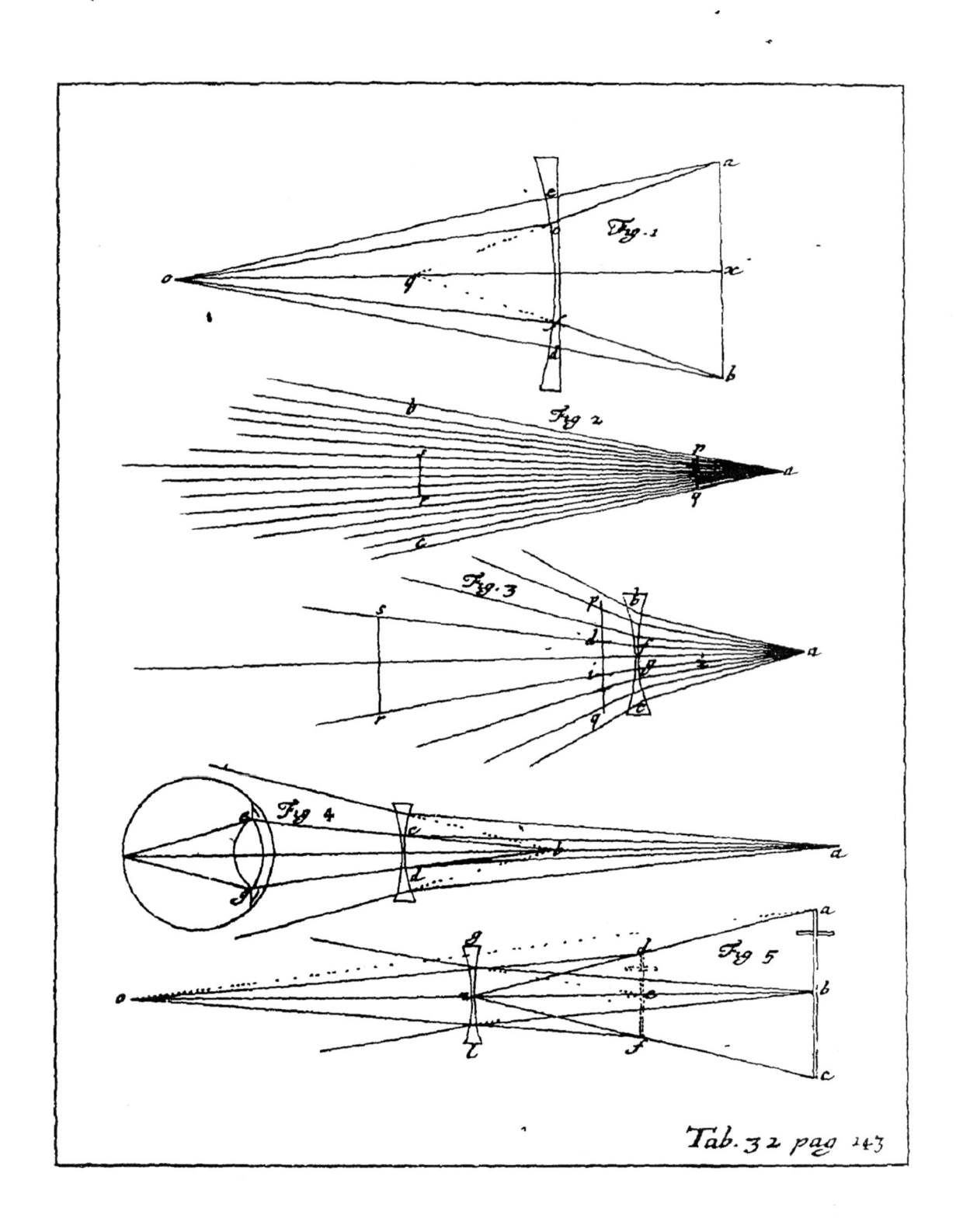

lection of the Rays proceeding from a single Point in the Object, into a single Point in the Representation; but Concave-Glasses do not *unite*, but scatter and dissipate the Rays. 'Tis true indeed, a Convex-Glass may cause a Distinct Base, notwithstanding a Concave placed behind it or before it (as we see in *Prop.* XV. XVII, XVIII.), but then this Distinct Base proceeds not from the Concave, but from the Convex: For the Concave exerts its scattering power even in this Case; and it protracts the Uniting of the Rays to a greater Distance from the Convex, as is manifest from the fore-cited *Propositions*.

I say also, *The Appearance of Objects through Concaves is diminish'd. Tab.* 32. *Fig.* 1. *a x b* is an Object, *o* the Eye. Draw *a e o*, *b d o*, directly strait from the Extremities of the Object to the Eye. The Angle comprised by the direct Rays *a e o*, *b d o*, that is, the Angle *a o b* is the Natural Optick-Angle. Let now the Concave-Glass *c f* be interposed; here, because the Rays *a e*, *b d*, would naturally concurr at *o*, now the Concave-Glass is interposed, their Concourse shall be protracted beyond *o*; wherefore the Eye at *o* shall not perceive the Extremities *a*, *b*, of the Object through the Glass by the Rays *a e*, *b d*, but by some *other Rays*, and these *other* Rays must either fall *without* (that is farther from the Axis *o x*, than) *a e*, *b d*, or they must fall *within a e*, *b d* : But they cannot fall *without a e*, *b d*; for if *a e*, *b d*, themselves be made by the Glass to concurr beyond the Eye at *o*, much more shall the Concourse of any other Rays that fall *without a e*, *b d*, be protracted beyond *o*, and consequently they cannot convey the Appearance of the Extreme Points *a*, *b*, to the Eye at *o*. Wherefore it remains, that the Rays that do this, must fall *within a e*, *b d*. Let us suppose these Rays to be *a c*, *b f*, which in their Natural direct Course, would concur at *q*, but by the Refractive Power of the Concave, are bent and made to proceed in *c o*, *f o*, their Concourse being protracted till they arrive

at

T 32 F 1.

at the Eye in *o*. Here the *Optick-Angle* through the Glass is *c o f*, which is less than the Natural *Optick-Angle a o b*, and consequently the *Appearance of the Object is diminish'd*. Which was to be proved.

PROP. XLIV.

Concerning the Distinct and Confused Appearance of Objects through Concaves; as also of their Faint or Obscure Appearance.

We are here to remember what before is laid down, concerning the *Virtual Focus* of a Concave exposed to *Parallel* or to *Diverging* Rays (in *Prop.* XI, XII, XIII. *& Corol. Prop.* XV.) We are likewise to take notice, that in Plain Vision, when the Rays from any single Point in an Object do not Diverge more than what the Refractive Power of the Coats and Humors of the Eye can correct; so that these Rays may be brought together in a Correspondent Point on the *Retina*; then the Appearance of that Point is *Distinct*. For instance, *Tab.* 32. F. 2 Let the Point *a* diffuse the Rays *a b*, *a s*, *a r*, *a c*. Suppose the Breadth of the Pupil were *p q*, and the Eye there placed, perhaps the Refractive Power of the Eye is not sufficient to correct the Divergence of the Rays *a p b*, *a q c* But if the Pupil (continuing of the same Breadth) recede to *r s*, then only the Rays *a s*, *a r*, fall into it; and these perhaps may be reduced by the Eye to determine in a Point on the *Retina*, because they do not Diverge *so much* as the former If therefore we suppose the Pupil in its former station at *p q*, but now only to be of the Breadth *t d*, so as to admit only the Rays *a d s*, *a t r*, then the Point *a* may be seen as distinctly as at *r s* This is manifest even by Experiment, for apply a Minute Object so near the Eye, that it appears very *confused*; then place before the Eye a very small Hole made with

[145]

a Pins end in a Paper; The Object shall now appear *Distinct*. For the Hole in the Paper serves to make the Pupil more *Narrow*. Which evidently proves what we have laid down.

The same may be shewn concerning Vision through a Concave Glass *Tab.* 32. *f.* 3. *a* is a Radiating Point, whose Rays *a b*, *a c*, fall on the Concave *b c*. These after passing the Glass Diverge more than before. Let *p q* be the Breadth of the Pupil, receiving the refracted Rays *a p*, *a q*, These Diverge *so much*, that 'tis not in the power of the Eye to reduce them, and form them into an inward Cone, determining its *Apex* on the Fund of the Eye. But let the Pupil continue of the same Breadth, and recede to *r s*, where it may only receive the Rays *a d s*, *a t r*; and then perhaps the Eye may prevail to reduce these; because they do not Diverge *so much* as the other Rays that fell on the Pupil at *p q*. Or otherwise, let the Pupil continue at *p q*, But let its Breadth be contracted to *d t*; so that it may receive no more Rays in this Posture, than (continuing of its natural Breadth) at *r s*. Here likewise the Appearance of the Point *a* may be *Distinct*. Of this likewise we may make a most convincing Experiment: For take a Concave of a small Sphere, and place it very near the Eye, and the Appearance of distant Objects through it is *Confused*. Remove it farther from the Eye, and the Appearance shall be more *Distinct*. But even in a Posture where the Appearance is *Confused*, contract the Pupil by placing before it a small Hole prick'd in a Paper, And the Object shall appear *more Distinct*, though *Obscure*, which upon the removal of the Hole, shall be again *Confused*, though more *Lightsome*. *Vid. Kepleri Dioptr. Prop.* C.

Wherefore if we have the Distance of a Radiating Point from a Concave, and the virtual *Focus* of the Concave, and the Distance of the Eye behind the Glass; we may easily by the foregoing Rules (*viz. Corol. Prop.* XV.) find the virtual *Focus* of these Rays. As suppose in the same *Fig.* the Rays flowing from *a*, after paſſing the Glaſs, Diverge as if they came directly from *z*. And conſequently, if in Plain Viſion the Eye at *r s* be able to ſee diſtinctly the Point *a*, if it were removed nigher, as at *z*, then it ſhall be able to ſee the Point *a* diſtinctly through the Glaſs. But whether any Particular Eye be able to do this, is impoſſible to be known by Rule; The *Strength* and *Weakneſs* of Mens Eyes being *infinitely various*. And therefore one Man may ſee a Point at a certain Diſtance *diſtinctly* through a Glaſs, which Glaſs to another Man would render it *Confuſed*; As 'tis Plain in the Caſe of *Myopes*, or *Short-ſighted* Perſons.

As to the *Strong* or *Faint* Appearance of Objects through Concaves; Becauſe the Concave (*Tab.* 32. *f.* 3.) ſcatters the Rays flowing from the Point *a*, inſomuch that now the Rays *a b*, *a c*, ſcape the Pupil *p q*, the Point *a* ſhall appear *more Faint* through the Glaſs than naturally. For *Strong* or very *Luminous* Viſion proceeds from a *greater* Quantity of Rays or Light entring the Pupil; And *Faint* or *Obſure* Viſion from a *leſs* Quantity of Rays.

T.32 F3

Scholium.

We may here conſider the *different* Effects of Convex and Concave Glaſſes. For when a Point appears *Confuſed* through a Convex, 'tis by Reaſon of the *Too great Convergence* of the Rays that fall on the Eye. And therefore, Becauſe the farther from the Glaſs towards the Point of Concourſe the Rays that fall on the Eye Converge the *more*, the Appearance is through *Them* ſtill the *more Confuſed*.

But in Concaves; Becauſe the *Confuſed* Appearance of a Point proceeds from the *Too great Divergence* of thoſe Rays that fall on the Eye; and becauſe the farther the Eye is from the Glaſs, the Rays that fall on the Eye Diverge *leſs* than thoſe that fell upon it when it was nigher the Glaſs; Therefore through Concaves,

caves, the *farther* the Eye is from the Glass, the *more Distinct* is the Appearance, but still *more Faint.*

PROB. XLV.

Concerning the Apparent Place of Objects seen through Concave Glasses.

Tab. 32. *f.* 4. If the Point *a* Radiate on the Concave Glass *c d*, and the Rays after passing the Glass Diverge as if they came directly from the Point *b*. And the Eye *e g* receive all or part of the Rays, and thereby perceive the Radiating Point *a*, the Point *b* is the *Locus Apparens* of the Point *a*. That is, the Point *a* is seen by the Eye, as if it were at *b*.

By which we may Observe, that the *Apparent Place* of Objects seen through Concaves is brought *nigher* the Eye. And hence 'tis manifest, why they help their Eyes, who are short-sighted, or can only see *nigh* Objects. For these Glasses make *distant* Objects seem *nigh. Vid. Dechales Dioptr. Lib. 2. Prop.* XXXIX.

Here also by the way we shall Note, That suppose a *Purblind* Person, that can Read distinctly or see Objects at the distance of a Foot from his naked Eye. A Concave Glass, whose virtual *Focus* is a Foot distant from it, makes such a Person see *distant* Objects *distinctly*. Wherefore knowing the Distance at which a *Purblind* Person Reads distinctly, 'tis easie to assign him a proper Glass for his Eye, to see distant Objects. *Vid. second Part C.* 3.

Tab 32 *f.* 5. Is in all things Correspondent to the Doctrine laid down in *Prop.* XXXI. *Sec.* 7. and marked with the same Letters; so that the very Words of that Section may be applied to the Concave, as well as to the Convex. Only the *Imaginary* Focus *e* for the Concave is to be determin'd by *Prop.* XI, XII, XIII. XV. and *Corol. Prop* XV. &c I shall not therefore Repeat, but refer to that Section.

Prop. XLVI. Probl.

To determine the visible Area, and the Optick Angle or Apparent Magnitude of an Object seen through a Concave from these Data, The Power or Focal Length of the Glass; The Distance of the Object from the Glass; The Distance of the Eye from the Glass, and the Breadth of the Glass.

T 33. F 1.   *Tab.* 33. *f.* 1. *g z l* is a Concave Glass, whose virtual *Focus* is given. Likewise *g z* the half Breadth of the Glass is given also. *a b c* is an Object, whose Distance from the Glass *b z* is given. And the Distance of the Eye *o* from the Glass, *o z*, is also given.

Let us now conceive the Point *o* an Object or *nigh Radiating* Point, sending its Rays *o g*, *o z*, *o l*, on the Concave Glass; These (by the foregoing Doctrine of Concaves) after passing the Glass *Diverge* more than before their Entrance, and proceed in *g a*, *l c*, as if they came *directly* from a certain Point *f* This Point *f* or the Line *f z*, is easily determin'd by *Prop.* XI, XII, XIII. XV. and *Corol.* thereof. Wherefore having *f z*, we may say, As $fz : zg :: fb \ (= fz + zb) \ ba$. Which is half the *Visible Area*.

As to the Optick Angle through the Glass, *g o z*, 'tis easily obtain'd in the right-angled Triangle *g o z*, having *g z* and *z o*.

Draw *a o* directly, The Angle *a o b* is the natural Optick Angle, under which the Object would appear to the Eye, were the Glass removed; This we obtain in the right-angled Triangle *a b o* by having *a b* and $bo = bz + zo$.

Scholium 1.

If instead of the Glasses Breadth, we have given the Breadth
T 33 F 2. of the Object *a b c* (*Tab.* 33. *f.* 2.) We may easily determine
the

Tab 33 pag. 148

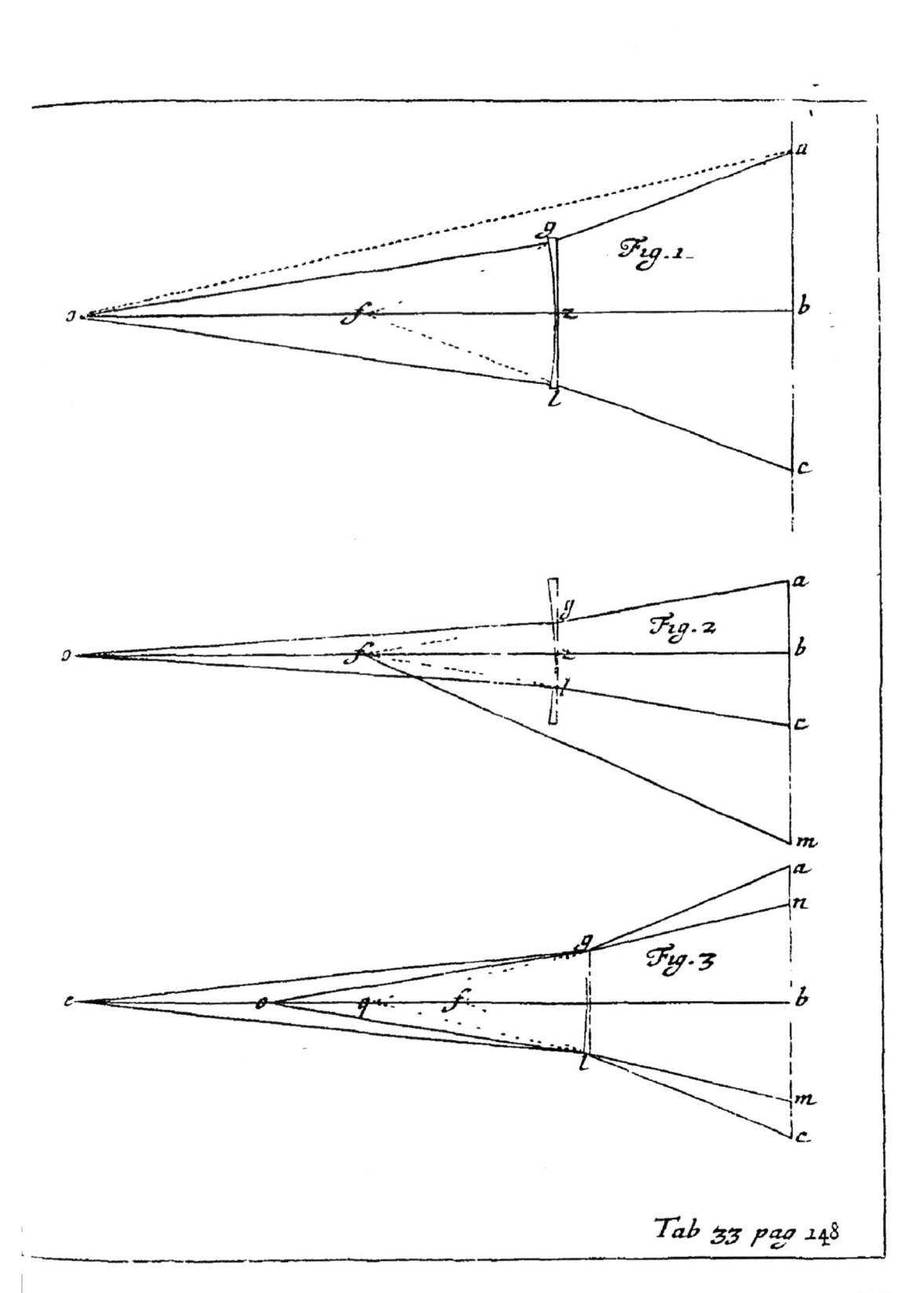

[149]

the Portion of the Glaſs through which this Object is ſeen. For from the Point f, draw fa, fc, Theſe Interſect the Glaſs in gl, I ſay gl is the Portion of the Glaſs, through which the Object ac is viſible.

And if the Line fm being drawn do not fall on the Glaſs, the Point m in the Object is not viſible through the Glaſs to the Eye at o.

Scholium 2.

The foregoing Problem, as it relates to the Optick Angle, may be ſolved another way by determining the *Locus Objecti*. But then to the former *Data*, inſtead of the *Breadth of the Glaſs*, we cannot add the *Breadth of the Object*.

This is Evident from *Tab* 32 f. 5. To which we may apply the Words of the Second *Scholium*, *Prop*. XLII. without further Repetition   T 32 F 5

Example of a Calculation according to *Prop*. XLVI. apply'd to *Tab*. 33. f 1.   T 33 F 1

```
Focus of the Glaſs    = — — — 4573.      ⎫
½ Breadth of the Glaſs = gz = 500         ⎬ Data.
Diſtance of the Object = bz = 10000       ⎪
Diſtance of the Eye   = zo = 20000        ⎭
    Half the Viſible Area = ab = ?        ⎫ Quæſit.
    Half Optick Angle  = goz = ?          ⎭
```

Firſt by *Corol. Prop.* XV. $zo +$ Fo. Glaſs : zo ∷ Fo. Gl : zf
That is in Numbers — — 24573 : 20000 ∷ 4573 . 3722.
Then — — — — $zf : gz ∷ bf (= bz + zf) : ab$
That is in Numbers — — — 3722 : 500 ∷ 13722 . 1843.

Laſtly in the right-angled Triangle goz, as zo : Rad ∷ gz : Tang. $\angle goz = 1° \ 25' \ 50''$.

Example Calculated according to the Method Propos'd in this Second *Schol. Prop.* XLVI. but the Letters refer to *Tab*. 32.   T 32 F 5
f 5.

Focus

[150]

$$\left.\begin{array}{l}\text{Focus of the Glass} = \text{———} = 4573. \\ \text{Distance of the Object} = bz = \text{———} 10000 \\ \text{Distance of the Eye} = zo = \text{———} 20000 \\ \text{Half Breadth of the Object as} \\ \text{Found in the foregoing Example} = ab = 1843\end{array}\right\} Data.$$

First by *Corol. Prop.* XV. $bz +$ Gl. Focus $: bz ::$ Gl. Fo $: ze$
That is in Numbers   14573 : 10000 : 4573 3138
Then ——————————— $zb : ba :: ze : ed$
That is in Numbers —— 10000 : 1843 . : 3138 · 578.

Lastly in the right-angled Triangle deo, as oe ($= oz + ze = 23138$) : Rad $:: ed$: Tang. $\angle doe = 1° 25' 50''$. agreeable to what was found by the immediately preceding Calculation.

I shall now shew, how by this Method of Demonstrating the Properties, Effects, and Appearances of Glasses, Some of the noted Propositions in Dioptrick Writers may be easily proved. In which the Authors have been very *Operose*, and in some very *Obscure*. And because I will not interrupt the Series of my Propositions, I shall give them in the following Order.

PROP. XLVII.

The further the Eye is removed from the Concave Glass, the Object appears the less. Zahn Telescop Fund. 2. Synt. 2. Cap. 5. Prop. *XXIII.* Dechales Dioptr. Lib. 2. Prop. *LII.*

T 32 F 5   This is manifest from *Tab.* 32. *f.* 5. For we are to Consider the Image def, in the virtual Focus, as the Object, and as look'd at without the Glass. For the Lines do, fo, which determine the Optick Angle, are drawn directly to the Eye at o. Wherefore if we conceive the Eye o removed farther from the Glass, the Angle dof must needs decrease, and consequently the Object appear *less*. What is here said of the Concave may be ap-
T 31 F 3 ply'd to the Convex in *Tab.* 31. *f.* 3.

PROP

[151]

Prop. XLVIII.

If a Concave Glass be removed from the Eye, so large an Area or space of the Object cannot be seen through it.

This is the 97th Prop. of *Kepler's Dioptricks*. Wherein he seems to make no Distinction between *removing the Glass from the Eye, and removing the Eye from the Glass*. Whereas there is a very great Difference between both Motions to be consider'd in *Dioptricks*. For in *moving the Glass from the Eye*, the Glass Approaches the Object, and the *Locus Apparens Objecti* is changed. But in *moving the Eye to or from the Glass*, the *Locus Apparens Objecti* never alters. *Prop.* XXXI. *Sec.* 7. And from his Proof of this Proposition 'tis manifest, that he should have expressed it thus,

If the Eye be removed from a Concave, so large a space of the Object cannot be seen through it.

Wherefore instead of the foregoing 48th. Proposition, I substitute this; Which is Evident by our foregoing Method from *Tab* 33. *f.* 3. Wherein *a b c* is an Object, *g l* a Concave Glass, *o* the Eye *nigh* the Glass, *e* the Eye *more Distant* from the Glass. Let the Point of Divergence, answering to the Station at *o*, be *f* (determin'd by the foregoing Doctrine): draw *f g a*, *f l c*, directly; the space visible at *o* is *a c*. Now, when the Eye is removed *from* the Glass to *e*, the Point of Divergence shall also be removed from the Glass, and determin'd by what foregoes, as suppose at *q* (till the Eye be at an infinite Distance, and then the Point of Divergence is as far from the Glass as 'tis possible, *viz* in the virtual Focus): draw *q g n*, *q l m*, directly; The space visible at *e* is *n m* less than *a c*. Which was to be Demonstrated.

T33 F3.

Or otherwise. *Tab.* 34. *f.* 1. *d e f* is the *Locus Apparens Object* *a b c* through the Glass *g l*, the Eye is at *o*, *o g*, *o l* produced directly meet the Image in the Points *d*, *f*. Wherefore exactly the whole Object *a b c*, and no more, is seen through the Glass *g l* by the Eye at *o*. Let the Eye be removed to *q*, If we draw *q d*, *q f*, these fall not on the Glass, and consequently the Extremities of the Object *a* and *c* shall not be perceived by the Eye at *q* through the Glass. (*Schol.* 1. *Prop.* XLVI.) Draw therefore *q g*, *q l*, and produce them directly to *n* and *m*, the Points in the Object *y x*, answerable to the Points *n*, *m*, are the *utmost Extremities* visible through the Glass *g l* to the Eye at *q* Which Points *y*, *x*, are easily determinable by what is laid down *Prop.* XL. *Sec.* 3. For from the Center of the Glass *z*, draw *z n y*, *z m x*, directly; *y*, *x*, are hereby determin'd.

As to this 48*th.* Prop. *viz. That if a Concave Glass be removed from the Eye, so large an Area or space of the Object cannot be seen through it.* 'Tis needless to enlarge thereon, after our 46*th.* Prop.

Prop. XLIX.

The farther a Concave Glass is removed from the Eye, The Objects are thereby the more diminish'd, as long as the Glass continues nigher to the Eye than to the Object.

This is the 98*th.* Prop. of *Kepler's Dioptricks*. We may find it also, In *Cherubin's La Dioptrique Oculaire* pag. 77. *Dechales Dioptrica* Lib. 2. Prop. *XXXVIII. Herigonii Dioptr.* Prop. *XXXI.* But in all of them obscurely and loosely proved.

The Proposition is universally True, as well in Convex as Concave Glasses, only with this Restriction in the Convex, *That the Object is to be nigher the Glass, than the Glasses Focal Length.* And then we may express the Proposition universally thus,

Tab 34 pag. 157.

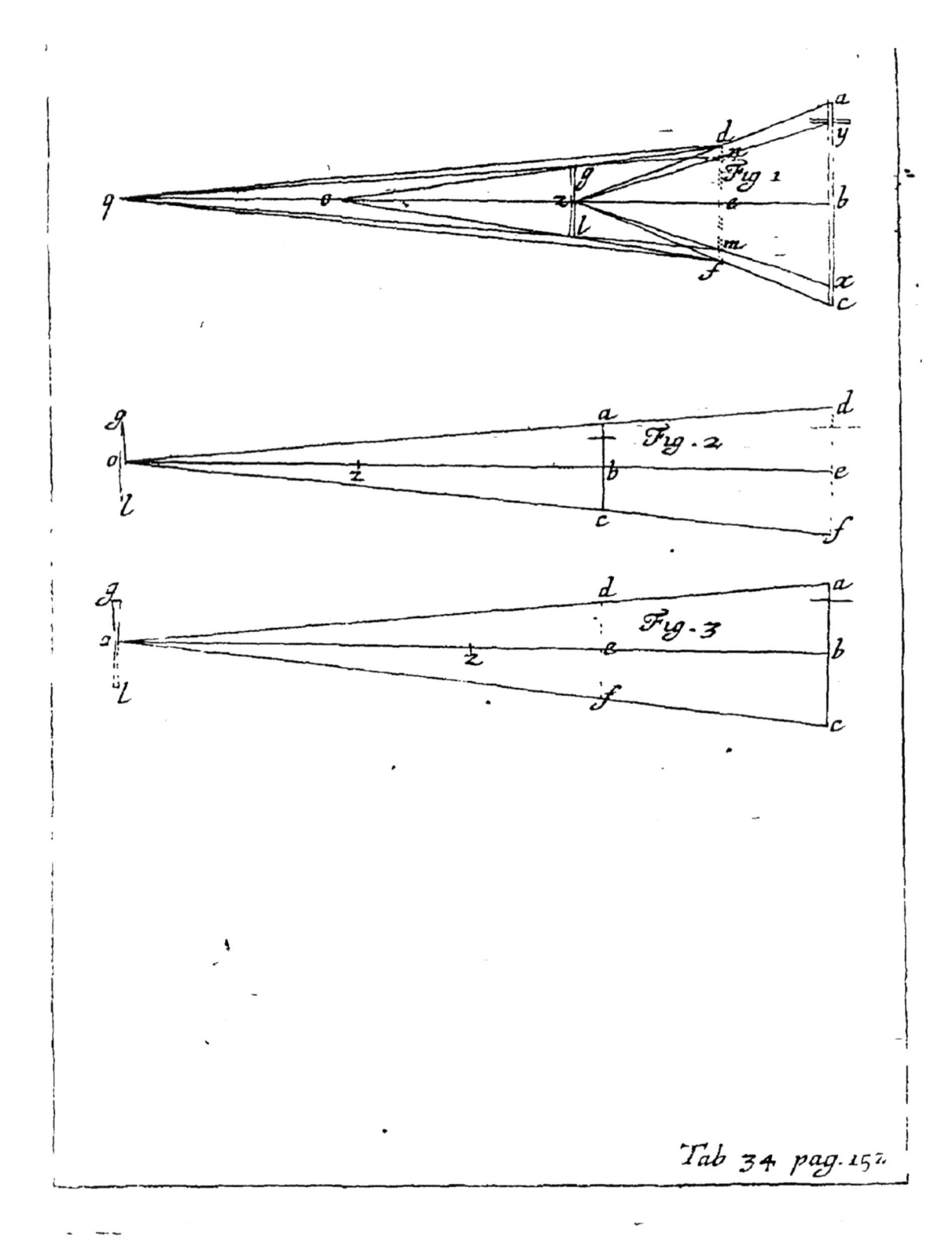

[153]

A Convex-Glass being equally Distant from the Eye and from the Object, renders the Appearance the most Magnified; and a Concave the most Diminished, that That Distance of Eye and Object will allow.

For the Proof hereof I need offer no more than the following Calculations (instituted according to the Doctrine Precedent) wherein we shall find (*Tab* 31. *f.* 3. and *Tab.* 32. *f.* 5.) the Angle *d o e*, (which is the Angle under which the Object appears through the Glass) in the second Case (wherein the Glass is equally Distant from the Eye and Object) to be *greater* for the *Convex*, and *less* for the *Concave*, than the same Angle in either of the other Cases. T 31. F 3
T 32. F 5

And by the same Calculations we may likewise observe in the first and third Cases, That when the Glass is *equally* removed from the *middle* towards the Eye, or towards the Object, the Appearance is *equally* magnified by the Convex, and diminish'd by the Concave; for we find in the first and third Cases, the Angles *d o e* equal.

I say, this may be sufficient for the Proof of the foregoing Position. But to this I shall add also this farther Consideration. That by the preceding Doctrine, the magnify'd Appearances of Objects through Convexes, and their diminish'd Appearances through Concaves, being deduced from the *Loci Apparentes* of Objects through those Glasses. We may easily conceive, That supposing the Convex-Glass *g l* (*Tab.* 34. *f.* 2.) or Concave *g l* (*Tab.* 34. *f.* 3.) to touch the Eye *o*, and that the Apparent Place of the Object *a b c* is *d e f*. The Eye perceives the Object under its own Natural Optick-Angle, neither magnify'd or diminish'd by one or t'other Glass. T 34 F 2
T 34 F 3.

Likewise if, in the same Figures, we conceive the Glasses (which are still supposed of the least thickness imaginable) to touch the Objects, the Object and *Locus Apparens* thereof are the *same*, and consequently, the Optick-Angle in this Posture can neither be *increased or diminish'd* by either of the Glasses.

X

Where-

[154]

Wherefore it remains, that seeing the Glasses do *not at all* Exert their Effects in either of the *Extremes*, that is, *either touching the Eye, or touching the Object*. And seeing they Exert their Effects *equally* being *equally* removed from the middle z between the Eye and the Object, It will follow, that they Exert their Effects *most powerfully* being placed just in the middle z between the Eye and Object, that is, the Convex by *Magnifying*, and the Concave by *Diminishing* the Appearance.

And thus much shall suffice concerning *single Glasses* apply'd to the *Eye*.

Here follow the Calculations.

T 31 F 3

Calculation for the CONVEX Tab. 31. F. 3.

Focus of the Glass = 10,000 ⎱ Given the same
Breadth of the Object = ab = 1,000 ⎰ in all the Cases.

First Case.	Second Case.	Third Case.
Wherein the Distance between the Eye and the Glass oz is given greater than the Distance between the Object and Glass bz	Wherein the Glass is equally distant from the Eye and Object, that is, $bz = oz$	Wherein the Distance between the Eye and the Glass oz is given less than the Distance between the Object and the Glass bz
Data $\begin{cases} bz = 3,000 \\ oz = 9,000 \end{cases}$	Data $\begin{cases} bz = 6,000 \\ oz = 6,000 \end{cases}$	Data $\begin{cases} bz = 9,000 \\ oz = 3,000 \end{cases}$
$ze = 4,286$ $ed = 1,429$	$ze = 15,000$ $ed = 2,500$	$ze = 90,000$ $ed = 10,000$
$oe = oz + ze = 13,286$ $\angle doe = 6° 8' 15''$	$oe = oz + ze = 21,000$ $\angle doe = 6° 47' 0''$	$oe = oz + ze = 93,00$ $\angle doe = 6° 8' 15''$

Calculation

[155]

Calculation for the CONCAVE Tab. 32. F. 5.		
Focus of the Glass = 10,000 Given the same		
Breadth of the Object = ab = 1,000 in all the Cases		

First Case.	*Second Case.*	*Third Case.*
Wherein the Distance between the Eye and the Glass oz is given greater than the Distance between the Object and the Glass bz.	Wherein the Glass is equally Distant from the Eye and Object, that is, $bz = zo$	Wherein the Distance between the Eye and the Glass oz is given less than the Distance between the Object and Glass bz.
Data $\begin{cases} bz = 3,000 \\ oz = 9,000 \end{cases}$	Data $\begin{cases} bz = 6,000 \\ oz = 6,000 \end{cases}$	Data $\begin{cases} bz = 9,000 \\ oz = 3,000 \end{cases}$
$ze = 2,308$ $ed = 0,769$	$ze = 3,750$ $ed = 0,625$	$ze = 4,737$ $ed = 0,526$
$oe = oz + ze = 11,308$ $L. doe = 3° 53' 20''$	$oe = oz + ze = 9,750$ $doe = 3° 40' 0''$	$oe = oz + ze = 7,737$ $L. doe = 3° 53' 20''$

Hitherto we have Treated of *single* Convexes and Concaves, apply'd to the Eye. I proceed now to the *Combination* of Convexes with Convexes, and Convexes with Concaves; Wherein the Properties, Effects, and Appearances of *Telescopes*, and *Microscopes*, of all kinds shall be declared.

Definitions.

The *Object-Glass* is the Glass next the Object.

The *Eye Glass*, simply so called, is the Glass *immediately* next the Eye. But if there be more than one, the *first Eye-Glass* is that *next* the Object-Glass; the *second* is that *next the first*, &c.

Prop. L.

The Telescope, consisting of a Convex Object-Glass and a Convex Eye-Glass of a less Sphere or greater Convexity, is explained.

T 35. F 1. *Tab.* 35 *f* 1. Let there be a Distant Object such as *A B C*; From whose *highest* Point *A* let the Rays *a a a*, mark'd by the long Pricks, proceed. And from the *middle* Point *B*, let the Rays expressed by the continued Lines *b b b*, proceed. And from it's *lower* Point *C*, the Rays mark'd by the round Pricks *c c c*. And so Rays from all the other Points in the Object. These falling on the Object-Glass *x y z*, are formed thereby into the Distinct Base *f e d*. Let now the Eye-Glass *g h l* be placed as far distant from this Distinct Base *f e d*, as is the Focus of this Eye-Glass, that is, Let *e h* be the Focal length of the Eye-Glass *g h l* (And consequently the Distance of the Glasses *y h* is the Aggregate of both their Focal lengths) And let the Eye *o* be placed as far distant (or rather a little more distant) from the Eye-Glass *g h l* as is the Focal length of the same Eye-Glass. I say the Eye shall perceive the Object *A B C, Distinct, Magnified,* and *Inverted*.

First, I say the Object is seen *distinctly*. For the Rays from each Point, being made by the Object-Glass to Converge towards the Distinct Base, proceed forward from the Distinct Base Diverging, and so fall on the Eye Glass. Thus the

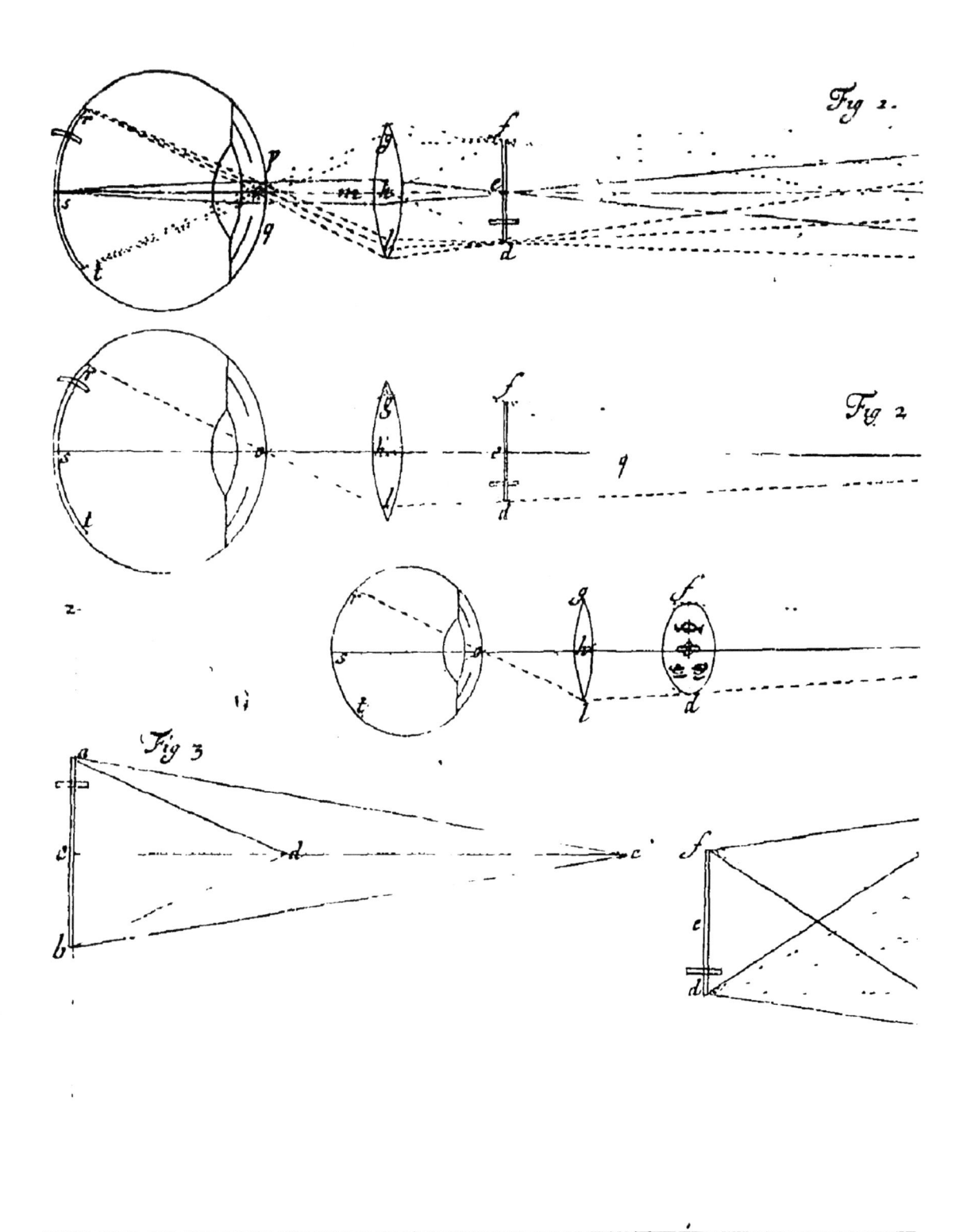

Fig. 1.

Fig. 2.

Fig. 3.

Fig 4.

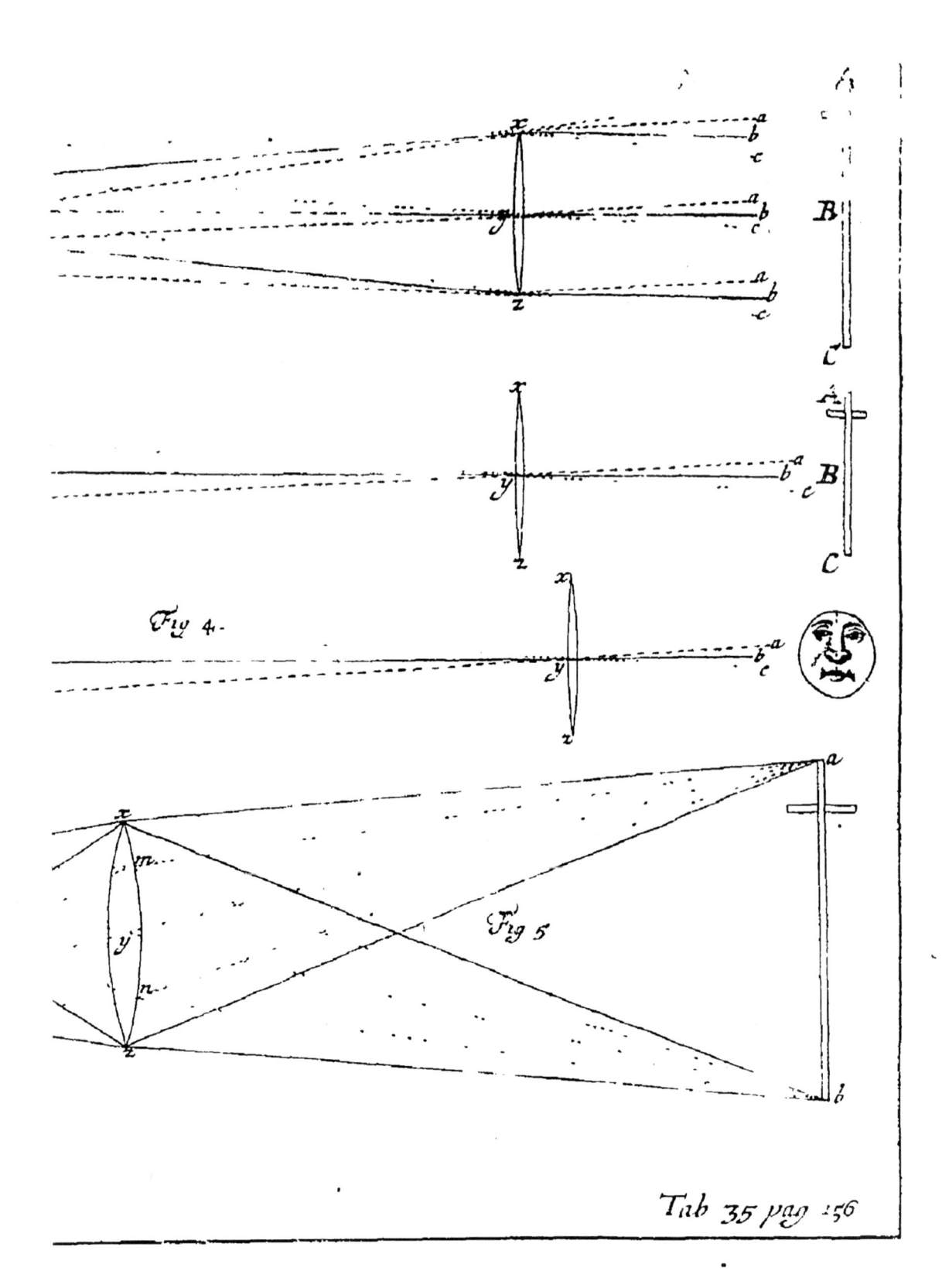

Tab 35 pag 156

Rays *b x*, *b y*, *b z*, from the middle Point of the Object *B*, are made to Converge into *x e*, *y e*, *z e*; And crossing at *e*, they flow forward, and fall on the Eye-Glass about *h* Diverging. Wherefore the Point *e* being now in the Focus of the Eye-Glass, the Rays that flow from it upon the Eye-Glass, after passing the Eye-Glass become parallel (*Prop.* VI.) and fall so on the Eye at *o*; By whose Coats and Humors they are refracted and brought together on the Point *s* on the *Retina* (*Prop.* XXVIII. *Sec.* 7.) there painting the lively Image of the Point *B* in the Object.

Secondly, In like manner may we conceive the Representation of the Collateral Points: thus the Rays *a x*, *a y*, *a z*, proceeding from the upper Point A of the Object, are by the Object-Glass *x y z* made to Converge towards the Distinct Base in *d*; From whence flowing forward they fall Diverging on the Eye-Glass at *l*; by which they are made to run parallel amongst themselves, and are bent towards the Focus at *o*, where falling on the Pupil parallel, they are by the Eye refracted and brought together in the Point *r* on the *Retina*. There painting the Representation of the Point A in the Object.

Thirdly, That the Rays flowing *Diverging* from each particular Point in the Distinct Base *f e d* are brought by the Eye-Glass to a *Parallelism* amongst themselves, is manifest from *Prop.* VI. And that the Rays from *f*, from *e*, and from *d*, are mixt and confused by the Eye-Glass in its Focus at *o* (or thereabouts) is manifest from hence, that we may conceive one Ray in the Cone of Rays *g f*, or in the Cone of Rays *z f x*, that runs parallel to the Axis *y e h o s*, or at least that would run so parallel, if the Breadth of the Object-Glass in respect of the Breadth of the Eye Glass will permit. This Ray, I say, by the known Properties of the Convex Eye-Glass, shall be refracted into its Focus at *o*, and all the other Rays of the same Cone *f g*, after passing the Eye Glass, shall

be

be refracted and made to proceed parallel to that single Ray, that is bent into the Focus *o*, because the Point *f* is supposed in t'other Focus of the Eye-Glass. Wherefore the Rays from all the Points in the Distinct Base are confounded together about the Focus of the Eye-Glass.

Fourthly, Or otherwise I shall explain this matter thus; If we conceive *y*, a Radiating Point, sending forth the Rays *y g*, *y h*, *y l*: And the difference between the Focal length of the Object-Glass and Focal length of the Eye-Glass to be very great (as suppose the Object-Glass to be twelve Foot, and the Eye-Glass three Inches) we shall find by *Prop.* V. the Point *o*, where the Rays *g o*, *l o*, cross the Axis or Perpendicular Ray *h o*, to be very nigh the Focus of the Eye-Glass (*viz.* in our Supposition *h o* shall be 3.063 Inches) and let the Focal lengths of the Object-Glass and Eye-Glass bear whatever Proportion, the Point *o*, where *g o*, *l o*, shall cross *h o*, may be determin'd by *Prop.* V. But then indeed the Rays that fall on the Eye *without* *g o*, or *within* it, do cross the Perpendicular Ray *h o*, *farther* from the Eye-Glass, or *nigher* to the Eye-Glass than *g o* it self, For they do not proceed from the same Point *y*; And *g o* is only the Refraction of the Ray *y g*. And therefore, unless the difference between the Focal lengths of the Object-Glass and Eye-Glass be *Considerable*, the Eye may move considerably *nigher* *to* the Eye-Glass, or *farther from* the Eye-Glass than the Point *o*, and not perceive any Alteration in the Appearance of the Object. But if the said Difference be *Considerable*, (as it always is in Telescopes) the Eye can move but very little either *farther from* or *nigher to* the Eye-Glass than *o*, but it shall perceive a great Alteration in the Appearance (that is, in the Visible Area) of the Object. As shall be manifested more plainly hereafter.

From all which it appears, That the Pupil of the Eye at *o*, being in the place of the *greatest Confusion*, where the Rays from

from all Points in the Object are mixt together, and the Rays from each single Point fall parallel amongst themselves; The Appearance of the Object must needs be *Distinct*. By *Prop.* XXVIII. *Sec.* 3.

Fifthly, I say likewise the Object is *magnified*. If the naked Eye were in the place of the Object-Glass at *y* (*Tab.* 35. *f.* 2.) the Object would appear to it under the Angle $ayc = fyd$. That is, the Object would appear to the Eye at *y*, under the same Angle as the Distinct Base *f e d*, were it an Object, would appear to the same Eye at *y*. Wherefore let us now consider the Distinct Base *f e d* as the Object. This appears to the Eye at *o* through the Eye Glass under the same Angle *g o l*, as were the naked Eye viewing it at *h*, by *Prop.* XXXIII. Make *e q* equal to *e h*, and draw *h f*, *h d*, and *q f*, *q d*. The Angle *f h d* by *Prop.* XXXIV. is equal to *g o l*, the Optick-Angle through the Telescope, and the same Angle *f h d* is equal to *f q d*. But *f q d* is much greater than *f y d* = *a y c* the Natural Optick-Angle to the Eye supposed at *y*. and yet much greater than the Natural Optick-Angle would be to the Eye at *o*. Because *o* is yet further from the outward real Object than *y* by the whole length of the Telescope. Wherefore the Object is *Magnified*.

Lastly, I say the Object appears *Inverted*. This is manifest from the very Scheme (*Tab.* 35. *f.* 1.) without farther Explication. For the Object is *Inverted* in the Distinct Base, and the Eye-Glass does not return it again before it arrive at the Eye, but is painted on the *Retina* r s t *Erect*; wherefore by *Prop.* XXVIII *Sec.* 4, 5. the Object appears Inverted. See also *Prop* XXXIX. *Sec.* 4, 5.

Scholium.

The *Locus Apparens* of an Object through this Glass is the Distinct Base *f e d* (*Prop.* XXXI.) as is manifest from this Ex-

Experiment. Stretch an Hair exactly in this Distinct Base, it shall appear as it were fixt to the very Object. *Vid. Chap.* 5. *Sec.* 3. of the Second Part.

PROP. LI. LEMMA.

If the Eye directly approach to or recede from an Object; it shall be, as the Tangent of the Semioptick-Angle of one Station: to the Tangent of the Semioptick-Angle of t'other Station:: So (reciprocally) the Distance of the Eye from the Object in this latter Station: to the Distance of the Eye from the Object in the Former Station.

T 32. F. 3. *Tab.* 35. *f.* 3. Let abc be an Object, from whose middle Point c erect ce Perpendicular to ab. Let the first Station of the Eye be at e, and its second Station at d; and draw ad, ae; I say therefore, As ce: to cd:: so Tangent of the Angle adc: to the Tangent of the Angle aec.

Demonstration.

Produce ca infinitely towards z, draw ez parallel to ad. The Angle zec is equal to the Angle adc (29. 1. *Eucl.*) then ec being put Radius, zc is the Tangent of the Angle $zec = adc$; And ac is the Tangent of the Angle aec. And it shall be, As ce: to cd:. so zc: to ac: (2. 6. *Eucl.*) which was to be Demonstrated.

This is the 31 *Prop.* of *Gregorii Opt. Promot.* but there otherwise Demonstrated.

PROP.

PROP. LII. LEMMA 2.

If the Eye directly approach to, or recede from an Object, its apparent Bigness increases or diminishes, as the Tangents of the Semioptick-Angles at one and t'other Station.

This is manifest, for the Eye at d (*Tab.* 35. *f.* 3.) sees ac as big as the Eye at e would see zc, by *Prop.* XXVIII. *Sec.* 6. Because the Angles adc, zec are equal; and *Quæ sub æquali Apparent Angulo, Æqualia videntur.* So that the Eye advancing from e to d, sees ac as much bigger, as if, continuing at e, the Object ac had increased to cz.

Corollary.

From this and the last Proposition it follows, that if the Eye directly approach to or recede from an Object, its apparent Magnitude increases or diminisheth, as the Distances of one and t'other Station reciprocally, that is, the apparent Magnitude of ac to the Eye at d: is to the apparent Magnitude of ac to the Eye at e :: as ce : to cd.

PROP. LIII.

The apparent Diametral Magnitude of an Object viewed through the Telescope of Prop. L. Is to the apparent Diametral Magnitude of the Object viewed by the naked Eye at the Station of the Object-Glass :: *As the Focal length of the Object-Glass* : *to the Focal length of the Eye-Glass.*

This is the *great Proposition asserted* by most Dioptrick Writers, but hitherto *proved* by none (for as much as I know)

[162]

they offer indeed Experiments and Methods of Tryal to confirm the Truth thereof, but proceed no farther.

Vid. *Cherubin Diop. Oculaire Part. II. Prop. XXI. LIX. LX. LXII. Kepleri Dioptr. Prop. CXXIV. Galilei Nuncius Sidereus pag.* 12. *Edit Lond.* 1653. 8*vo.*

Honoratus Faber in his *Synopsis Optica Prop. XLIV.* for the Telescope consisting of a Convex Object Glass and Concave Eye-Glass; and in *Prop XLV.* for the Telescope consisting of a Convex Object Glass and Convex Eye-Glass, indeavours at something, which he calls a *Demonstration* of this Property. But whether that which he there offers will amount to clear Satisfaction, I leave to their Judgments, who shall Read him.

Dechales in *Prop* LIV. *Lib. II. Dioptr.* thinks this Proposition so far from *Demonstrable*, that he takes it to be *False*; and says, He never met with any Demonstration thereof, that did not include manifest *Paralogisms.* Perhaps he may be right in this latter part of his Assertion; but the Reason he gives for his concluding it a False Proposition is manifestly Weak and Erroneous: And that on the account of an inartificial kind of Notion and Method, that he takes for Explicating the Magnifying of Telescopes; especially of the *Telescope* furnish'd with a Concave Eye-Glass, which he explains after his manner in *Prop.* LIII.

It were needless to inlarge in this matter, I shall therefore pass it over, and hasten to the *Demonstration* of this *Proposition.*

T 35 F 2. *Tab.* 35. *f.* 2. Let the Object-Glass xyz Project the Image of the Object ABC in the Distinct Base fed, ghl is the Eye-Glass, he the Focal length of the Eye-Glass, to which let eq be made equal. Draw hf, hd, and qf, qd. And let the Eye at o be placed in the Exteriour Focus of the Eye-Glass. The Rays yfg, ydl, are refracted by the Eye-Glass, and cross at o. Wherefore gol is the Angle under which the Object appears through the Telescope. But the Angle gol is equal to the

the Angle fhd (as well by what foregoes in *Prop.* L. *Sec.* 3. & 5. as by *Prop.* XXXIV.) And the Angle fhd is equal to the Angle fqd.

Wherefore were the naked Eye at y the Station of the Object-Glass, it would perceive the Object under the Angle $fyd = ayc$. But now being armed with the Telescope, it sees the Object under the Angle fqd. Let us take their halfs fye, fqe; and consider fe, half the Distinct Base, as the Object viewed by the naked Eye at the Stations y and q. I say (by *Lemma* 2.) The apparent bigness of the Object fe at the Station q: Is to its apparent bigness at the Station y :: As the Tangent of the Angle fqe: To the Tangent of the Angle fye. But (by *Lemma* 1.) the Tangent of the Angle fqe: Is to the Tangent of the Angle fye :: As ey: To eq. Therefore the apparent bigness of the Object fe at the Station q: Is to its apparent bigness at the Station y :: As ey: To eq: that is, As the Focal length of the Object-Glass: To the Focal length of the Eye-Glass. But the Angle goh, under which the Eye sees half the Object through the Telescope, is equal to the Angle fhe or fqe. Therefore the apparent Diametral bigness of an Object viewed through a Telescope: Is to the apparent Diametral Magnitude of the Object viewed by the naked Eye at the Station of the Object-Glass :: As the Focal length of the Object-Glass: To the Focal length of the Eye-Glass. Which was to be *Demonstrated*.

The same may be declared otherwise. Thus, *Tab.* 35. *f.* 2. Let us suppose the naked Eye at h to view the Object Inverted by means of the Distinct Base fed; The Inverted Object shall appear under the Angle fhd (by *Prop.* XL.) But the Eye at o through the Glass perceives the Inverted Image of the Object under the Angle gol equal to fhd, (by *Prop.* XXXIII.) and fhd is equal to fqd, and consequently (as in the foregoing Demonstration) the Proposition is manifest.

I shall now mention the common Method for trying the Truth of this Proposition by Experiment. Having the Focal length of an Object Glass (for Instance) 144 Inches, and the Focal length of an Eye-Glass three Inches. A Telescope composed of these, shall make the apparent Diametral Magnitude of an Object: To the apparent Magnitude of the same Object viewed by the naked Eye :: As 144: To 3 :: or 48 : To 1. Wherefore, such a Glass is said to Magnifie 48 times in the Diameter of the Object, and 2304 (= square of 48) in the Surface of the Object. The Superficies of like Figures being to each other, as the Squares of their Diameters, or Homologous Sides.

Wherefore from a convenient Scale take one part, and therewith describe a Circle, And from the same Scale take 48 parts, and describe another Circle. Let these two Circles be cut out in Paper, or other Conspicuous Material, and placed at three or four Foot from each other, on a Wall at such a Distance as will require the length between the Glasses in the Telescope but just 147 (= 144 + 3) Inches, to shew these Objects distinctly; Then with one Eye through the Telescope observe the smaller Circle, and at the same time with t'other Eye naked look upon the greater Circle; these two Circles shall appear equal to both Eyes.

Perhaps it may be objected, That the Comparison is not fair between both Appearances. For the Proposition supposes the naked Eye at the Station of the Object-Glass; But this Experiment sets the naked Eye Distant from the Object-Glass the whole length of the Telescope. This would be a material Objection against this Method of Tryal, were not the Distance of the two Circles from the Eyes vastly greater than the length of the Telescope, so that the Telescopes length may not bear any sensible Proportion thereto. And such we suppose it in this Experiment, by advertising that this Distance is

to

to be so great, that the Distance between the Glasses may be no longer than for viewing a Distant Object, *viz.* the just Aggregate of the Focal lengths of the Glasses, that is, 144 + 3 = 147 Inches, that is, $ye + eh = yh$.

I shall now give an Example of a Calculation according to this Proposition. Wherefore in *Tab.* 35. *f.* 4. let us take the Moon ABC for our Distant Object, and let us suppose its Diameter to subtend an Arch of a great Circle of Heaven of 30′ Minutes. Let the Ray ayd proceed from its upper Limb, bye from its Centre, cyf from its lower Limb. These cross in the Vertex y, or middle Point of the Object-Glass xyz, making the Angle $fyd = aye$, equal to 30′ Minutes. Let the Focal length of the Object-Glass ey be given twelve Feet = 144 Inches, or 144,00 Parts: And the Focus of the Eye-Glass he be given three Inches, or 3,00 such Parts. Let the Distinct Base, wherein the Image of the Moon is Projected by the Object-Glass be fed, and draw fh, dh. It is shewn before that the Angle goh is equal to the Angle fhe.

Wherefore in the Right-angled Triangle fey, we have ey = 144,00, and the Angle $fye = 15′$, to find $fe = 0,63$.

Then in the Right-angled Triangle feh, we have $he = 3,00$, and $fe = 0,63$, to find the Angle $fhe = 11° 51′ 40″$.

Wherefore the Semidiameter of the Moon, which by the naked Eye would be seen under the Angle of 15′ Minutes, is seen through this Telescope under an Angle of 11° 51′ 40″.

Let us now enquire, whether the Object appearing under an Angle of 15′ Minutes, and being afterwards made to appear under an Angle of 11° 51′ 40″, doth not thereby appear 48 times bigger than naturally. (for so much, by what foregoes, does this Glass Magnifie).

And for shewing this, let us imagine fe increased 48 times its length 0,63, And then inquire what Angle fye would be. Wherefore fe is now supposed = 30,24 = 48 times 0,63; Then in the Right-angled Triangle fey, we have $fe = 30.24$, and $ey = 144.00$, to find the Angle $fye = 11° 51' 40''$. Which shews that the Semidiameter of the Moon, being made by the Glass to appear under an Angle of $11° 51' 40''$, is seen by the Eye as big, as if the Semidiameter of the Moon it self were really increased 48 times, and viewed by the naked Eye. Which is the proposed Design of this Calculation.

Corollary 1.

From hence it follows, That the same Object-Glass being at one time combined with an Eye-Glass whose Focus is 1. And at another time with an Eye-Glass whose Focus is 2. The first Telescope Magnifies twice as much as the latter.

Corollary 2.

Supposing two Telescopes of different lengths; If the Focus of the Eye-Glass of the shorter bears the same Proportion to the Focus of its Object-Glass, as the Focus of the Eye-Glass of the longer bears to its Object-Glass: These two Telescopes Magnifie *equally*.

And hereupon perhaps it may be enquired, To what end then is all the Pains and Trouble in forming and managing Telescopes of 30. 40. 50. 100. 200. 300, &c. Feet; When Objects may be Magnified as much by smaller Object-Glasses, or Object-Glasses of shorter Focal lengths, combined with Proportional Eye-Glases?

I answer First, That Object-Glasses of a shorter Focus will not bear proportionably Eye-Glasses of such short *Foci*, without coloring the Object and rendring it dark, as Object-Glasses of longer *Foci*. For Instance, let us suppose that an excellent Object-Glass of twelve Foot Focus will receive an Eye-Glass

Glass of no shorter a Focus than three Inches with Clearness and Distinctness. I say an Object Glass of 24 Foot Focus of the same Perfection shall receive an Eye-Glass of less than six Inches Focus with equal Clearness and Distinctness. And perhaps it may take an Eye-Glass of five or four Inches Focus. And then an Object-Glass of twelve Foot with an Eye Glass of three Inches Magnifies but 48 times. But an Object Glass of 24 Foot with an Eye-Glass of four Inches Magnifies 72 times, viz. ½ more than the former, which is a great Difference, and of vast Advantage, when it may be obtained with the same Clearness and Distinctness. I confess the longest Telescopes do generally render the Objects more Dark and Obscure, yet when shorter Glasses have proportionably as short Eye-Glasses, and as close Apertures, they are more Obscure, than the longer Telescopes.

I answer Secondly, That the Image of the Moon or other Object in the Distinct Base of an Object-Glass of 24 Foot is twice as long as the Image in the Distinct Base of an Object-Glass of twelve Foot. And consequently we shall not wonder, that the Picture in the former, should be much more Distinct and Perfect, than in the latter, As 'tis much more easie to represent every Feature and Line of a Face in a large Piece, than in a small Piece of Miniature.

Corollary 3.

And if the Object-Glass be formed on a less Sphere than the Eye-Glass (as suppose the Object-Glass formed on a Sphere of six Inches Radius, and the Eye-Glass on a Sphere of twelve Inches Radius) hereby the Appearance of the Object shall be Diminished. And the Appearance through the Glass shall be to the naked Appearance as six to twelve, or ½ the Natural Appearance.

Scholium.

Scholium.

From hence it is manifest, how requisite it is in relating any *Phænomena* observed by the Telescope (or even by the Microscope) to mention not only the length of the Tube in general, But to specifie the particular Focus of the Eye Glass, as well as of the Object-Glass; as also the Aperture of the Object-Glass. For by this means, they that intend to observe the same *Phænomena*, may understand how to adapt their Telescopes proper for the Observation. This the *Learned and Ingenious Monsieur Hugens in his* Systema Saturnium *puts down exactly, pag.* 4. Where also we find this Passage. *Illud in Dioptricis Nostris Demonstratum invenietur, Speciei per Tubum visæ ad eam quæ Nudo Oculo percipitur, hanc secundum Diametrum esse Rationem, quæ Distantiæ Foci in Exteriori vitro (Objectivo Scilicet) ad illam quæ in Interiori sive Oculari vitro est Foci Distantiam.* But hitherto we are so unhappy as to want that excellent Persons Dioptricks. In the mean time, let that which I have given in the foregoing *Prop.* LIII. serve till a better be offered.

Prop LIV. Probl.

To Determine the Angle received by a Telescope of the foregoing Combination. The Rule is, as the Distance between the Object Glass and Eye-Glass: To half the Breadth of the Eye-Glass .. So Radius: To the Tangent of half the Angle received.

T 35 F 2 *Tab.* 35 *f.* 2. The Distance of the Glasses is *h y*. Let half the Breadth of the Eye-Glass be *g h*. Then, as *h y*: To *g h* :: So Radius: To the Tangent of the Angle *g y h*, which is half the Angle *g y l*, the Angle received. That is, the Eye at *o* shall perceive no more of the Object, than subtends this Angle before the Object-Glass.

Schol.

Scholium 1.

But if the Eye Approach *nigher to*, or recede *further from* the Eye-Glass *g h l* (*Tab.* 35. *f.* 1.) than its Focus at *o*, it shall perceive a lesser *Area* of the Object, though what it sees shall be as Distinct as at *o*. For let us suppose the Pupil of the Eye at *m*, The Rays *g o*, *l o*, do not enter the Eye, and consequently the Points in the Object answerable to *f*, *d*, in the Distinct Base, shall not be visible. The same may be conceived if the Eye recede farther from the Eye-Glass than *o*; because all the Rays from the several Points in the Object are mixt together, and intersect at *o*, in the Focus of the Eye Glass, and thence flowing forward they separate and Diverge. But then the Eye at *m* receives the Rays, that do enter it, *Parallel* or at least a very little *Diverging*, and consequently the Vision is *Distinct*.

Scholium 2.

From hence also 'tis manifest, that the Angle received, or Visible *Area* of the Object, is not increased or diminished, by the greater or lesser Aperture of the Object-Glass. For the Angle *g y l* continues the same, though the Object-Glass were all covered to the very middle Point *y*. All that is effected by this *greater* or *lesser Aperture* is the more *Bright* or *Obscure* Appearance of the Object. But of this more fully in the next Proposition.

PROP. LV.

Concerning the Apertures of Object Glasses.

By the *Aperture* of a Glass I mean, that part of the Glass which is left open and uncovered. And this ought to be various according as we would have more or less Light admitted. It also varies according to the various Focal lengths of the Object Glasses. For a ten Foot Object-Glass shall bear a greater Aperture than an Object-Glass of one Foot; and a twenty Foot Glass yet greater than a ten Foot Glass.

But at what Rate or Proportion the Apertures of Glasses alter in respect of their lengths, is not yet well setled.

Monsieur Auzout, (*Phil. Transact.* N. 4. P. 55.) Tells us, that he finds, *That the Apertures, which Glasses can bear with Distinctness, are in* (about) *a Subduplicate Ratio to their lengths*: Or as the Square Roots of their lengths. Whereof he intends to give the Reason and Demonstration in his *Dioptrica* (which we yet want.) But this Ingenious Person should have told us, when he speaks of the Apertures of Glasses, whether he designs them for Objects on the Earth or in the Heavens. And if in this latter, whether for the *Moon, Mars, Jupiter,* or *Venus*. For each of these Objects will require a different Aperture of the same Glass. Because the Strength of their Light is different. For to view *Venus* there is requisite a much smaller Aperture, than to view the *Moon, Saturn* or *Jupiter*.

However till some better Rule can be found for settling the Apertures of Object-Glasses (which at present I shall not pretend to) I shall here Present you with Mr. *Auzout*'s Table, as 'tis to be found in the fore-cited *Philosophical Transaction*, *Numb.* 4. Noting only, that his Feet are *Parisian Feet* (which is to the *London* Foot as 1068. to 1000) and each Inch (which is the part of his Foot) is subdivided into twelve Lines. For it had not been worth our Pains to have reduced the whole Table to our *English* Measure. *Vid. Tab.* 36.

I have said before (*Schol.* 2. *Prop.* LIV.) That the Angle received, or Visible *Area* of an Object, is not Increased or Diminished by the greater or lesser Aperture of the Object Glass, all that is effected thereby is the Admittance of more or less

Rays;

A TABLE of the Apertures of Object-Glasses.
The Points put to some of these Numbers denote Fractions.

Length of Glasses	For Excellent ones	For good ones	For ordinary ones	Lengths of Glasses	For excellent ones	For Good ones	For ordinary ones
Feet Inches	Inch Lines	Inch Lines	Inch Lines	Feet Inches	Inch Lines	Inch Lines	Inch Lines
4	4	4	3	25	3 4	2 10	2 4.
6	5	5	4	30	3 8	3 2	2 7
9	7	6	5	35	4 0	3 4.	2 10
0	8	7	6	40	4 3	3 7	3 .
1 6	9	8	7	45	4 6	3 10	3 2
2 0	11	10	8	50	4 9	4 0	3 4.
2 6	1 0	11	9	55	5 0	4 3	3 6.
3 0	1 1	1 0	10	60	5 2	4 6	3 8.
3 6	1 2	1 1	11	65	5 4	4 8	3 10
4 0	1 4	1 2	1 0	70	5 7	4 10	3 .
4 6	1 5	1 3	1 .	75	5 9	5 0	4 2.
5 0	1 6	1 4	1 1.	80	5 11	5 2	4 5
6	1 7	1 5	1 2	90	6 4	5 6	4 7.
7	1 9	1 6	1 3	100	6 8	5 9	4 10
8	1 10	1 8	1 4	120	7 5	6 5	5 3
9	1 11.	1 9	1 5	150	8 0	7 0	5 11
10	2 1	1 10	1 6	200	9 6	8 0	6 9
12	2 4	2 0	1 8	250	10 6	9 2	7 8.
14	2 6	2 2	1 9.	300	11 6	10 0	8 5
16	2 8	2 4	1 11.	350	12 6	10 9	0 0
18	2 10	2 6	2 1	400	13 4	11 6	9 . 8
20	3 0	2 7	2 2.				

The feet here express'd are Paris-feet, and a Line is the 1/12 part thereof. The Paris-Foot is to the London-foot as 1068 to 1000

Tab. 36 pag. 170

rious according as we would have more or less Light admitted. It also varies according to the various Focal lengths of the Object Glasses. For a ten Foot Object-Glass shall bear a greater Aperture than an Object-Glass of one Foot; and a twenty Foot Glass yet greater than a ten Foot Glass.

But at what Rate or Proportion the Apertures of Glasses alter in respect of their lengths, is not yet well setled.

Monsieur Auzout, (*Phil. Transact.* N. 4. P. 55.) Tells us, that he finds, *That the Apertures, which Glasses can bear with Distinctness, are in* (about) *a Subduplicate Ratio to their lengths:* Or as the Square Roots of their lengths. Whereof he intends to give the Reason and Demonstration in his *Dioptrica* (which we yet want.) But this Ingenious Person should have told us, when he speaks of the Apertures of Glasses, whether he designs them for Objects on the Earth or in the Heavens. And if in this latter, whether for the *Moon, Mars, Jupiter*, or *Venus*. For each of these Objects will require a different Aperture of the same Glass. Because the Strength of their Light is different. For to view *Venus* there is requisite a much smaller Aperture, than to view the *Moon, Saturn* or *Jupiter*.

However till some better Rule can be found for settling the Apertures of Object-Glasses (which at present I shall not pretend to) I shall here Present you with Mr. *Auzout*'s Table, as 'tis to be found in the fore-cited *Philosophical Transaction, Numb.* 4. Noting only, that his Feet are *Parisian* Feet (which is to the *London* Foot as 1068. to 1000) and each Inch (which is the $\frac{1}{12}$ part of his Foot) is subdivided into twelve Lines. For it had not been worth our Pains to have reduced the whole Table to our *English* Measure. *Vid. Tab.* 36.

I have said before (*Schol.* 2. *Prop.* LIV.) That the Angle received, or Visible *Area* of an Object, is not Increased or Diminished by the greater or lesser Aperture of the Object Glass; all that is effected thereby is the Admittance of more or less

Rays,

A TABLE of the Apertures of Obiect-Glasses.
The Points put to some of these Numbers denote Fractions.

Length of Glasses. Feet, Inches	For Excellent ones. Inch.Lines	For good ones. Inch.Lines	For ordinary ones. Inch Lines	Lengths of Glasses. Feet Inches	For excellent ones. Inch Lines	For Good ones. Inch Lines	For ordinary ones. Inch Lines
4	4	4	3	25	3 4	2 10	2 4.
6	5	5	4	30	3 8	3 2	2 7
9	7	6	5	35	4 0	3 4.	2 10
0	8	7	6	40	4 3	3 7	3 .
1 6	9	8	7	45	4 6	3 10	3 2
2 0	11	10	8	50	4 9	4 0	3 4.
2 6	1 0	11	9	55	5 0	4 3	3 6.
3 0	1 1	1 0	10	60	5 2	4 6	3 8.
3 6	1 2	1 1	11	65	5 4	4 8	3 10
4 0	1 4	1 2	1 0	70	5 7	4 10	3 .
4 6	1 5	1 3	1 .	75	5 9	5 0	4 2.
5 0	1 6	1 4	1 1	80	5 11	5 2	4 5
6	1 7	1 5	1 2	90	6 4	5 6	4 7.
7	1 9	1 6	1 3	100	6 8	5 9	4 10
8	1 10	1 8	1 4	120	7 5	6 5	5 3
9	1 11.	1 9	1 5	150	8 0	7 0	5 11
10	2 1	1 10	1 6	200	9 6	8 0	6 9
12	2 4	2 0	1 8	250	10 6	9 2	7 8.
14	2 6	2 2	1 9.	300	11 6	10 0	8 5
16	2 8	2 4	1 11.	350	12 6	10 9	0 0
18	2 10	2 6	2 1	400	13 4	11 6	9 8
20	3 0	2 7	2 2.				

The feet here express'd are Paris-feet, and a Line is the 1/12 part thereof. The Paris-Foot is to the London-foot as 1068 to 1000.

Tab. 36 pag 170

Rays, and consequently the more Bright or Obscure Appearance of the Object. *Tab.* 35. *f.* 5. Let the greater Aperture of the Object-Glass *x y z* be *x z*; And the lesser Aperture *m n*. *a b* is a Remote Object Projected in the Distinct Base *d e f*. The Cone of Rays *x a z* is Projected in the Cone of Rays *x d z*; And consequently the Cone of Rays *m a n* (as being a part of the former *x a z*) shall be Collected at *d* in the Cone *m d n*. But then by this latter Aperture *m n*, all the Rays that fall on the outward Ring of the Glass, here expressed by *x a m*, *z a n*, are excluded, and consequently the Point *d* shall not be illustrated with so much light as were the Aperture as wide as *z x*. And therefore (supposing an Eye-Glass behind this Object-Glass, so as to constitute a Telescope) such a vigorous Light from each Radiating Point in the Object will not be brought into the Eye.

We have the exact Natural Resemblance hereof in the Eye it self: whose Pupil is contracted and dilated, according as the Light of an Object is more or less Intense.

Another Particular, wherein this Contraction or Dilatation of a Glasses Aperture is requisite, is this: An Object may be so nigh a Glass that the Rays from each single Point, falling upon the whole Breadth of the Glass, may Diverge so much that the Glass is not able to Correct the Divergence of those Rays that fall towards its outward Borders, so as to reduce them to Determine or Unite in the Distinct Base with those Rays, that fall nigher the middle of the Glass (as before is noted after *Prop.* III.) And then 'tis requisite to contract the Aperture of the Glass, so as to exclude these Exorbitant Rays. A notable Experiment of this we may make by holding a Minute Object very nigh the Pupil of the Eye, the Object shall appear very *Confused*. But by applying a Paper with a small Pin-hole before the Pupil, it shall reduce the Appearance to much more Distinctness than before.

[172]

Prop. LVI.

The Telescope Consisting of a Convex Object-Glass, and Three Convex Eye-Glasses is Explained

I have shewn in *Prop* L. *&c.* the Nature and Properties of the Telescope consisting of a Convex Object-Glass, and Convex Eye Glass. I have shewn how the Image of the Object being formed in the Distinct Base of the Object-Glass *x y z* (*Tab.* 35. *f* 1.) by the Rays from each single Point of the Object there uniting, and flowing forward on the Eye-Glass, are thereby all collected together and confounded in its outward Focus at *o*

*T*35. F 1.

Now (in *Tab.* 37. *Fig.* 1.) Let us Combine two other Eye-Glasses *k*, *l*, with the said Telescope of *Prop.* L. And place them so, that the Distance between the first Eye-Glass *h*, and the second Eye-Glass *k*, may be the sum of their *Foci* Also that the Distance between the second Eye-Glass *k*, and the third Eye-Glass *l*, may be likewise the sum of their *Foci*. So that all the Glasses are Distant from the next adjacent Glasses, the sum of their *Foci* Only here it may be noted, that to cause Distinct Vision through this Telescope, 'tis not absolutely necessary that the second Eye-Glass *k* be exactly Distant from the Focus *o* of the first Eye-Glass *h*, the just length of its own Focus ; For it may be more or less, but then the Visible *Area*, and Magnified Appearance of the Object shall be altered. As will be manifest after we have explained this Glass to those that consider it.

*T*37. F 1.

It is then evident that the first Eye-Glass *h* mixes all the Rays from different Points in the Focus at *o* ; from whence they flow forward, and fall upon the second Eye-Glass *k*, each parcel of Rays parallel amongst themselves : And by the Glass *k* are

formed

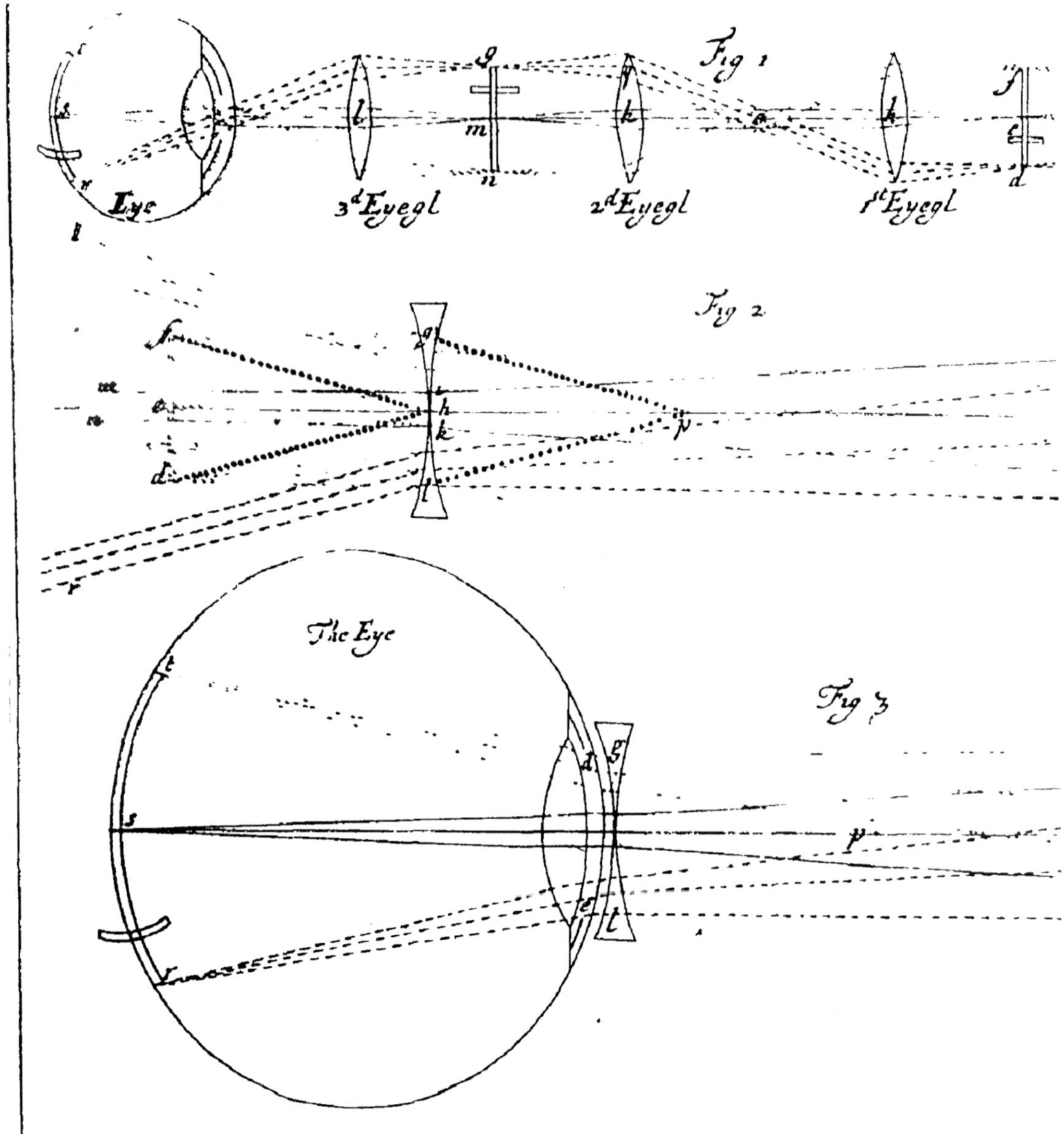
Fig 1
Eye
3d Eyegl
2d Eyegl
1st Eyegl
Fig 2
Fig 3
The Eye

Tab 37 pag. 172

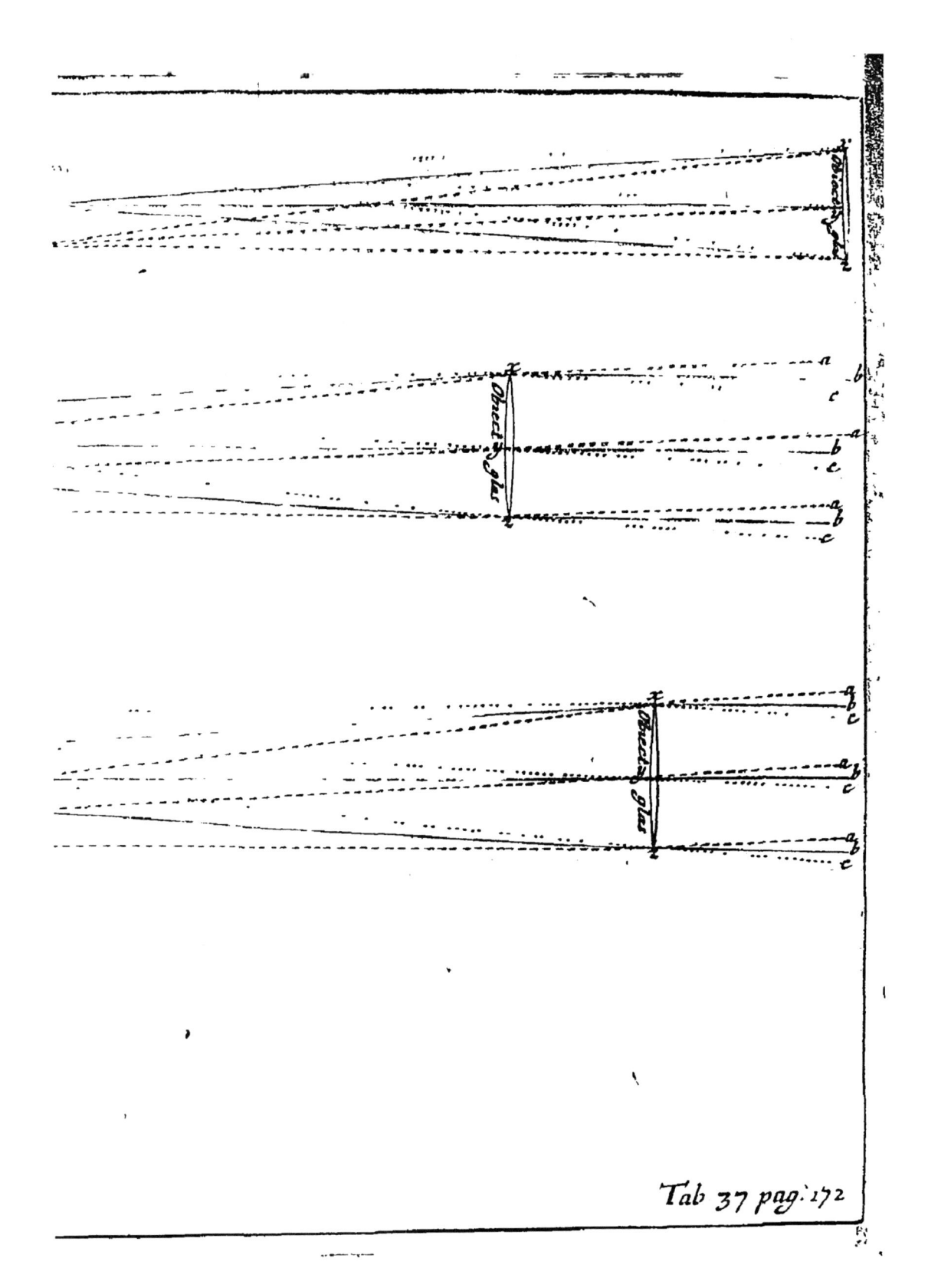

formed into the second Distinct Base gmn. For we may imagine the middle Ray oq to proceed directly from o, the Focus of the Glass k; wherefore oq shall be refracted by the Glass k, and be made to run in qg parallel to its Axis km. And then all the other Rays that are parallel to oq before they enter the Glass k, after they have passed the Glass k, do unite with qg in the Focus of the Glass k, and so the second Distinct Base gmn is formed.

Or otherwise. We may conceive the Glass k to be the Crystalline of the Eye, looking through the Telescope of *Prop.* L. *by*. And as the Crystalline in that Case does by means of the Glass h form in its Focus on the *Retina* the Image of the Distinct Base fed; So may we imagine the Glass k to form in its Focus gmn, by means of the Glass h, the Image of the Distinct Base fed.

Then from the second Distinct Base gmn the Rays proceed as is expressed in the Scheme, and fall on the third Eye Glass l; By whose means we may imagine the Distinct Base gmn projected distinctly on the *Retina* of the Eye rst, in the same manner as is shewn before in the Telescope of *Prop.* L.

And here we may observe that the Image on the *Retina* rst is *Inverted*, therefore the Object shall appear *Erect. Prop* XXVIII. *Sec* 4, 5.

And we may conceive this sort of Telescope as a double Telescope of *Prop* L. For the Glasses h, y, make one Telescope, And the Glasses k, l, another. And as the former by it self *Inverts* the Object; so the latter with the former *Reverts* the *Inverted* Image, and consequently makes the Object appear *Erect*. Yet it has been lately Publish'd in the *Journal des Scavans* 17. *Sept.* 1685. as a very difficult Problem in Dioptricks, why four Glasses in this kind of Telescope represent Objects *Erect*? I think I have solved this Problem to satisfaction, and my Answer is Publish'd *Num.* 187. of the *London Philosophical*

phical Transactions. As also in the *Bibliotheque Universelle & Historique de l'Annee* 1688. *Tome* 3. *pag.* 329. But the Learned Author of this latter in his Translation has mistaken my Sense in one Particular. I shall therefore give it here again in the Second Part of this Work *Chap.* 2.

<small>*Dioptrick Problem solved in the Second Part of this Treatise Chap. 2.*</small>

Concerning the Magnifying Power of this Telescope; our *Prop.* L. will direct us how to Calculate it. For by that Proposition 'tis manifest, that if the several Eye-Glasses h, k, l, be of equal *Foci*, and the Distance between h and k be the sum of both their *Foci*, that then the apparent Diametral Magnitude of an Object through the Glass, is to the Diametral Magnitude viewed by the naked Eye, as the Focus of the Object-Glass, to the Focus of any one of the Eye-Glasses. But if the *Foci* of the Eye-Glasses h, k, l, be different, or the Distance between h and k different from the sum of their *Foci*, then to obtain the magnified Appearance, we must have Recourse to Calculation. Wherein the Cases are so very various, that to insist on them all would be very tedious, and infinitely laborious. For the Focus of h may be greater, equal, or less than of k or of l; and so of k than of l or h; and so of l than of k or h; As likewise the Distance between k and h may be infinitely varied. I shall therefore pass this over, A little Consideration of the several Varieties will make any of them plain, and shew how they may be easily Calculated by those versed in the foregoing Doctrine. For 'tis but considering, how the Distinct Base $g\,m\,n$ is Projected, whether equal to, greater or less than the Distinct Base $f\,e\,d$, And how the Eye-Glass l conveys this Distinct Base $g\,m\,n$ to the Eye.

In like manner, by *Prop.* LIV. may the Angle received, or Visible *Area* of an Object through this kind of double Telescope, be Determined, as in the single Telescope; Respect being had to the several Apertures, *Foci*, and Distances of the several Eye-Glasses h, k, l.

Scholium.

Scholium.

From the Explication of this kind of Telescope, and of that in *Prop.* L may we easily apprehend the Theories of the various Combinations of Convex-Glasses in the Compositions of divers Telescopes of 3, 4, 5, 6, 7, 8, *&c.* Glasses.

Wherefore in explaining any kind of Telescope, we are first to obtain (by some Practical Rules to be deliver'd hereafter *Part* II *Chap* 4. *Sec.* 3.) the Focal length of each particular Glass by it self. Then we are to consider the Distances of each of these Glasses (as they lye in the Tube) from the Glasses before and behind it. Afterwards we are to consider, where the Distinct Base, or Distinct Bases are formed by these several Glasses, and how they are Projected as to Amplification or Diminution, which is easily found by the Doctrine before delivered. And then how the Eye-Glasses affect these Distinct Bases; As how they Confound them, Rectifie them, Invert or Magnifie them.

For the Result of all is this, that the Rays from the several Images in the several Distinct Bases, shall be Confounded on the Pupil of the Eye, in order to be rectified by the Crystalline, which (as has often been intimated) we may consider as a Convex-Glass, whose Focus is on the *Retina*. And from a due Consideration of the Premisses, it will appear why some Telescopes consisting of Convex-Glasses represent the Object *Erect*, others Inverted; in some *one* Glass is to be taken as *one*, in others two Glasses perform the Effect but of *one*.

And thus all the Combinations of Glasses expressed in the 8, 9, 10, 11, 12. *Iconisms* of *Zahn Telescop. Fund* 2. *Syntag.* 3. *Cap.* 6, 7, 8, 9. are easily explained, with a thousand other Varieties.

PROP.

Prop. LVII.

The Telescope Composed of a Concave Eye-Glass, and Convex Object-Glass of a larger Sphere is Explain'd.

The Posture of the Glasses in this Telescope is this; The Distance of the Glasses is to be the *Difference* of their *Foci*, that is, the Concave Eye-Glass is to be placed so much nigher the Object-Glass than the Focal length of this Object-Glass, as is the virtual Focus of this Eye-Glass. And the Eye is to be placed as nigh the Eye-Glass as possible.

Note. I shall call the *virtual Focus* of the Concave, simply its *Focus*, it being well known that a Concave has no *other Focus*, but a *virtual Focus*.

I shall now shew, that through this Glass the Object appears *Distinct*, *Erect*, and *Magnify'd*. And shall shew the *Angle received* or *visible Area*, according to the several Postures of the Eye.

Only premising in this Proposition (as I have done in several former) that we suppose the Glasses of the least thickness imaginable; and especially the *Concave-Glass* in its middle Point is supposed of no thickness at all, but the two Surfaces to touch.

To explain this Glass the better, I shall express the Figure very large, *Tab. 37. f. 2.* Wherein we shall first consider the Telescope it self separate from the Eye. Wherefore, let some Distant Object (as suppose a *Cross*) send the Rays *a a a* from its upper Point, *b b b* from its middle Point, and *c c c* from its lower Point. These falling on the Object-Glass *x y z* are formed thereby into the Distinct Base *f e d*. Let now the Concave-Glass *g h l*, be placed between the Distinct Base *f e d*, and the Object Glass *x y z*, so far distant from the Distinct Base, as is the Focus of this Concave, that is, let *e h* be the virtual Focus

cus of the Concave Eye-Glass. Then the Rays (for Instance) from the middle Point, *x i*, *y h*, *z k*, falling on the Concave and Converging towards its Focus *e*, after passing the Glass become Parallel (*Corol Prop.* XIII.) and run onwards in *i m*, *h e*, *k n*. The same may be conceived of the Rays from the Collateral Points; which Converge towards the Focus in *f* and *d*; *viz.* that these also after passing the Concave Eye-Glass, do proceed onwards Parallel amongst themselves.

But concerning these Rays from the Collateral Points, we must note also; That, as it is shewn before in *Prop.* L. *Sec.* 3, 4. Concerning the Convex Eye-Glass *g h l* (*Tab.* 35. *f.* 1.) that it brings the Rays of the Collateral Points *f g*, *d l*, Parallel amongst themselves into its Focus at *o*. So the Concave Eye-Glass *g h l* (*Tab.* 37. *f.* 2.) for the same Reasons expressed before in *Prop.* L. *Sec.* 3, 4. *Mutatis Mutandis*, makes the several parcels of Rays from the Collateral Points, after passing it, to *Diverge*, as if they proceeded directly, from the Point *p*; *p h* and *h e* being equal, and each equal to the Focal length of the Concave Eye-Glass. These things being fully considered; we proceed in the Explication of this Telescope. And therefore now let us apply the Eye thereto, And this also in a large Figure, *Tab.* 37. *f.* 3. T 37 F 3

T 35 F 1.

T 37. F 2

I say first, the Object appears through this Glass *Distinct*; For by what foregoes the Rays from each single Point, do fall on the Eye *Parallel* amongst themselves; And therefore each Point (by *Pr.* XXVIII.) is *distinctly* represented on the Fund of the Eye.

I say secondly, the Object appears *Erect*. For 'tis manifest by the Inspection only of the Scheme, that the Rays flowing from the *lower* Point of the Object, are Terminated at *t* the *upper* Part of the Retina. And the Rays from the *upper* Point of the Object are Terminated at *r* the *lower* Part of the Retina. So that the Image is painted *inverted* on the Retina. And therefore by *Prop.* XXVIII. the Object appears *Erect*.

Y a

I say

I say lastly, the Object is *Magnified* by this Glass. For the Proof of this we are to remember, what foregoes in *Prop.* XXXVII. 'Tis there declared, that if an Object be Projected by a Convex-Glass *x y z* (*Tab.* 37. *f.* 2.) in the Distinct Base *f e d*; And the Eye be placed any where between the Glass and the Distinct Base, as suppose at *h*, draw *f h*, *d h*, and the Object appears under the Angle *f h d*, which is much greater than *f y d*, the natural Optick-Angle. The same will hold, though we interpose the Concave-Glass *g l*; for the Ray *x g* from the Objects lower Point, that runs Parallel to the Axis *b y h e*, is Refracted into *g t*, as if it came directly from the Point *p*. And so the Ray *z l* from the Objects upper Point, that runs Parallel to the Axis *b y h e* is Refracted into *l r*, as if it came directly from the same Point *p*. If therefore we suppose the Rays *x g f*, *z l d*, Parallel to the Axis; then *g l* shall be equal to *f d*; And *p h* being by Supposition equal to *h e*, *p g t* shall be Parallel to *b f*; And *p l r* shall be Parallel to *h d*. And consequently the Angle *g p l* shall be equal to the Angle *f h d*. Wherefore the Object through this Glass appears under the same Angle, as we may imagine the *Apices* of the Pencils *f*, *d*, would appear to the naked Eye at *h* (the Concave Eye-Glass being removed) And consequently the Object appears *Magnified*.

The *Visible Area*, or *Angle Received* by this Glass, is Determined by the *Aperture* or *Breadth* of the Eyes Pupil. For 'tis manifest, from *Tab.* 37. *f.* 3. That if the Pupil *d e* of the Eye were not large enough to receive the Rays from the extreme Points of the Object, it would not perceive the *whole* Object through this Glass. Wherefore by the *Breadth* of the Pupil given, as also by the Focal Distances of the Object-Glass and Eye-Glass being given, we may easily obtain the *Visible Area*, or *Angle Received*. For let us suppose that we find from these Data, that the whole Object Projecting the Distinct Base *f e d* (*Tab.* 37. *f.* 2.) would be Projected in the breadth of the Pupil,

Pupil, at the Distance *by* from the Object-Glass. Then find the Angle *fyd* (as is easie from these *Data*, and the preceding Doctrine) and we have the *Angle Received*.

Corollary 1.

In the XXXI. *Prop. Sec.* 9. We have considered the *Locus Apparens* of an Object, Projected in the Distinct Base by a Convex-Glass, to the Eye placed between the Glass and Distinct Base. And if the *Affirmative* of the Quere, which I there propose, hold true; The *Locus Apparens* of the middle Point of the Object seen through the Glass of *Tab.* 37. *f.* 2. is at *p*. T.37 F 2

Corollary 2.

If we suppose a Convex Eye-Glass, whose Focal length is equal to the Focal length *ph* or *eh* of this Concave Eye-Glass, apply'd (as directed in *Prop.* L.) to this same Object-Glass *xyz* in *Tab.* 37. *f.* 2. It would magnifie the Object equally with this Concave: And from hence it follows, that the preceding Proposition LIII. concerning the Magnifying of a Telescope, may be apply'd to this sort of Telescope furnished with a Concave Eye-Glass. But then the Advantage of the Telescope in *Prop.* L. beyond that of this Proposition, is most signal in this particular, That it receives a very much greater Angle, or shews to the Eye a much greater *Area* of the Object. The *Area* in this being Determined by the breadth of the Convex Eye-Glass; But in that of a Concave Eye-Glass, the *Area* is proportioned to the breadth of the Pupil.

Corollary 3.

If the Eye recede from the Concave Eye Glass of this Proposition, it perceives not so great a space of the Object. This is manifest only by Inspection of the two Schemes (*Fig.* 2, and 3. *Tab.* 37.) For if the Breadth of the Pupil *d e*, be but just sufficient to receive the Rays from the extreme Points of the Object, after they have passed the Eye-Glass, and are thereby so much Divaricated; if the Eye recede, the Pupil shall not be broad enough; and consequently shall see less of the Object. Just as in the Telescope of *Prop* L.

Corollary 4.

If the Eye move upwards or downwards, or to one side, or t'other of the Eye-Glass (supposing the Eye-Glass much broader than the Pupil) it perceives *consecutively* different parts of the Object. Thus suppose in *Fig.* 2. *Tab.* 37. The Pupil placed before the middle of the Eye-Glass at *h,* and not broad enough to receive the Rays from the upper and lower parts of the Object: If the Eye move upwards, it will meet with the Rays *g t* from the lower Point of the Object, which before escaped it; and so moving downwards it meets the Rays *l r* from the upper parts of the Object.

Of MICROSCOPES.

Hitherto of *single* Glasses, and of Glasses *combined* for viewing Distant Objects. We come now to treat of Glasses for viewing *minute* and *nigh* Objects, commonly called *Microscopes*. The Theory of these does so depend on what foregoes, that we shall have no occasion of insisting long upon them.

And first for *Microscopes* consisting of a *single* Convex-Glass. In these the Object is usually placed either in the Focus of the Glass, or a little nigher the Glass than the Focus; And the Eye is placed in or about the Focus on t'other side the Glass.

In

Tab. 38 pag. 181

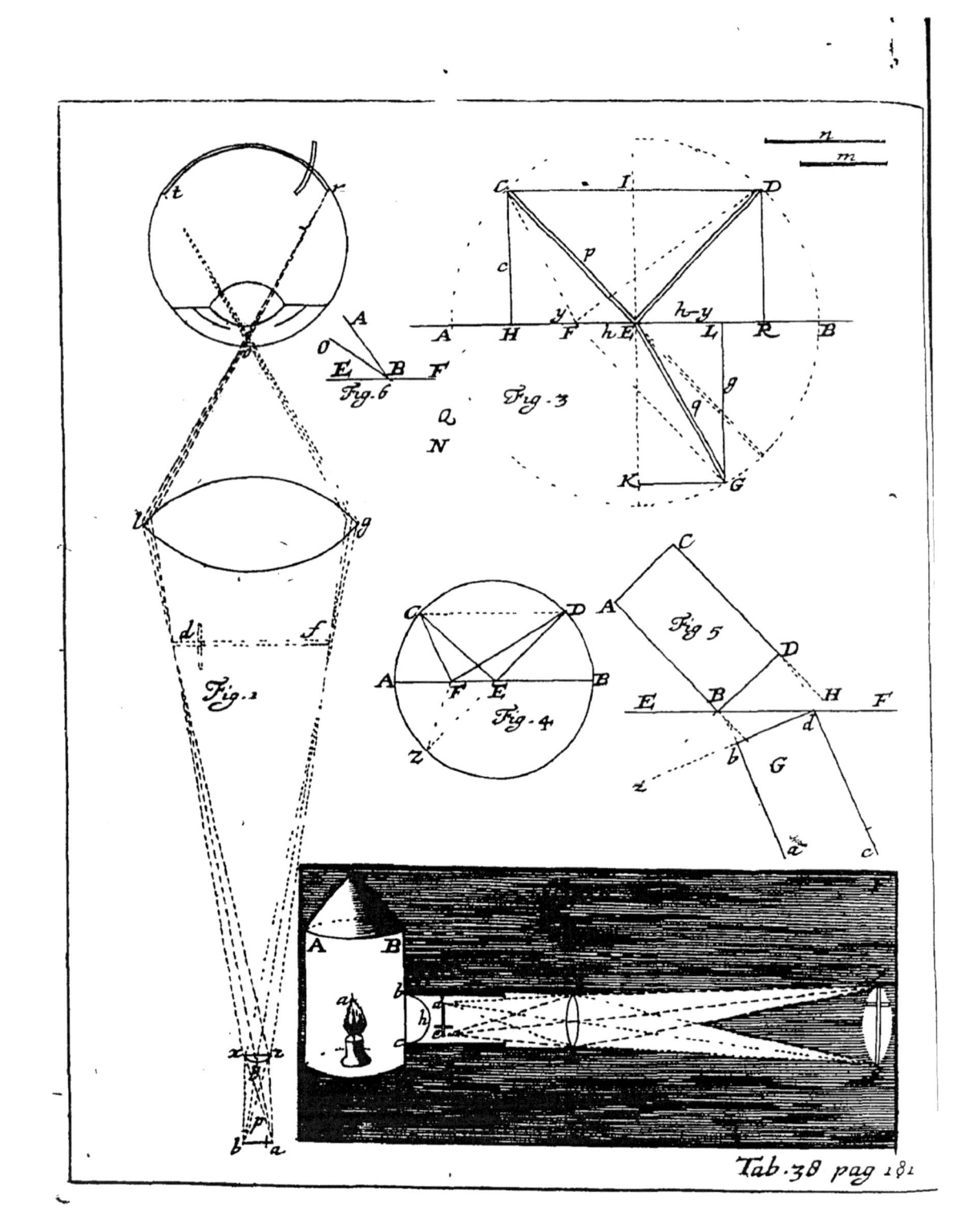

In which Cases the Appearances were already solved. *Prop.* XXXI, XXXII, XXXIII, XXXIV, XXXV.

As to *double* Microscopes, or Microscopes consisting of more than one Convex-Glass, wherein the Object is Projected in a Distinct Base, before it be conveyed to the Eye; I explain them as follows, observing the Series of the Propositions.

P R O P. LVIII.

The double Microscope composed of a Convex Object Glass, and Convex Eye Glass is Explained.

Tab. 38. *Fig.* 1. Let ab be a minute nigh Object exposed before the Object-Glass xyz, the Segment of a very small Sphere. Let the Focus of this Object-Glass be at p. Then the Object being something more distant from the Glass, than its Focal length yp, shall be Projected in the Distinct Base fd, somewhere on t'other side the Glass, according to the Doctrine before delivered *Prop.* V. And of what bigness the Image shall be Projected in the Distinct Base is determined by *Prop.* XXVI. Let the Eye-Glass lg be placed so far distant from the Distinct Base fd, as is the Focal length of this Eye Glass; And the Eye ort placed where this Eye-Glass confounds all the Rays go, lo, which shall be about the Focus of the Eye-Glass.

All things being thus combined, The Effects of this Microscope are explained in all things, as in the Telescope of *Prop.* L. As to the Magnified, Inverted, and Distinct Appearance of the Object. And therefore 'tis needless to inlarge farther thereon: To those versed in what is already delivered, the very Inspection of the Scheme is sufficient.

Only as to the extraordinary Magnifying of these Microscopes, we may farther Remark; that whereas for viewing a Minute Object, a well-constituted Eye does usually Approach thereto about the diſtance of eight Inches: could we approach the Eye thereto, and view it diſtinctly at the diſtance of half an Inch, the Optick-Angle would be wonderfully magnify'd by *Prop.* LI, LII. that is to ſay, the apparent Magnitude of the Object would be increaſed at the rate of ſixteen to one. Let us then ſuppoſe the Eye at *y*, viewing the Object *a b*, which would then appear under the Angle *a y b* equal to *d y f*; which is the ſame as were the Object increaſed to the bigneſs *d f*, and viewed by the Eye at the ſame diſtance from it as *y* in the figure is now removed from *d f*. Wherefore if by help of the Eye-Glaſs *g l*, the Eye can yet approach to the Diſtinct Baſe *d f* (which we may now repute the real Object) ſuppoſe ten times nigher than *y* is to *d f*; the apparent Magnitude of *d f* ſhall again be increaſed ten times more than before, by the nigh approach of the Eye (ſuppoſe at *y*): that is, the Object by all theſe helps ſhall be magnified 160 times in length, or Diametral Magnitude.

As to the Calculation of all theſe Angles, and apparent Magnitudes, it cannot be difficult to thoſe vers'd in what is before deliver'd.

There are various Combinations of Glaſſes in this kind of double Microſcopes, for in ſome there are two Object Glaſſes, that is to ſay, one Object-Glaſs of a very deep Convexity, and an other of a leſſer Convexity, placed nigher the former than the Projection of the Diſtinct Baſe (according to *Schol.* 1. *Prop.* XVI.) which ſometimes is called a Middle-Glaſs. In others there are two Eye-Glaſſes, &c. But the Theory of all theſe depends on, and is ſo manifeſt from what has been delivered, that 'tis needleſs to enlarge.

I ſhall conclude the Firſt Part of this Treatiſe with a Piece of *Dioptricks*, which though *Ludicrous* affords an Appearance ſurpriſing and pleaſant enough. The Explication thereof is much labour'd at by ſeveral, though it be very Obvious from what foregoes. 'Tis this,

P R O P.

PROP. LIX.

The Explication of the Magick Lantern, *sometimes called* Lanterna Megalographica.

The Contrivance is briefly this, *Tab. 38. f. 2. ABCD* is a Tin Lantern, from whose side there proceeds a square or round Arm or Tube *b n k c m l*, consisting of two Parts, the outermost whereof *n k m l* slides over the other, so as that the whole Tube may be lengthened or shortened thereby. In the end of the Arm *n k m l* is fixt a Convex-Glass *k l*: about *d e* there is a Contrivance for admitting and placing an Object *d e* painted in dilute and transparent Colours on a plain thin Glass; which Object is there to be placed *Inverted*. This is usually some Ludicrous or frightful Representation, the more to divert the Spectators: *b h c* is a deep Convex-Glass, so placed in the other end of the Prominent Tube, that it may strongly cast the light of the Flame *a* on the Picture *d e* painted on the plain thin Glass. And here 'tis to be noted, that the Glass *b h c* is only designed for the strong Illumination of the Picture *d e*, and has nothing to do in the Representation, and therefore in some of these Lanterns, instead of the Glass *b h c*, we shall find a *Concave-Speculum* so placed, that it may strongly cast the light of the Flame *a* on the Picture at *d e*.

Wherefore, Let us now consider the Picture *d e* as a very lightsome Object of distinct Colours and Parts. And let us conceive *d e* more remote from the Glass *k l* than its Focus. 'Tis then manifest, that the Distinct Image of the Object *d e* shall be projected by the Glass *k l* on the opposite white Wall *F H* at *f g*; And here it shall be represented *Erect*. For now the whole Chamber *E F G H* is dark, the Lantern *A B C D* inclosing all the Light, So that in Effect this Appearance of the *Magick Lan-*
tern

tern is no more than what is already declared concerning the Reprefentation of outward Objects in a dark Room by a Convex Glafs, after *Prop* IV (*vid Tab.* 14. *f* 1.) And here we may obferve, that if the Tube be *Contracted*, and thereby the Glafs *k l* brought *nigher* the Object *d e* ; the Reprefentation *f g* fhall be Projected fo much the *larger;* and fo much the more *Diftant* from the Glafs *k l*, according to the Rules before laid down. So that the fmalleft Picture at *d e* may be Projected at *f g* in any greater Proportion required, within due limits. From whence the Name of *Lanterna Megalographica*. And confequently, protracting the Tube and drawing the Glafs *k l* more diftant from the Object *d e*, will diminifh the Reprefentation *f g*, and Project it *nigher* the Glafs *k l*.

As to the Mechanick Contrivance of this Lantern, the moft convenient Proportion of the Glaffes, *&c.* This is fo ordinary amongft the common Glafs-Grinders, that 'tis needlefs to infift farther thereon in this place. 'Tis fufficient to me that I have explained the Theory thereof.

Scholium.

On this depends the Theory of the *Optick* Experiment propos'd by Mr. *Hook* Num. 38. Pag. 741. *Philofoph. Tranfact.* For reprefenting ftrange Vifions and Appearances.

The End of the Firft Part.

DIOPTRICKS.

THE
SECOND PART,

Containing

Various Dioptrick Miscellanies.

THE CONTENTS.

Chap. 1.	Of Refraction and Light.	Pag. 191
Chap. 2.	A Dioptrick Problem.	Pag. 203
Chap. 3.	Of Glasses for defective Eyes.	Pag. 207
Chap. 4.	Of Mechanick Dioptricks.	Pag. 214
Chap. 5.	Of Telescopick Instruments.	Pag. 228
Chap. 6.	Of the Invention of Optick-Glasses, Discoveries made by them, and other Applications of them.	Pag. 251
Chap. 7.	An Optick Problem of Double Vision.	Pag. 287
Chap. 8.	An Appendix.	Pag. 295

To My esteemed Friend

Henry Osborn

OF

Dardys-Town in the County of *Meath*

ESQUIRE.

THE *Respect which I have ever had for you since our first Acquaintance, and which on all Occasions I have expressed in private, I have now an Opportunity of declaring to the Publick: And that too so very apposite, that it would be unpardonable in me to omit it at this time; by presenting the following Sheets to you, Dedicating them to your Name, and Devoting them and their Authour to your Use and Service.*

You may well remember the frequent Discourses we have had on several Subjects treated of in the following Chapters, and on account whereof I first set on this Dioptrical Work: And particularly, I think, our Dis-

quisitions

Dedication.

quisitions concerning the Justness of Telescopick Sights adapted to Astronomical Instruments, and our Considerations of the Micrometer, were the first Occasion of my Thoughts turning this Way; And therefore the ensuing Discourses belong to you of Right. But if to this I add, the Advantage I have received by your Acquaintance, and the repeated Satisfaction I have had in your agreable Conversation; I am bound by indispensible Tyes to make this Acknowledgment.

I cannot but admire your prudent Choice of a private, retired Life; notwithstanding your great Advantages both of Nature and Fortune, that render you capable of the most publick and weighty Imploy. By this Course, you have an Opportunity of enjoying your self, and improving your Philosophical Thoughts beyond the common pitch: You can look on unconcern'd, and securely observe the froathy Sea of Business, wherein Men fluctuate; and some are shipwreckt, sink, and perish.

And because you seem careless of propagating your Name the common ways; suffer me to erect this slight Monument to it: Though I am certain at the same time, that, if you pleased, you may raise a lasting Mausolæum to your Memory; but you seem above these Desires, yet you'll permit

Dedication.

mit your Friend to Honour it as far as he can; and if the Materials or Workmanship do not seem to promise a long Duration to Posterity, this only reflects on my Abilities, (which I shall never vindicate) but cannot lessen the sincere Intention of

April 17.
1690.

Your most affectionate

Humble Servant,

WILL. MOLYNEUX.

DIOPTRICKS.

DIOPTRICKS,

PART II.

CHAP. I.

Of Refraction and Light.

(1.) *This Discourse promised.* (2.) *Leibnutz's Universal Principle in Opticks,* &c. (3.) *On Occasion whereof; Of Final Causes.* (4.) *Farther Explication of Refraction.* (5.) *Light a Body, from several Arguments.* (6.) *From its being resisted in its passage through Diaphanous Mediums.* (7.) *Its Requiring time to move from place to place.* (8.) *Impossible to be increased, but by robbing some other Place of its Light.* (9.) *Therefore impossible to be augmented uniformly.*

(1.) IN the second Experiment of *Part* I. I had occasion to mention the *Natural Cause of Refraction*; or why the Rays of Light passing through different Mediums are refracted at their Immersion or Emersion. I then avoided any farther enquiry into the reason thereof, as being more of a *Physical* than *Mathematical* Consideration. But at the same time, I promised a farther Disquisition thereon, to be borrowed from a most Learned Author, whose reason we shall find briefly comprehended in this, That the Different Resistance that a Ray of Light finds in passing (for instance)

(1.) *This Discourse promised.*

stance) through Air and Glass, is the cause, why 'tis bent from its direct Course. But how this Refraction comes to be *from* the Perpendicular, in proceeding *from a Dense to a more Rare Medium*; or *towards* the Perpendicular, when *from a Rare to a more Dense Medium*; we shall more fully apprehend by the Discourse it self, which I here subjoyn from the *Acta Erud. Lipsiæ*, Ann. 1682. *pag*. 185.

(2) Leibnutz universal Principle in Opticks.

(2.) *One Universal Principle of Opticks, Catoptricks, and Dioptricks. By the Learned and Ingenuous G. G. Leibnutzius.*

The chief Hypothesis common to all these Sciences, and by which the Progress of all Rays of Light is geometrically determined, may be thus laid down. *Light proceeds from the Radiating Point, to the Point to be enlightned, that way, which is of all the most easie*; *and this is first to be Determined in respect to plain Surfaces, and then is accommodated to Concave or Convex Surfaces, by considering the Planes, that are Tangents to these Surfaces*. But here I take no notice of some *Irregularities*, which perhaps may conduce to the Generation of Colours, and to some other extraordinary *Phænomena*, which in practical Opticks are not at all considered.

Hence, *In plain or simple Opticks*, Tab. 38. Fig. 3. *The direct Ray proceeds from the Radiating Point* C, *to the Point to be illustrated* E, *by the shortest direct way*, the same Medium continuing all along, *that is, in the Right Line* C E.

In Catoptricks the Angle of Incidence C E A, *and of Reflection* D E B *are equal*. Let C be a Radiating Point; D the Point to be illustrated, and A B a *Plain Speculum*: 'Tis required to find in the *Speculum* the Point E, that reflects the Ray to D. I say, that it shall be such a Point, that the whole Progress, Way or Journey of the Ray C E+E D, may be the *least* or *shortest*, that is possible; or less than C F+F D, supposing that we take any other Point F in the *Speculum*. And this shall be obtained, if E be taken such, that the Angles CEA, DEB,

DEB, may be equal; as is manifest from Geometry. *Tab.* T 38 F 4.
38. *Fig.* 4. Produce D E to Z, and joyn F Z.

Then A Z = (D B =) A C. And F Z = F C.

Therefore C E + E D (= D Z) is less than C F or F Z + F D.

Ptolomy and other Antients insist on this Demonstration; and 'tis extant both elsewhere, and also in *Heliodorus Larissæus*.

In *Dioptricks*, * *The Sines* E H, E L, *of the Angles of Incidence* C E I, *and Refracted Angle* G E K *are to each other reciprocally as the Resistances of the Mediums.* Let I E be Air, and E K Water, Glass, or any other Diaphanous Medium more Dense than Air, C a Radiating Point in the Air, G the Point to be illustrated under the Glass: 'Tis inquired, by what Way or Path shall C radiate to G, or 'tis required to determine, in the Surface of the Glass A B, the Point E, which refracting the Ray that comes from C, sends it to G. Here this Point E must be taken such, that the Way, which the Ray takes, may be of all ways the *easiest*. But now in different Mediums, the Difficulties of the Way or Progress are in a Ratio compounded of the *Length* of the Way, and of the *Resistance* of the Mediums. Let the Right Line *m* represent the Resistance that Light finds in its passage through Air, and *n* the Resistance of its Passage through Glass. The *Difficulty* of the Way from C to E shall be as the Rectangle under C E and *m*, and from E to C as the Rectangle under E G and *n*. Therefore that the *Difficulty* of the *whole* Way C E G may be the *least* possible, the Sum of the Rectangles C E ׀ *m* + E G * *n* ought to be the least of all possible, or less than C F ׀ *m* + F G * *n*, supposing any other Point F taken besides E. The Point E is now required. Wherefore, seeing the Points C and G, and also the Right Line A B are given by Position, therefore the Lines C H, G L, Perpendiculars to the Plain A B, and the Line H L, are given also. Let us call C H, *c*, and G L, *g*, and H L, *h*, but the sought

T 38 F 3

* *Here I transfer according to the 2,4 Defnit of Part I and not according to the Author*

Line E H, let us call y; then E L shall be $h-y$, and C E shall be $\sqrt{cc+yy}$, which we shall call p; and E G shall be $\sqrt{gg+yy-2hy+hh}$, which we shall call q.

Wherefore $m * \sqrt{cc+yy} + n * \sqrt{gg+yy-2hy+hh}$ (or $mp + nq$) ought to be the least of all those Quantities that can possibly be so expressed; and 'tis required to determine y, that so it may be. By my Method *De Maximis & Minimis* (Vid. Act. Lips. Ann. 1684. pag. 467. 472) which, beyond all that are hitherto known, does wonderfully shorten the Calculation, it is manifest at the first sight, almost without any Calculation, That mqy shall be equal to $np + \overline{h-y}$, or that $np. mq :: y. h-y$, that is, the Rectangle of C E $*$ n shall be the to Rectangle of E G $*$ m :. As E H to E L. Therefore C E and E G being put equal, n the Resistance of Glass to Light shall be to m the Resistance of Air to Light :: As E H the Sine of the Angle of Incidence in Air C E I : To E L the Sine of the Refracted Angle in Glass G E K. Or these Sines shall be to each other reciprocally as the Resistances of the Mediums. Which was the Assertion to be proved.

Wherefore, if in one Example or Experiment E L be found $\frac{2}{3}$ of E H, the same Proportion shall hold in all other Experiments, wherever C and G be taken, that in Air, this in Glass. If C be in Air, and G in Water, Experiment shews, that E L shall be about $\frac{3}{4}$ of E H.

Thus far this ingenious Author. The rest of his Discourse is chiefly employed in rectifying *Des-Cartes* Notion of Refraction, which tho founded on the same Principle here expressed, yet has this peculiar, that he makes Water, or Glass, or any other more Dense Medium, resist the Progress of Light less than Air. But in this particular he is abundantly rectified by *Leibnutzius*, who shews the Incongruity of that Supposition.

Des Cart Notion of Refraction rectified.

(3.) One thing more there is remarkable in the Learned *Leibnitzius* Difcourfe, which I cannot here pafs over, and that is, A pious Reflection which he makes on this occafion, concerning *Final Caufes*. For 'tis manifeft, that the Ray proceeding from C, does not confult with it felf, how it may with the greateft eafe arrive at the Point E, or D, or G, neither is it carried by it felf to thofe Points. But the *Great Creator* of all things, has fo made *Light*, that this moft beautiful, orderly, and admirable Event fhould refult from its very Nature. Wherefore they are in a great Error, who reject *Final Caufes* in Natural Philofophy, which, befides affording us occafion of admiring and adoring the *Divine Wifdom*, do often difcover to us a curious Principle of finding out the Properties of thofe things whofe inward Nature is not *fo clearly* known by us, as that we can explain the immediate *efficient Caufes* and *Inftruments*, which the *Almighty Mover* imploys in producing thofe *Effects*, and obtaining thofe *Ends*.

Indeed I fhould think it an Attempt worth the Thought of fome profound Philofopher, to give an Account of thofe admirable, orderly, and beautiful Appearances in Nature, whereof we can moft plainly apprehend the *Defigns* and *Final Caufes*, but can hardly proceed to any farther Knowledg of them. (Thus for inftance, fuppofe it were asked, *What is the caufe of Refraction?* Were it not much fatisfactory to anfwer, *That thereby the Ray may proceed the eafieft way poffible*) This furely might be able to convince the moft obftinate Oppofers of *Divinity*: For certainly, if we can rely upon *any Deduction or Confequence* drawn out by the *Mind of Man*, we may affuredly reft fatisfied in this; that fo many *Phænomena*, ftupendous and furprifing for their *defigned Contrivance*, could not proceed but from an *Omnipotent* and *Defigning Being*. But if after all, they will arrive to fuch an height of Extravagance, as to fay, We cannot rely on thefe Conclufions, as being *all* in the *dark*, and

Remark on Final Caufes.

Final Caufes highly deferve our notice

knowing nothing; let them look to the hazard of their own Principles, who endanger their *eternal Happiness* on confidence of their own Arguments. But to resume our Subject.

<small>Fermat demonstrates the same</small>

The Famous Monf. *Fermat* has written a long Demonstration of this same Principle in *Dioptricks.* 'Tis publish'd amongst the French Letters, at the end of his *Opera Mathematica. Tolosæ* 1679. Pag. 158. To which I refer the Reader.

<small>Farther Explication of Refraction from D Barrow T 38 F 5</small>

(4.) But after all, perhaps it may not be amiss, to illustrate this Business of Refraction, by some more familiar and sensible Instance. Wherefore *Tab. 38. Fig. 5.* Let the Parallelogram A B C D represent a Ray of Light of this breadth, and let it fall on the plain Surface of the Glass E F, this in some measure does stop its Course, and the Point B entering the Glass, shall endeavour (but slower) to proceed onwards directly to G in the Line A B produced. But all this while the Point D, continuing yet in the Air, shall continue its former motion in the Right Line C D H, but now 'tis impossible for *both* the Points to obtain what both endeavour; for each cannot perform his *direct* Motion, one *flower*, and t'other *quicker.* And therefore that they may *both* come nighest to what *each* endeavours, they shall *both* be turned about some certain Point Z in the Right Line D B produced So that whilst the Point D in the *thinner* Medium proceeding *quicker* describes the greater Arch D *d*, the Point B, proceeding more slowly in the more *Dense* Medium, describes the lesser Arch B *b*; and when they have thus run through both these Arches, the Right Line B D shall obtain the Posture *b d*. And now that the Point D also is emerged into the more Dense Medium at *d*; and it also is now as much retarded as *b*, these circular Motions shall now cease, for D is not now carried quicker than B, and therefore describes not, as before, a greater Arch. Wherefore forsaking, as soon as they can, their former Progress, they shall both proceed in *d c*, *b a*, the Tangents to

their

their Arches. And the whole Ray A B C D thus bent, and brought into the Posture *a b c d* proceeds onwards directly in that Course. And here 'tis to be noted, That whatever Inclination A B has on E F, the Arches D *d*, B *b*, or their Semidiameters Z D, Z B, have always the same Proportion, to wit, such a Proportion, as the *peculiar* Difference in the Resistance or Density of one and t'other Medium does require (which is to be determined by Experiment): For *Tab.* 38. *Fig.* 6. Let us suppose the Point B thrust forwards towards Q or N, and that the Medium below E F is perfectly *Homogeneous*, that is, equally resisting in all Parts thereof; there is then no reason, why this Point should not be carried with an equal Celerity towards whatever Part, that is, it shall tend equally quick towards Q in the Right Line O B Q (supposing its direction lye that way) as towards N in the Right Line A B N. And therefore the Rays of Light A B, O B, however differently inclined, shall find an *equal* Resistance; and the Point B, whether it tend towards Q or N, shall be equally retarded. And also seeing the Point D (*Tab.* 38. *Fig.* 5.) continues in the first Medium, it shall be thrust forwards with the same Celerity, whatever is its Inclination. Whence 'tis manifest, that these Motions, or Paths passed over in the same time, to wit, the circular Arches D *d*, B *b*, shall always observe the same Proportion, that is, the Proportion of their Semidiameters Z D, Z B, or Z *d*, Z *b*; which Proportion therefore principally and chiefly measures and determines the Refractions of Rays in the same two Mediums. And this is the same Proportion, as is between the Sines of the Angles opposite to Z *d*, Z B, in the Triangle Z *d* B, that is, of the Angles Z B *d*, (or Z B E) and Z *d* B. But Z B E is the Complement of the Angle A B E, and therefore (by *Def.* 2. *Part.* I) Z B E is the *Angle of Incidence* or *Inclination* of A B to E F; and the Angle Z *d* B is the Complement of the Angle F *d c*, and therefore Z *d* B is the

Refracted

Refracted Angle (by *Def.* 3. *Part.* I.). From hence is manifest what we assert in the 7 *Experiment*, *Part* I. And here we shall note, that according to *Exper.* 6. *Part* I. Z D shall be to Z B :: As 300 To 193; or as 14 to 9.

Light a Body

(5.) And thus much concerning *Refraction*. The Consideration whereof does naturally suggest unto us, That *Light is a Body*. For however the Antient *Aristotelians* defined it, *Actus perspicui quatenus perspicuum*, which is perfectly unintelligible; yet so much we may perceive hereby, that they designed to exclude it from all *Corporeal Notion*. But the various Properties of Light, that do necessarily belong to a Body, are so many and evident, that they leave no room for any farther doubt in this matter. I shall mention but a few.

From its being refracted in its passage through Diaphanous Mediums

(6.) And first, by this *Affection* of being *refracted*, 'tis manifest that Light, in its passage through this and t'other Diaphanous Body does find a *different Resistance*. Now tis unconceivable, how any thing, but Body, should suffer Resistance; but we may conceive the Resistance, that Light suffers in its passage through different Diaphanous Bodies, to proceed from the Medium Hindering of the *Diffusion* or *Distribution* of Light through *more* of the Parts of this Medium, and consequently it may be said to be *less illuminable*. For the Nature of Light endeavours to *diffuse* it self. And on the contrary, by how much *Light* does more equably or uniformly affect the Parts of the Medium, which it enlightens, or by how much it communicates its *Energy* to *more* of the *Particles* of the enlightened Space; that Medium may be said to be by so much the *more illuminable*, or *less to resist* the Progress of Light. Whence it is, that by how much the affected Parts of the Medium are *more solid* and *small*, and admit between them the *less Space* for any other *Heterogeneous* Matter, that suffers not by *Light*; by so much the Medium is said to be *more enlightened*. But leaving these *Philosophical Refinements*, 'tis manifest

nifeſt that Reſiſtance muſt proceed from *Contact* of two *Bodies*. And *Contact*, either *Active* or *Paſſive*, belongs *only to Body*; according to that of the Philoſophick Poet, *Tangere enim & Lucretius tangi niſi Corpus nulla poteſt Res*. And our *Saviour* himſelf, the Fountain of all Wiſdom and Philoſophy, Divine and Natural, ſeems to confirm this Notion, when to prove himſelf *a True Body* after his Reſurrection, He commands his Diffident Diſciple *To Touch Him*.

(7.) The Second Property, that confirms *Light* to be a *Body*, and a *Body* moved or thruſt forward, is, That it requires *time* to paſs from one place to another, and does it not in an *inſtant*, but is only of all Motions the *quickeſt*. For the Experiment proving this, we are obliged to the Ingenious Monſ. *Romer*, who has demonſtrated beyond all Contradiction, from the Obſervations of the *Immerſions* and *Emerſions* of the Satellits of *Jupiter*; *That Light requires the Time of one Second to move the ſpace of* 3000 *Leagues, or* 9000 *Miles, which is near the Earths Diameter*. He that requires a farther Account hereof, may conſult the *Journal des Scavans* 1676. Decemb. 7. *Philoſoph. Tranſact.* Num. 136. Or Mr. *Newton*'s Incomparable Piece, *Philoſophiæ Natur. Princ Mathem* Lib. I. Schol. Prop. 96. Where 'tis aſſerted, That Light requires about ten Minutes time to come from the Sun to the Earth. And 'tis moſt evident, without this Allowance for the Time ſpent in Lights Motion, the Appearances of the *Satellits* Eclipſes and Emerſions are not to be explicated by any *Excentricity* or other Hypotheſis. But by this Allowance, they anſwer to the greateſt exactneſs. And this is a Part of Aſtronomy the moſt correct and accurately determined, as well as the moſt uſeful, of all others. For hereby Geography may be rectified, the Longitude determined, and Navigation made more eaſie and ſecure. For a Confirmation of all which, I appeal to the Labours of the Ingenious Mr. *Flamſteed* and Mr. *Halley*, to whom

Requiring time to move from place to place

whom the Learned World is for ever obliged by their Advancements of Astronomy.

Light not to be increased but by robbing some other place of its Light

(8.) A third proof that Light is a Body, is; That it cannot by any Art or Contrivance whatsoever be *increased* or *diminished*; that is to say, we cannot magnifie (for instance) the Light of the Sun or a Candle, no more than we can magnifie a Cubick Inch of Gold, or make it *more* than a Cubick Inch. But in this particular I desire to be rightly understood, lest I seem herein to advance a *Paradox*. I say therefore, Whenever we see Light increased, 'tis by Robbing of some other part of the Medium of its Light; or, by bringing the Light, that naturally should have been diffused through some other part, to the more enlightened place. Thus for Example, In a Burning-Glass, by which the Light of the Sun is highly encreased in its *Focus*, or Burning-Spot: We are first to consider, that in this Focus the Image of the Sun is projected, as being the Distinct Base of the Glass. And secondly we may observe all round about this bright Spot of the Suns Image, there is cast the strong Shadow of the whole breadth of the Burning-Glass. For all the Rays from the Sun, that would have fallen on this broad shaded space, are now brought together and crowded close in this bright Spot, there raising a vigorous *Light* and violent *Heat*. This is abundantly confirmed by an easie Experiment. For cover all the Burning-Glass, except one small round space in its middle, just the bigness of the bright burning Spot in its Focus; and tho there be a shaded space round the bright Speck, as before, yet we shall not be sensible of any *Increase* either of Light or Heat, which plainly shews, that this *Increase* of Light (when the Glass is all bare) proceeds from the crowding together of those Rays that would have fallen on the rest of the Glass, and which (were not the Glass interposed) would have fallen on the shaded space round about the bright Speck.

There

There seems but one Objection againſt what is here laid down; and that is, that Light is *increaſed* by Reflection, without depriving any place of the Light it would otherwiſe receive; or, without bringing to the enlightned part any Light that would otherwiſe eſcape it, or never come at it. But if we conſider the matter more attentively, we ſhall find it otherwiſe. For let us ſuppoſe an *Hole* of a Foot ſquare in the ſide of a Chamber, and that a Candle were placed cloſe to, and juſt before the middle of this Hole; there is but half this Candle that now enlightens this Room, the other half of the Rays proceeding directly out at the Hole: Let now a Looking-Glaſs be placed, ſo as juſt to fill up this Hole; the Rays which before would have gone out at the Hole, are now reflected into the Room; ſo that the Hemiſphere without the Chamber, which was enlightened whilſt the Hole continu'd open, is now robb'd of its Light, and all this Light is now reflected into the Room; whereby the *averſe* ſide of the Flame is made to enlighten, as well as the ſide *directly* expoſed to the Chamber. What is ſaid of this Caſe, may be accommodated to all: For ſo a Looking Glaſs lying Horizontal, and reflecting the Sun-Beams to the Ceiling of the Room, does plainly hinder the direct progreſs of the Rays to ſome other part, and conſequently robs that part of its Light. This is evident, by ſuppoſing an Hole behind the Glaſs, as in the former Caſe.

(9) From all which tis manifeſt, how vainly they attempt, who offer at *increaſing Light Uniformly*, that is, *equally* throughout the whole Sphere of a Luminous Body, or Radiating Point. Such are the Pretences of thoſe that would perſwade the World of Contrivances for making the ſmall Flame of a Lamp enlighten *ſtrongly* a whole Chappel, Hall, or Court, by being hung up in the midſt thereof. For theſe things are *impoſſible* to be effected in Nature, and they had as well pretend to *create Light*, for there is no other way of *increaſing* it, un-

Light not to be increaſed uniformly.

less by robbing another part of its Light; and then 'tis not *uniformly increased.* We have a very sensible Instance of this in the *New-invented Lanthorns,* now much used in *London*; which by the Convex-Glasses in their sides, do strongly throw those Rays along the Walks of the Passengers, which would otherwise (were the Glasses away, and the round Holes left open) be spent on parts of the Streets not frequented, whereby the untrodden parts of the Streets are robb'd of their Light, more strongly to supply and enlighten the Paths where Light is requisite.

I have insisted the longer on this particular, because there is nothing more commonly pretended, than this Invention of *increasing Light uniformly,* by those that do not consider how vain the Attempt is. I must confess, could the thing be effected, it would be a piece of *Oeconomick Philosophy,* the most pleasant and useful imaginable, and equivalent to the *perpetual Lamp* (if ever there was any such thing, as I very much doubt). The Student in his Closet, the Merchant in his Shop, the Housewife in her Offices, would find a great and pleasant Advantage therein. But above all, the *dark Northern Climates,* who are many Days, Weeks, and Months deprived of the Sun, would be infinitely obliged to the Inventor, who could make the Flame of a Lamp, no bigger than a Barly-Corn, supply the Presence of that *glorious Body.*

CHAP.

Chap. II.

Dioptrick Problem.

Why Four Convex-Glasses in a Telescope shew Objects Erect.

I Was unwilling to burden the First Part with Digressions, and therefore in *Prop.* LVI. thereof, I promised this Discourse in this place.

In the *Journal der Scavans.* For *Monday* 17. *Septemb.* 1685. Pag. 466. *Amst. Edition* We find this Passage.

'As Perspectives of *One* Convex-Glass make Objects appear
'*upright*, which those of *Two* Convex-Glasses *invert*; and again
'those of *Three rectifie*: So it should seem, that those of *Four*
'ought to *invert*. And yet Experience shews us that Objects
'appear *upright* through these Glasses. The singularity of this
'*Phænomenon* obliges all skill'd in *Dioptricks*, to enquire the
'reason thereof; but hitherto they have found none. Monf.
'*Regis*, who applies himself particularly to this Part of *Natural Philosophy*, believes that he has hit upon the Reason, and
'makes us hope that he will suddenly publish it.

Thus far the *Journal*: But does not tell us whose Remark this is: I am apt to believe, 'twas written by Monf. *Regis* himself, to the Publisher of the *Journal*.

To me this *Phænomenon* appears very easily explicable from the consideration of placing the Glasses in a Telescope. And I wonder that any one, who pretends to Skill in *Dioptricks*, should make a Difficulty of it. The posture of the Glasses in the Tube is thus; After the Object-Glass, the first Eye-Glass is placed so much distant (towards the Eye) from the Focus of the Object-Glass, as is this Focus of the Eye-Glass;

then the second or middle Eye-Glass is placed so much distant from the Focus of the first Eye-Glass, as is the Focus of this middle Eye-Glass. Lastly, the nearest or third Eye-Glass is placed so much distant from the Focus of the middle Eye-Glass, as is the Focus of this nearest Eye-Glass; and the Eye, looking through them all, is placed in the Focus of this nearest Eye-Glass.

I say therefore first, that *one single Convex-Glass*, cannot properly be said *by it self*, to shew Objects *erect* or *reverse*, but only *in respect of placing the Eye* that looks through it; and *in respect of the Objects Distance from it*. For if the Eye that looks through such a single Convex Glass, be placed nigher thereto than the Glasses Focus or *Distinct* Base, distant Objects appear *erect*: If the Eye be placed just in the Focus or Distinct Base, distant Objects are neither *erect* or *reversed*, but all in *Confusion between both*. And if the Eye be placed *farther* from the Glass than the Focus or Distinct Base, distant Objects are *reversed*.

This being laid down, I assert, secondly, That the Object-Glass of a Telescope, consisting of a Convex Object-Glass and Convex Eye-Glass, *reverses* the Object, both to the Eye-Glass, and to the Eye that looks through it. For the Eye-Glass is placed *farther* from the Object-Glass, than is the Focus of the Object-Glass. And the Eye-Glass does nothing towards the *rectifying* or *reversing*. Thus we see the *reversing* of Objects in a Telescope of two Convex Glasses, proceeds wholly from the *Object-Glass* and its *Position*; and the Eye-Glass has nothing to do in the Affair: For were the *Eye* it self in the place of the *Eye-Glass*, it would see the Object *inverted* through the single *Object-Glass*.

I come now to consider the second Eye-Glass placed after the first Eye-Glass. And here it is manifest, that placing this as it ought in a Telescope; if we place our Eye nearer to this middle Eye-Glass than its Focus the Eye sees the Object in-

verted

verted and *confused*: Place the Eye in the *Focus*, it sees the Object all in confusion, neither *erect* nor *reversed*. For here again, there is a distinct Representation of the Object to be received on a piece of Paper, as in the Focus of the Object-Glass; and the Eye being placed at any time in this place, being in the *Distinct Base*, sees all in confusion, (all which is manifest from the First Part, and therefore but lightly touch'd here). But then let the Eye be placed farther from this middle Eye-Glass than its Focus (for so is the third or immediate Eye-Glass, it being always distant from the middle Eye-Glass, the Aggregate of both their *Foci*), it perceives the Object *erect* and *confused*.

Lastly, the third or immediate Eye-Glass does nothing towards the *erecting* or *reversing* the *Species*, which it receives *erect* from the middle Eye-Glass, no more than, in a Telescope of two Convex-Glasses, the Eye-Glass does to the *Species* it receives from the Object-Glass; as is shewn before. All which will be manifest from inspection only of *Tab.* 37. *Fig.* 1.

Wherefore we are to consider the Telescope consisting of a Convex Object-Glass and three Convex Eye Glasses, as *two Telescopes*, each consisting of two Convex-Glasses. The first consists of the Object-Glass and first Eye-Glass, and this *inverts* the *Species*; that is, the *Species* is *inverted* in the *Distinct Base* of the Object Glass, and is so brought to the Eye. The *second Telescope* consists of the two *immediate Eye-Glasses*, and this *erects* what the former *inverted*; that is, the *Species* in the Distinct Base of the middle Eye Glass is *erect*, and is so brought to the Eye, by the Eye Glass. The Eye-Glasses themselves, in *either* Case, having nothing to do with the *erecting* or *inverting*, but merely in *representing* in the same posture the Image immediately before them.

The *French* Problem should not therefore have broken a Telescope of four Convex Glasses into *four Pieces*, but into *two*; and the Case would then have been plain; whereas, by breaking it into *four* Perspective-Glasses, that is attributed to *two* of them, which *neither* of them does, *viz. Inverting* and *Erecting*.

Therefore I say lastly, That *one* Convex-Glass (that is the Object-Glass) as posited in this Telescope, *inverts*: The *second* (that is the *first* Eye-Glass) does nothing towards *erecting* or *reversing*, but *represents* the Image as it is in the *Distinct Base* of the Object-Glass before it, that is, *inverted*. The *third* Glass *erects*, or rather *restores* what was before *inverted*. The *fourth* represents the Image, as it receives it from the *Distinct Base* of the *third*, that is, *erect*.

And this I think a sufficient and easie Answer to what the *French* Man makes a great Difficulty.

As a Corollary to what has been laid down in this Chapter, we may deduce this Practical Rule for combining or putting together a Telescope of *Prop.* LVI.

Take the two first Eye-Glasses, and combine them by Tryals, so as to make a Distinct Inverting Telescope of *Prop.* L.

Then take the Object-Glass and first Eye-Glass, and by Tryals combine them likewise.

Lastly, take both these Telescopes, and without altering the Distances of their Glasses in either of them singly, by Tryals combine both these Telescopes, till the Appearance be clear and distinct.

What is here done by Tryals, may be effected by actual Mensuration, or designing out the Distances of the Glasses from each other by knowing their Focal Lengths.

Chap. III.

Of Glasses for defective Eyes.

(1.) *Spectacles for old and pur-blind Men an Invention in Dioptricks of great use.* (2.) *Some Rules for choosing Spectacles both for old and pur-blind.* (3.) *Observations on Mr. Hook's Invention for helping Myopes by Convex Glasses.* (4.) *Telescopes and Microscopes adapted to defective Eyes.*

(1.) Were there no farther Use of *Dioptricks* than the Invention of *Spectacles* for the Help of defective Eyes, whether they be those of *old Men*, or those of *pur-blind Men*, I should think the Advantage that Mankind receives thereby, inferiour to no other Benefit whatsoever, not absolutely requisite to the support of Life. For as the *Sight* is the most noble and extensive of all our Senses; as we make the most frequent and constant use of our Eyes in all the actions and concerns of human Life; surely that Instrument that relieves the Eyes when decay'd, and supplies their Defects, rendring them useful, when otherwise almost useless, must needs, of all others, be esteemed of the greatest Advantage. In what a miserable condition do we count those, in whom it hath pleased the *great Contriver of the Eyes and Sight*, to shut those two little Windows of the Soul? And we may imagine, that they, in whom these Lights are but *partly* obscured, do in some measure partake of the Misery of the blind. How melancholy is the condition of him, who only enjoys the Sight of what is immediately about him? With what Disadvantage is he ingaged in most of the Concerns of human Life? Reading is to him troublesome, War more than ordinary dangerous, Trade and

Spectacles for old and pur-blind Men, an Invention of great use.

Condition of old Men deplorable without Spectacles.

and Commerce toilsome and unpleasant. And so likewise, on the other hand; How forlorn would the latter part of most Mens Lives prove, unless *Spectacles* were at hand to help our Eyes, and a little form'd piece of Glass supply'd the Decays of Nature? The curious Mechanick, engaged in any minute Works, could no longer follow his Trade than till the 50th. or 60th. Year of his Age: The Scholar no longer converse with his Books, or with an absent Friend in a Letter. All after would be melancholy Idleness, or he must content himself to use another Man's Eyes for every Line. Thus forlorn was the state of most *old Men*, and many *young*, before this admirable Invention, which, on this very account, can never be prized too highly.

Rules for Choosing Spectacles both for old and pur-blind

(2.) And because in the First Part hereof, *Prop* XXVIII and XLV. I have but slightly touched on the proper Method for helping *defective Eyes*; I think it convenient to prosecute that matter more fully in this place. Always supposing what foregoes in the First Part as understood.

First therefore for helping the Eyes of *old Men*, as being more frequently and universally requisite than the Relief of pur-blind Eyes.

In the First Part (*Prop.* XXVIII. Sec. 8. and *Prop.* XXXI) we learn, that a *Convex-Glass* is here to be used: For these seeing *distant* Objects *distinctly*, and *nigh* Objects *confusedly*, must use such Glasses for reading, &c. as make *nigh* Objects appear *as distant*, or, which bring the Rays from each single Point in a *nigh* Object, as if they came from a more *distant* Point. Or thus, seeing the Crystallines of *old Men* are *too flat* for *nigh* Objects, that is, want *Convexity*; we are to help them by adding to them an artificial or adventitious Convexity of a Glass. But then our enquiry must be, What is a *Proper* Convexity to this or that *particular* Eye? And because reading, or working curious small Works, as being engaged upon *nigh* Objects, are

the

the chief Imployments wherein *Spectacles* are requisite. I shall suppose our Enquiry chiefly designed for this purpose. And indeed, tho there can hardly be any Rules laid down, *strictly* to determin this matter; for *distinct* Sight may consist within a *great* Latitude: Yet if we observe the following Directions, we shall be apt to err less, and to fit our Eyes better with *Spectacles*, than if we observed no Rule at all, but chose at a venture.

First, When we first find our selves begin to require *Spectacles*, let us make choice of the *flattest Convexities*, that will possibly help our Eyes. These are usually called *Young Spectacles*. There are many ways of finding out and trying *such*, but none more ready, obvious, and easie, than trying with which one can read a small Print distinctly, with the Book *farthest* from the Eyes; or try which *Spectacles* burn at the greatest distance, for these *Spectacles* are the most proper for those Eyes to use, and shall prejudice the Sight less, and preserve it longest of any.

We may note likewise, that the distance of the Print, or Object from the Eye continuing the *same*, a Convex-Glass may be said to be *older* or *younger*, according as it is removed *farther from* or *nigher to* the Eye or Object. This is manifest from the Doctrine in the First Part, concerning the *Locus Apparens* of an Object through such a Glass. To which therefore I refer.

Secondly. If your naked Eyes can read a moderate Print at the full extent of your Arms, or at the distance of about two Feet or two and an half; and you desire a Pair of *Spectacles* to read with, at the usual Distance of reading, *viz.* about a Foot or little more: Procure a Pair of Glasses of such a Convexity, that an Object being exposed before them at the Distance of about a Foot, they may have their *Imaginary Focus*, or the *apparent Place* of the Object, distant from them about two, or two Feet and an half. All which may be easily obtained and effected by the Doctrine in the First Part.

Barrow, Lect Opt 14 p 103.

E e

In the next place, for relieving the Eyes of the *short-sighted*, *pur-blind*, or *Myopes*. We must consider, that these, laboring under the contrary Defect with *old Men* (for they see *nigh* Objects *distinctly*, but *distant* Objects *confusedly*), must be relieved with a Remedy of a contrary effect; and therefore they are helped by *Concave-Glasses*, which bring the Rays of *distant* Objects into the Eye, as if they were *nigh*. And because we may conceive the Crystallines of these Eyes as too *protuberant* or *convex*, therefore we are to take off from this too great *Convexity*, by adding an adventitious *Concavity*. But then, there is nothing so universally complained of by those who are thus affected, as the Difficulty they find in fitting proper Glasses to their Eyes. For the removal whereof, the following Rules may be observed.

First, That for viewing *distant* Objects, according to what is noted in the First Part, *Prop.* XLV. If a *short-sighted* Person can read distinctly, or see Objects at the distance of a Foot from his naked Eye; a *Concave Glass*, whose *Virtual*-Focal-Length is a Foot, makes such a Person see distant Objects distinctly. And so of any otherwise disposed Eye. So that knowing the Distance at which a pur-blind Person reads distinctly with *unarmed* Eyes, 'tis easie, by the Doctrine in the First Part, to assign him a proper Glass for his Eye to see *distant* Objects.

Secondly, For Glasses proper for *Myopes* to *read* by, or to see Objects at the distance of about a Foot and half. Let us suppose Eyes so affected, as not to be able to read, but at the distance of Four Inches, and that we desire Glasses for these Eyes to read by, at the ordinary distance of about a Foot and half. Let us form such *Concave*-Glasses, which, being exposed to an Object at the distance of a Foot and half, may have their *Virtual respective* Focus at the distance of four Inches. And so likewise for any other Distance. All which is easily performed by those versed in the First Part of this Work.

Barrow,
Lect Opt
14 p 102

Thirdly,

Thirdly, We are to note, that *Myops* shall require *different* Glasses for viewing Objects at *different* Distances. But the visive Faculty not being contained within such strict and determined Limitations; that Glass which is useful at an Object an hundred Foot distant, shall serve likewise at an Object distant fifty Foot; but then 'tis not so helpful at one distant five Foot. But another may be had proper even for this Distance, and not so useful at an Object distant an hundred or fifty Foot. All which is manifest from the Doctrine in the First Part.

Fourthly, There are some Eyes so ill conformed, that no Glasses whatever will relieve them. Of this I have often heard a very ingenious Man and great Philosopher Sir *William Petty* often complain in his own particular. But then this proceeds not from a *too little*, or *too great* a Convexity in the Crystalline; but from some other Indisposition or ill Configuration, not to be relieved by Glasses.

Lastly, Persons *pur-blind* labour under this great Inconvenience, that the Glasses which relieve them in one particular, do hinder their strong Vision of distant Objects in another particular. For as Concave-Glasses do order the Rays from any one single Point, properly to be received by the Eye of a *Myops*: So at the same time, they *diminish* the Appearance of the whole Object. And from hence it is, that tho these sort of Eyes may be well enough relieved for *Reading* and *Writing* at a *convenient* distance, and for seeing pretty large Objects at the distance of 100, 200, or 500 Foot, yet for Objects *much farther*, unless they be very *large* indeed, they are not so easily supply'd.

(3.) And here I cannot but take notice of an ingenious intimation of Mr. *Hooks* (to whom the World is certainly much obliged for his curious Contrivances in *Mechanicks*, and his other Philosophick Indeavours) published in *Num.* 3 of the *Philosophical Collections*. Lond. 1681. which he calls *Myopibus Juvamen*.

M Hook's Contrivance for helping Myopes considered.

'Tis briefly this, That some sort of *short-sighted* Persons, who cannot be relieved by *Concave* Glasses, may perhaps find some help in *Convex*-Glasses; their Eyes being removed at a convenient distance farther from these Glasses than their *Distinct Bases*. As for reading by these Glasses; the Book must be *inverted*, and then the Image in the *Distinct Base* shall be *erect*, and the Eye shall perceive it *erect*. As for Writing, the Difficulty is greater than mentioned by the *Learned Author*: For the *Myops* must not only learn to write *inverted*, but also *retrograde*, *viz.* from the Right to the Left Hand; and, what is yet more inconvenient, from the bottom towards the top of the Page; which is hardly practicable on account of blotting the wet Writing. As for viewing *distant Objects* with these Glasses, I acknowledg with the ingenious Author, that much of the Disagreableness of the *inverted Prospect* is taken off by use and custom, as I my self have experienced by my frequent use of inverting Telescopes. But yet I cannot go so far with the Author, as to assent to his Deduction from hence; which is, that 'tis only use and custom that makes us judge Objects *erect* that are perceived by an *inverted* Image on the Fund of the Eye. For then a Man *standing on his Head*, should judge the Trees and other Objects he sees *inverted*, which no one in his Senses will do, but rather judge what is right, *viz.* that he himself is *inverted*, whilst the circumjacent Objects continue *erect*. This will be more evident to us, by considering the case of an adult Person, who has been blind from his Birth, and now suddenly restored to his Sight: He is not prejudiced by custom, and yet (doubtless) would judge as is usual. But lastly, an other great Difficulty that will attend the use of these Spectacles for *Myopes*, is, that they must be carried at such a *distance* from the Eyes, that it will be very troublesom to manage them commodiously. And if to this again we add the distance requisite for the Object, I question whether some Mens Arms will be long enough to manage a Pen for Writing, or turning the Leaves of a Book.

I have been the longer on this Proposal; becauſe the *Worthy Author* does candidly invite all, to communicate to the Publick, what real Benefit by it, or Objections againſt it, they ſhall find

(4) I ſhall conclude this Chapter with the way of Adapting *Teleſcopes* and *Microſcopes* to *defective Eyes*. Which is briefly thus,

Adapting Teleſcopes and Microſcopes to defective Eyes.

A Teleſcope compoſed of a *Convex* Object-Glaſs and *Concave* Eye-Glaſs, being apply'd to an *old* Eye, the Eye-Glaſs may be a little *farther* removed from the Object-Glaſs than ordinarily: On the contrary, in ſuch a *Teleſcope* for the Eye of a *Myops*, the Eye Glaſs may be removed a little *nigher* to the Object-Glaſs; the reaſon hereof is manifeſt from what has been delivered in the Firſt Part. But then, *how much farther*, or *nigher* they are to be removed, is only to be determined by Experiment, and by every ones fitting the Glaſs to his own Eye.

And ſo likewiſe in Teleſcopes compoſed of a *Convex* Object-Glaſs, and *Convex* Eye-Glaſs: For the Eye of an *old Man*, the Eye-Glaſs may be removed a little *farther* from the Object-Glaſs, or from the *Diſtinct Baſe*. And for the Eye of a *Myops* a little *nigher* to the Object Glaſs, than for Eyes *naturally* and *orderly* affected.

In like manner for *Microſcopes*, Firſt the ſimple or ſingle Convex for an *old* Eye, is to be removed a little *farther* from the Object, and for a *Myops*, a little *nigher* the Object, than the uſual poſture.

And ſo in *Double Microſcopes*. For an old Eye, the Eye-Glaſs is to be a little *farther* from the Object-Glaſs or *Diſtinct Baſe*, and for a *Myops*, a little *nigher* the Object-Glaſs or *Diſtinct Baſe* And becauſe in theſe, the *Diſtinct Baſe* is brought nigher to, or farther from the Eye-Glaſs (without altering the

Diſtance

Diſtance of the Eye-Glaſs and Object-Glaſs), only by removing the whole Microſcope *nigher to* or *farther from* the very Object: This latter Motion effects the ſame as the former, and therefore may be uſed for *old* or *ſhort* Sights inſtead of the former.

Chap. IV.

Of Mechanick-Dioptricks,

(1.) *Chief Authors that have treated of Grinding or Forming Optick-Glaſſes.* (2.) *For trying whether a Glaſs be not plain.* (3.) *For finding the Focal Lengths of Glaſſes.* (4.) *Concerning the Centre of a Glaſs.* (5.) *For trying the Regularity and Goodneſs of an Object-Glaſs.* (6.) *Managing great Glaſſes, and the Author's Treating thereof.* (7.) *Proportioning Glaſſes in Teleſcopes* (8.) *Mr. Hooks's Contrivance for making an Object-Glaſs of a ſmall Sphere ſerve a long Tube.*

Authors treating of Glaſs-grinding

(1.) I Deſign not in this Chapter to deliver at large the ſeveral ways of Grinding and Forming *Optick Glaſſes*, the manner of making the *Forms*, *Tools*, or *Diſhes* wherein they are ſhaped; or the various *Machines* contrived by ſeveral ingenious Heads for this purpoſe: For this may juſtly require a particular Treatiſe by it ſelf. And becauſe nothing of this kind has ever yet appeared in Engliſh, according as I find the preſent Work accepted, I may perhaps hereafter attempt ſomething in this way, for the ſatisfaction of ſome ingenious *Engliſh* Spirits, who may be inclinable to offer at theſe Exerciſes. In the mean time, they that are Maſters of the Languages wherein they are written, may apply themſelves to *Pere Cherubin's Dioptrique Oculaire*, and *Zahn's Oculus Artificialis*; wherein they will find an abundance on this Subject. But after all that can be writ concerning it, Practice and Experience will find out many

Cherubin
Zahn

many Conveniencies and Inconveniencies, which can hardly be committed to Words, or described; and therefore this is at last the best Instructour. But here I shall mention the chief Modern Authors that have contrived *Engines* for Grinding Glasses, that those who please may consult them. Mr. *Hook* in his *Micrographia* describes an Engine for this purpose. *Hevelius* in his *Selenographia, Chap.* I, II. describes another for Modelling the Forms or Dishes for Grinding Spherick Glasses. And in the First Part of his *Machina Cœlestis, Chap.* XXIII. describes one for Grinding *Conick-Glasses*. *Ant. Mar. Schyrleus de Rheita* in his *Oculus Enoch & Eliæ, Lib.* IV. has a Machine for *Conick-Glasses*. *Maignan* at the end of his *Perspectiva Horaria* describes Machines both for Spherick and Conick-Glasses. *Des-Cartes* in his *Dioptricks* has another for *Conick-Glasses*. Monſ. *Borelly* has given the World the Secret of his manner of Grinding great Glasses in Cypher, *Journal des Scavans, Ann.* 1676. *July* 6. but has not yet obliged us with the Discovery: Tho he be a Person of the greatest Candor and Freedom, and the most communicative, as I am obliged to express with much Gratitude for his Civilities shew'd me in *Paris* 1685. at which time he gave me an Object-Glass formed by this way for a Telescope 24 Foot long. The celebrated Monſ. *Fatio de Duillier* (of whom Dr. *Burnet* gives deservedly so excellent a Character in his Letters of Travails) in the *Journal des Scavans, Ann.* 1684. *Novemb.* 20. describes an Invention of his own, for exactly forming the Dishes for Grinding Spherick Glasses; which indeed is very ingenious, and perfectly new. But I cannot tell how easily it may be practised, without some farther Improvement; for his Contrivances of the Block *c*, and of the Screws *d, g*, (I refer to his Figure) seem not to have all the Motions requisite, to keep the Point *e* exactly *true* to the Axis of the little Telescope *h k*.

The

Wren. The Incomparable Sir *Christopher Wren*, our *English Archimedes, Apollonius, Diophantus,* proposes his Contrivance for Forming *Hyperbolick* Glasses, Num. 48. and 53. of the *Philosophic. Transact.*

Conick-Glasses not better than Spherick From Mr Newton But all farther Endeavours for Forming *Conick-*Glasses, which have hitherto been wholly frustrated and unsuccessful, may now be put to a full stop, when we hear in this matter the Opinion of as great a Philosopher and Mathematician, as this or any Age could ever boast of, *The Celebrated Mr.* Newton *of* Cambridge, who in his profound Treatise, *Philosophiæ Naturalis Principia Mathematica,* has fathom'd the greatest Depths of Nature, and laid a Foundation for Posterity to raise an infinite Superstructure. Thus he, in the First Book, *Schol. ad Prop.* XCVIII. *Ad usus autem Opticos, &c.* In *English* as follows, *But for all Optick Uses, Spherick Figures are the most commodious. If the Object-Glasses of Telescopes were composed of two Spherick-Glasses containing Water between them, perhaps the Irregularity of the Refractions that are made on the Surfaces of the Glasses towards their edges, may be accurately enough corrected by the Refractions of the Water. And such Object-Glasses are preferable to Elleptick or Hyperbolick Glasses; not only because they are easier and more accurately to be formed; but also because they refract more accurately those Pencils of Rays that are* (collateral or) *out of the Glasses Axis. But the different Refrangibility of different Rays, will for ever hinder us from perfecting Opticks by Glasses either of Spherick, or any other Figures whatsoever. And unless we can correct the Errors that arise from hence, all our Labour is lost in other Corrections.*

And indeed if we consider it right, we shall find it impossible, by whatever Figures to render the Appearance of the *Collateral* Parts of an Object so *distinct* as the *direct*; for the very natural Eye does it not; and therefore we are forced to apply it successively *directly* before the Parts of any Object we design to view: And we may well despair to perform by Art,

more

more than what the Almighty Framer of the Eye has given us a Pattern for.

What this *Great Man* means by the *Different Refrangibility of Different Rays*, We may find, *Num.* 80. *p.* 3075. *N.* 83. *p* 4059. *N.* 84. *p.* 4087. *N.* 85. *p* 5004. *N.* 88. *p.* 5084. *N.* 110. *p.* 217. *N.* 121. *p.* 499. *N.* 123. *p.* 556. *N.* 128. *p.* 692: of the *Philosoph. Transactions*; wherein he lays down a perfectly new and most ingenious Theory of *Light*. {*Different Refrangibility of Rays.*}

In the same Tracts, *Num.* 81, 82, 83. we may find an Account of a new *Cata-Dioptrical Telescope*, invented by this same excellent Person. {*Cata-Dioptrick Telescope.*}

(2.) All that I shall offer at more in this Chapter, is, to lay down some practical Rules for finding the *Foci* and *Centres* of Glasses; with some other *Accidental Remarks*, that may be requisite to the clearer understanding and performance of some Precepts delivered in this Treatise. {*Trying whether a Glass be not plain.*}

The Object-Glasses of Telescopes are generally of so little Curvity on their Superficies, that by *looking on* them or by *feeling* them, it cannot be discovered, whether they are *plain* or of a *Spherick* Figure; or which is formed on a Sphere of a *greater*, which of a *lesser* Radius. To find this (as I have said before, in *Schol. Prop.* XXXI. *Part* I.) we are to shake the Glass nimbly at our Arms length before the Eye; and if the Objects seen through it seem to *dance* or *move*, the Glass is not plain. And that Glass which makes the Objects seem the most to move is formed on the *less* Sphere, whether *Convex* or *Concave*.

(3.) When we have thus found our Glasses to be *Spherick*. Then supposing them *Convex*, there are several Methods for finding their *Foci*. I shall lay down some of the plainest and most certain. {*For finding the Foci of Glasses.*}

First, for Glasses of pretty deep Convexities (that is, of small Spheres), apply them to the end of a Scale of Inches and Decimal Parts, and expose them before the Sun; and upon the

F f Scale,

Scale, we shall find the bright Intersection of the Rays exactly measured out. Or expose them in the Hole of a dark Chamber; and where a white Paper receives the distinct Representation of *distant* Objects, there is the Focus of this Glass. This is an universal and certain way for all Convexes. For a Glass of a pretty long *Focus*, observe some distant Objects through it, and recede from the Glass, till the Eye perceive all in *confusion*, or till the Objects begin just to appear *inverted*; here the Eye is in the Focus. If it be a Plano-Convex Glass, make it reflect the Sun against a Wall; we shall on the Wall perceive two sorts of Light, one more *bright* within an other more *obscure*; withdraw the Glass from the Wall, till the *bright* Image is at its smallest; the Glass is then distant from the Wall about the fourth part of its *Focal* Length. If it be a double Convex, expose each side to the Sun in like manner, and observe *both* the Distances of the Glass from the Wall: The first Distance is about half the Radius of the Convexity turned from the Sun, and the second Distance is about half the Radius of t'other Convexity likewise: Thus we have the Radii of the two Convexities; whence the Focus is determined by *Prop.* III. *Part* I. The reason hereof depends on the Doctrine of *Catoptricks*.

But the most exact way of determining the just Focal Length of the Object-Glass of a Telescope, is what I shall lay down in *Chap.* V. *Sec.* 4. of this Part, which, because I must necessarily deliver in that place, I will not here anticipate.

Foci of Concaves   The Foci of Concaves are obtained by *Reflection*; for as a *Concave Mirror* or *Speculum* burns at the distance of about half the Radius of the Concavity; so a *Concave Glass* being supposed a *Reflecting Speculum*, shall unite the Rays of the Sun, at the distance of about half the Radius of the Cavity.

Concerning the Centres of Glasses   (4.) Before we proceed to the *Centration* of Glasses, we are to recollect the 18th. *Definition* of the First Part, wherein we define the *Axis of a Glass*. I say therefore, when the *Axis* of a Glass passes directly through the Centre of the Glasses Breadth, or roundness of its Aperture, that Glass is said to be *truly centred*. And this will always be so when the Glass is *equally thick* round the edges of its *Aperture*. But this will be more intelligible by a Scheme *Tab.* 40. *Fig.* 1. Let *a g d e a* be a Plano-Convex. T.40.F.1. Glass, much thicker towards the Edge *d e*, than towards *a*; let *a g* be equal to *g d*, *g* is the *Centre* of this Glass, for 'tis the middle Point of its Aperture or Breadth. But then this Glass is not *truly centered*: For, to *l* the Centre of the Convexity *a g d* draw *g l*, I say *g l* is not the Axis of this Glass; but if there may an other Line *l k* be drawn, whose Portion within the Glass *i k* is greater than *h g* (as in this Case it may easily be demonstrated. For *l k* = *l g* and *l h* more than *l i*. For ∠ *l i h* = Rect. therefore *h g* less than *k i*) and which being perpendicular to the plain Surface *a e*, as well as to the Convex Surface *a k d*; *l k* must consequently be the Axis of this Glass. Wherefore *k* is the *true Centre* of this Glass. And because, to compleat this Glass, there is wanting the Portion *d f e*; therefore to make the true Centre of the Glass *k*, coincident with the middle Point of its Breadth or Aperture; we are to make *k b* equal to *k d*; and then we are to cut off, or to cover the Portion of the Glass *b a c* equal to *d f e*; and so we obtain the *compleat* and *truly Centered* Glass *c b k d e c*. The same may be understood of *double Convexes*, without farther Explication.

But because in Object-Glasses of even moderate Lengths, 'tis impossible by the Eye, or any Admeasurement of their Thickness, to know whether they be *truly Centered*: Therefore we must have recourse to some other Methods, that may shew this. And these are various.

First, Holding the Glasses at a due distance from the Eye, let us observe the two reflected Images of a Candle; and where these two Images *unite* or *coalesce*, there is the *true Centre* of the Glass; if this be in the *middle* of the Glasses *Breadth*, the Glass is *truly Centred*; if not, we are to rectifie it, shall be declared hereafter.

A second way is, By presenting the Glass before the Sun, and making it reflect the Light on a Plain nighly parallel to its Surface, at a proper distance; and we shall perceive two sorts of Light reflected; one *smaller*, but much more *strong* and *vigorous*, within another more faint and large. Then by a due posture of the Glass (found by Tryals) both these Lights are to be projected as round as possible; and at a proper distance from the Wall on which they are reflected; the *round brightest* Spot is to be brought into the smallest compass that it can (Tryal will make all this plain). When the Glass is in this posture, if the *bright* Spot be projected just in the middle of the fainter Light, the Glass is *well centred*. If it be projected to the Left Hand of this middle, the Glass is thickest towards the Left Hand Edge. And so to whatever side of the faint Light, this bright Spot is projected, on *that side* is the Glass *thickest*; and on *that side* lies the *true Centre*. The reason hereof I shall explain in a Plano-Convex-Glass, and is the same in a double Convex; *mutatis mutandis*. For the bright Spot is the Image of the Sun projected by the curve Surface of the Glass consider'd as a *reflecting Speculum* (whereof more hereafter), and the faint Light is the Reflection of the Sun from the other plain Surface. *Tab. 40. Fig. 2. a d e* is a Plano-Convex-Glass, thicker towards the side *d e* than towards *a*. Let the Curvity *a d* (whose Centre is *c*) be exposed directly to the Sun: By the known Laws of *Catoptricks*, the Parallel Rays (from the middle Point of the Sun, for instance) falling on the Curvity (which parallel Rays in the Figure are expressed by continued Lines), are united in the Focus at *f*, distant from the Curvity about half its Radius, there causing a brisk Light and Heat. In the mean time these parallel Rays do fall on the plain Surface *a e* obliquely, and

and are reflected thereby alongst the prickt Lines; and these are they which cause the *faint* Light. Now 'tis manifest, that if a Plain at *f*, parallel to the plain Surface *a e*, received these two Reflections, the *bright* Light at *f* would not be found in the middle of the *faint* Light: For here we see the *faint* Light is thrown much to one side. And the *bright* Light *f* is projected upwards from the middle of the *faint* Light; for the Glass is thickest upwards towards its Edge *d e*.

The third Way of Examining the *Centres* of Glasses is yet more *compleat* than the former; for it does not only discover the Fault (if there be any, as in long Object-Glasses 'tis very rare but there is; especially if they be wrought in the Form by the unguided Hand, and not by Engine), but withal, it rectifies the Fault. 'Tis thus; Cover the Surface of the Glass with a thin piece of Paper, in which there is cut a round Hole of about an Inch diameter, and round about this Hole there are to be struck two or three Concentrick Circles; move this Paper upon the Glass, till you see, on the plain that receives the reflected Light, that the *bright* Spot is exactly in the middle of the other fainter Light round it. This also one may measure by a Pair of Compasses, having, to that end, slightly fixed the Paper to the Glass, that we may more nicely determine, whether this *bright* Spot be exactly in the middle. This therefore being carefully adjusted by gently sliding the Paper on the Glass (if it be requisite), we are, without the least altering this *true* Position of the Paper, to fix it more firmly *to* the Glass. And laying it thus on a Table, let us mark on the Glass (by the Point of a Diamond) three Points in one of the Circumferences Concentrick to the round Hole in the Paper. And sticking a small piece of Cement on the Glass about the middle of the round Hole; by means of the three marked Points, let us find the exact Centre of this round Hole. Then uncovering the whole Glass (except only the Cement

ment in which the Centre is marked), with a Diamond-pointed Compass, let us strike as large a Circle on the Glass, as its Breadth will bear. Then *round* the Glass according to this Circle, and 'tis as exactly *centred* as the Sense can judge.

But note, That whereas I have said that the *brighter* Spot is smaller than the *fainter;* and that the *brighter* Light is to be reflected *into* the *middle* of the *fainter.* This is to be understood, supposing the Breadth of the Glass will *allow* it. For the Glass may be so narrow, that the Projection of the bright Image of the Sun may be *broader* than the Breadth of the Glass. But this happens so seldom in Practice, that I pass it over.

Pere Cherubin, who is often very nice in matters of little moment, and loose enough in those of greater weight and absolute necessity, describes an implicated Contrivance for true Centring of Glasses. *Vision Parfait.* Tom. II. p. 109.

For trying the Regularity and Goodness of an Object-Glass.

(5.) The same Frier lays down a Way of Examining the Regularity and Goodness of an Object-Glass, *pag.* 25. which it may not be amiss here to insert. After we have *centred* the Object-Glass as well as we can, by the foregoing Method: To try the Regularity of its Form to the greatest exactness, *says he,* We must do thus. On a Paper strike two Concentrick Circles; one whose Diameter is the same with the Breadth of the Object-Glass; t'other of half that Diameter. This inward Circumference divide into six equal Parts, by the known way of applying the Radius six times in the Circumference, and making six fine small Holes therein with a Needle. Let us cover one side of the Glass with this Paper; and then exposing it to the Sun, we are to receive the Rays that pass through these six Holes on a Plain at a just distance from the Glass. And by withdrawing or approaching this Plain from or to the Glass, we shall find, whether the Rays that pass through these six Holes unite exactly together at any distance

from

from the Glass; if they do, we may be assured of the Regularity of this Glass, that is, of its *just Form*. And at the same time we obtain exactly the Glasses *Focal Length*.

But after all, there is no better way for trying the Excellency of an Object-Glass, than by placing it in a Tube; and trying it with small Eye-Glasses at several distant Objects. For that Object-Glass that represents the Objects the *brightest* and most *distinct*, and bears the *greatest Aperture*, and *most* Convex or Concave Eye-Glass, without colouring or Haziness, is surely the best. The most convenient Object to try them at, is the *Title Page* of a large Book; wherein there are generally Letters printed of divers Magnitudes, and therefore affords variety of small Objects; whereby the comparative Excellency of Object Glasses may be nicely estimated. This the Celebrated Monsf. *Cassini*, the *French* King's Astronomer, shew'd me when I visited him at the *Observatory* in *Paris*, *Ann.* 1685. who tryed all his Glasses by the large Title-Page of a Book, fixt inverted on the Jaume of a Steeple Window more than ½ of a Mile distant from the *Observatoire*.

(6) The next Piece of *Mechanick-Dioptricks*, which I shall mention, is, The *Managing Great Glasses*. And herein I shall not swell this Volume with describing those sumptuous Contrivances and costly Machines invented for this purpose: It shall suffice me to refer the Reader to the Original Authors, where he may find them described at large. *Managing great Glasses.*

Hevelius in his *Machina Cœlestis*, Part. I. Cap. 19, 20, 21, 22. describes the Engines he used for his Telescopes. And amongst others, a Contrivance for managing his Tube of 60 Foot, and another of 150 Foot long. *Hevelius.*

The deservedly Celebrated Monsf. *Hugens*, one of the chief Mathematick Luminaries of the present Age, has publish'd a small Tract, *Astroscopia Compendiaria*, designed only for Describing his way of Managing great Glasses with very little trouble *Hugens.*

ble, and without a Tube. This I am sure is no barren Speculation of the Ingenious Author's, but succesfully practised by him; as I can gratefully testifie, having had the favour of being shewn the whole Contrivance by the Excellent Author himself in his Garden at the *Hague*, Ann. 1685. at which

Planetary Clock time I had the happiness also of seeing his *Planetary Clock*, or *Moving Ephemeris*, a Machine that cannot be sufficiently admired.

Cusset. Monsi. *Cusset*, an ingenious *French Man* of *Lions*, has publish'd his Contrivance for managing great Glasses, in the *Journal des Scavans*, Ann. 1685. May 18.

Monsi. *Cassini*, when I was with him at the *Observatoir* in *Paris* (amongst other Curiosities, which according to his usual Candour and Civility he communicated to me) shew'd me two very pretty Contrivances for managing great Glasses; which, because not yet publick, I shall describe as well as I can by Memory at this distance of time. The first was a plain Piece of Clock-work, moved by a Spring and regulated by a Pendulum Vibrating half Seconds. This carried an Arm that stood something prominent from the Body of the Work; which Arm at its extremity carried the Object-Glass fixt in a Ring. This Arm and the Object-Glass, by means of graduated Arches in the Clock-work could be turned *ad Libitum* directly to any Star. Thus suppose *Saturn* were to be observed; by a common *Ephemeris*, knowing his Longitude and Latitude, together with the Time of Day or Night, the Arches of the Clock being put to such and such Divisions, and the Machine it self placed with such or such a part horizontal or perpendicular; the Object-Glass was of course directly exposed to the Star. Then the Pendulum being put in motion, the Machine kept the Glass constantly exposed directly to the Star in its diurnal Motion. This whole Machine then, being placed upon an Height, carried the Object-Glass in its due position; and the *Observer below* managed

the

the Eye-Glass by his free Hand, assisted with a *Rest*. Tho I cannot retain so exact a Remembrance of this Engine, as to venture at a Scheme of the particular Parts; yet this Description perhaps will be sufficient to give the ingenious Astronomer an Idea thereof, so as to apprehend the Contrivance in general. Something much of the same kind may we find described in Mr. *Hooks Animadversions on Hevelius Mach. Cœlestis.* p. 66, 67, 68, *&c.*

The other Contrivance he mentioned to me, if I forget not, he or Monf. *Borelly* told me, was due to Monf. *Azout*. It is thus, From the Tube of a small Telescope there stands out an Arm perpendicular to the side of this smaller Tube: This Arm carries the great Object-Glass, then an Observer upon an Height manages this small Telescope, following therewith the Motion of a Star; by which means the great Object-Glass (being parallel to the Object Glass of this lesser Telescope) is kept constantly in prosecution of this same Star: Then the other Observer *below* manages the Eye-Glass as before.

These two Contrivances are indeed pretty Thoughts; but I cannot promise that they can be so easily practised; unless the Machines that carry the great Object-Glass be made to *rise* and *fall* at pleasure, as the Star rises or sets. For otherwise, the Observer that manages the Eye-Glass, shall soon lose the sight of his Object; unless he have the opportunity of *rising* and *falling*, by some such Contrivance as the forementioned Monf. *Cusset* proposes in the fore-cited place. But this is vastly chargeable.

'Tis now above seven Years since Monf. *Boffat* of *Tholouse* has promised the World his Contrivance for managing great Glasses, of which he has given a small Specimen in the *Journal des Scavans* 1682. Dec. 28. but we hear nothing farther of it; perhaps because the Contrivance requires *reflecting Speculums*, which much weaken the light of the Object, and are therefore found useless.

Proportioning of Glasses in Telescopes and Microscopes

(7.) I may reckon another Piece of *Mechanick Dioptricks*, The *proportioning* of the Glasses in Telescopes and Microscopes. We have said before, that, of two or more Object-Glasses of the same Focal Lengths; that is the best, which will bear an Eye-Glass of the greatest Convexity (this is usually called the Deepest Charge). But yet there are some Proportions to be observed, which Experience has found out, as the most convenient and best adapted for most Mens Eyes, that are well disposed. For so a good Object-Glass of 12 or 13 Feet, will bear a *Charge* of 3 Inches, better than a *Charge* much *deeper* or *shallower*.

But moreover, In adapting an Eye-Glass to an Object-Glass, respect is likewise to be had to the *Object* we contemplate; for Objects of a sedate Light, as *Saturn, Jupiter, &c.* will allow deeper *Charges,* than those of a more brisk and strong Light, as *Venus, &c.*

Wherefore this whole Affair being only the Subject of Experiment, to that I shall refer, and only hint by the bye; That for Telescopes of three Convex Eye-Glasses, *Cherubin* advises (*Dioptrique Oculaire,* III. *Par. Sec.* 2. *Cap.* VII. *pag.* 188.) that, of the three Eye-Glasses, that next the Object-Glass should be of the *deepest* Charge, the middle Eye-Glass ought to be something *shallower,* and the immediate Eye-Glass the *shallowest* of all.

For Proportioning Glasses in *double* Microscopes, we may consult the same Author. But 'tis tedious to transcribe.

The LV. *Prop.* of the First Part, relates to the *Apertures* of Object-Glasses. After which, we have nothing to add in this place; which otherwise might have been challenged by a Discourse thereon, as being of a *Mechanick* Consideration.

M Hooks Contrivance to make a Glass of a small Sphere serve a long Tube

(8.) The last Piece of *Mechanick Dioptricks* I shall mention, is an ingenious Thought of Mr. *Hooks,* for making a short Object Glass perform the part of one formed on a much larger Sphere.

'Prepare

"Prepare (says he) two Glasses, the one exactly flat on "both sides, the other flat on the one side, and Convex on "the other, of what Sphere you please. Let the flat Glass be "a little broader than tother. Then let there be made a "Cell or Ring of Brass very exactly turned, into which these "two Glasses may be so fastened with Cement, that the plain "Surfaces of them may lye exactly parallel, and that the Con-"vex-side of the Plano Convex-Glass may lye inward, but "so as not to touch the flat of the other Glass. These being "cemented into the Ring very closely about the edges: By a "small Hole in the side of the Brass Ring or Cell, fill the "interposed space between these two with *Water, Oyl of Tur-*"*pentine, Spirit of Wine, Saline Liquors, &c.* then stop the Hole "with a Screw: And according to the differing Refraction of "the interposed Liquors, so shall the Focus of this compoud "Glass be longer or shorter. *Vid. Philosoph. Transf. Num.* 12. *pag.* 202.

This, I must confess is an ingenious Hint: But I doubt the desired Effect will not be so successfully attained thereby, so as to constitute an Object-Glass for a Telescope. For certainly, were it effectual; 'tis so easie and withal so useful, that before this time it would have obtained, and been practised *universally*. And this makes me question, whether it would be of any better effect, than a *Meniscus-Glass*, or a Combined Glass of *Prop.* XVII. *Part.* I.

Chap. V.

Of Telescopick-Instruments.

(1) *Controversie between* Hevelius *and* Hook *concerning Telescopick Sights.* (2.) Hevelius's *Objections against them. His Mistake concerning them.* (3.) *Their Fabrick or Contrivance.* (4.) *Adjusting them to plain Rulers or Tubes.* (5.) *To Quadrants, Sextants, &c.* (6.) *Dioptrick Reason of their Performance.* (7.) *Adapting the* Micrometer *to a* Telescope.

Controversie between Hevelius and Hook concerning Telescopick-Sights.

(1.) THE Fame of *Johannes Hevelius, Consul of Dantzick,* is deservedly celebrated by all that delight in Astronomy. His Performances herein are highly extoll'd by all; and the sumptuous Volumes of his Labours and Studies, which he has published, have procured him an immortal Name of Honour amongst the Literate. But notwithstanding all his commendable Endeavours, he has not yet arrived at the height of perfection, but something is yet wanting and deficient even in his most costly Machines. Whoever peruses the large and elegant Volume of his First *Machina Cœlestis,* will admire at the vast Treasure he has expended on Astronomical Instruments of all sorts, when he sees even the very *Description* of them so very sumptuous. And yet, at the same time, whoever peruses a small Book of *Animadversions on this Machina Cœlestis,* by the ingenious Mr. *Hook,* will find one grand *Defect* does attend the noble *Hevelius* Instruments, which renders them (I will not say, useless, faulty, or no better than *Ticho's,* yet) not so compleat and perfect, as otherwise they had been by the Addition of *Telescopick Sights.* For *Hevelius* wholly used *Plain Sights,* which certainly are not so accurate as Telescopick

Tab. 30. pag. 128

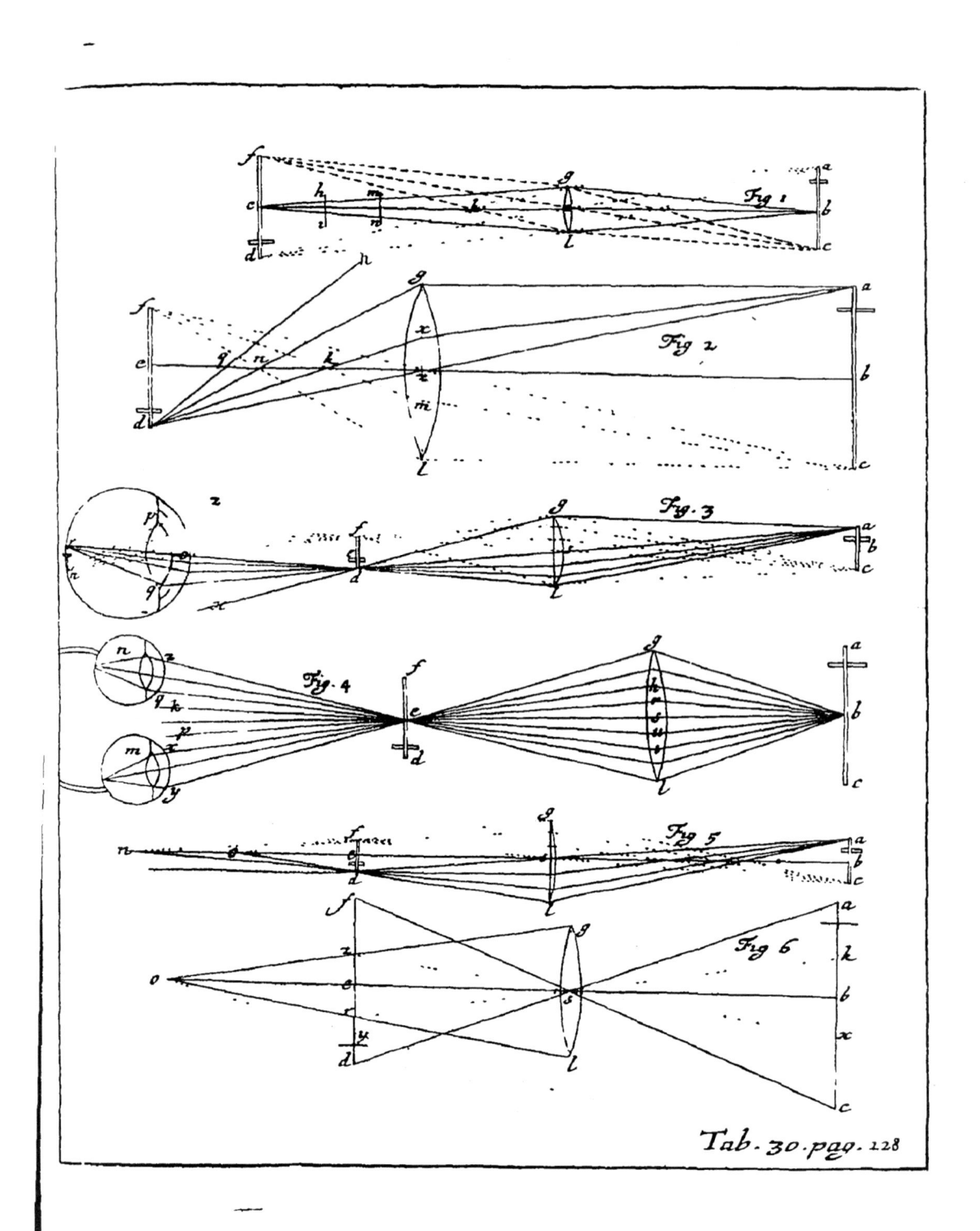

copick. And tho I muſt confeſs ingeniouſly, that this renowned Aſtronomer, by his extraordinary Diligence, great Care, and perpetual long-continued Practice, but chiefly by his peculiar ſharpneſs of Sight, had arrived to a great exactneſs of Obſervation by plain Sights (as I find by comparing the Obſervations made by the moſt curious Aſtronomers of our Age, *Flamſteed, Halley, Caſſini, &c.* by Teleſcopick Sights, with thoſe Obſervations made by *Hevelius,*) yet this we are to attribute more to the peculiar acuteneſs of his Eye, and to his extraordinary Diligence and Care in Obſervation, than to the exactneſs of *plain Sights.* For to me it ſeems manifeſt, from what the Learned Mr *Hook* lays down in the forementioned Book, that the naked Eye cannot ordinarily perceive an Angle (or Object that ſubtends an Angle) leſs than a Minute, or half a Minute at the ſmalleſt. For tho we perceive Stars of that magnitude that their Diameters are not half a Minute; yet this is by a ſort of *adventitious* or *glaring* Light, that is cauſed by the Refraction of their Rays in the Air, which makes them appear to us much bigger than really they are; as is manifeſt, when we come to look at them with a Teleſcope that takes off this *glaring* Light

(2.) The want therefore of Teleſcopick Sights is what Mr. *Hook* chiefly inſiſts upon, as defective in *Hevelius* coſtly Aſtronomical *Apparatus*: But yet, in his whole Book of *Animadverſions,* he takes no notice of the chief Objections, which *Hevelius* uſes againſt them. And I am perſwaded the Candour of that Noble Aſtronomer (whoſe Memory muſt now be ſacred) was ſo great, that upon the removal of theſe Difficulties, he would have given up the Cauſe, for it ſeems the Controverſie was long agitated between them. *Hevelius Object ors againſt them*

Theſe Objections we ſhall find in the Firſt Part of the *Machina Cœleſtis, Cap.* XIV. *pag.* 296. *Accedit, ſi quando Obſervator non æquè directè & preciſè ſemper, ut ſæpius, crede, contingeret,*

[230]

tingeret, per *Centra lentium collineat, facile diversitas aliqua aspectûs observationibus possit induci, quæ suo tempore Cœli scrutatores jugiter seduceret. Cæterum, cum Acus vel Fila adeo prope lentem Ocularem ad observatoris oculum vix in remotione aliquot digitorum subsistunt; dubito an Dioptra hæc oculo tam propinqua, multo accuratius Stellas quasvis minimas, quam Pinnacidia nostra, ad sex novemve pedes ab invicem remota, possit detegere. Nam etiamsi objectum distinctius videas; in eo tamen, quod Dioptra tua oculo propius adhæret, plus à vero deflectere poteris, quam nos circa nostra Pinnacidia, quæ tanto spatio ab invicem removentur. Ut taceam, quod intersectio filorum minimas Stellas tibi tegat, &c.*

For English Readers thus,

"Add to this, That if at any time the Observator chances
"not to look directly and precisely through the midst of the
"Glasses (as believe me it may often happen) some Varieties
"may easily intermingle with the Observations, which in time
"may egregiously deceive the Astronomer. Moreover, seeing
"the Needle or cross Threads, do stand so close to the Eye-
"Glass, and near the Eye of the Observator, I question whe-
"ther these Sights, so near the Eye, can discover the smallest
"Stars much more accurately, than our plain Sights, which
"are distant from each other Six or Nine Feet. For, tho by
"these Telescopick Sights, one may see the Object more di-
"stinctly; yet because they are so nigh to the Eye, one may
"err, more than 'tis possible by our plain Sights, that are so
"far asunder; so that I shall take no farther notice of another
"Inconvenience, which is, that the Intersection of the Threads
"shall cover the smallest Stars from your Sight.

His Mistake concerning them. Thus far the Learned *Hevelius*. Which shews plainly, that he had no right apprehension of the Nature of these Sights. And therefore the best way of reconciling him to them, had been, fairly to have laid down the *Dioptrical Reasons* of their Performance and Exactness. Upon a right understanding whereof,

Fig. 2

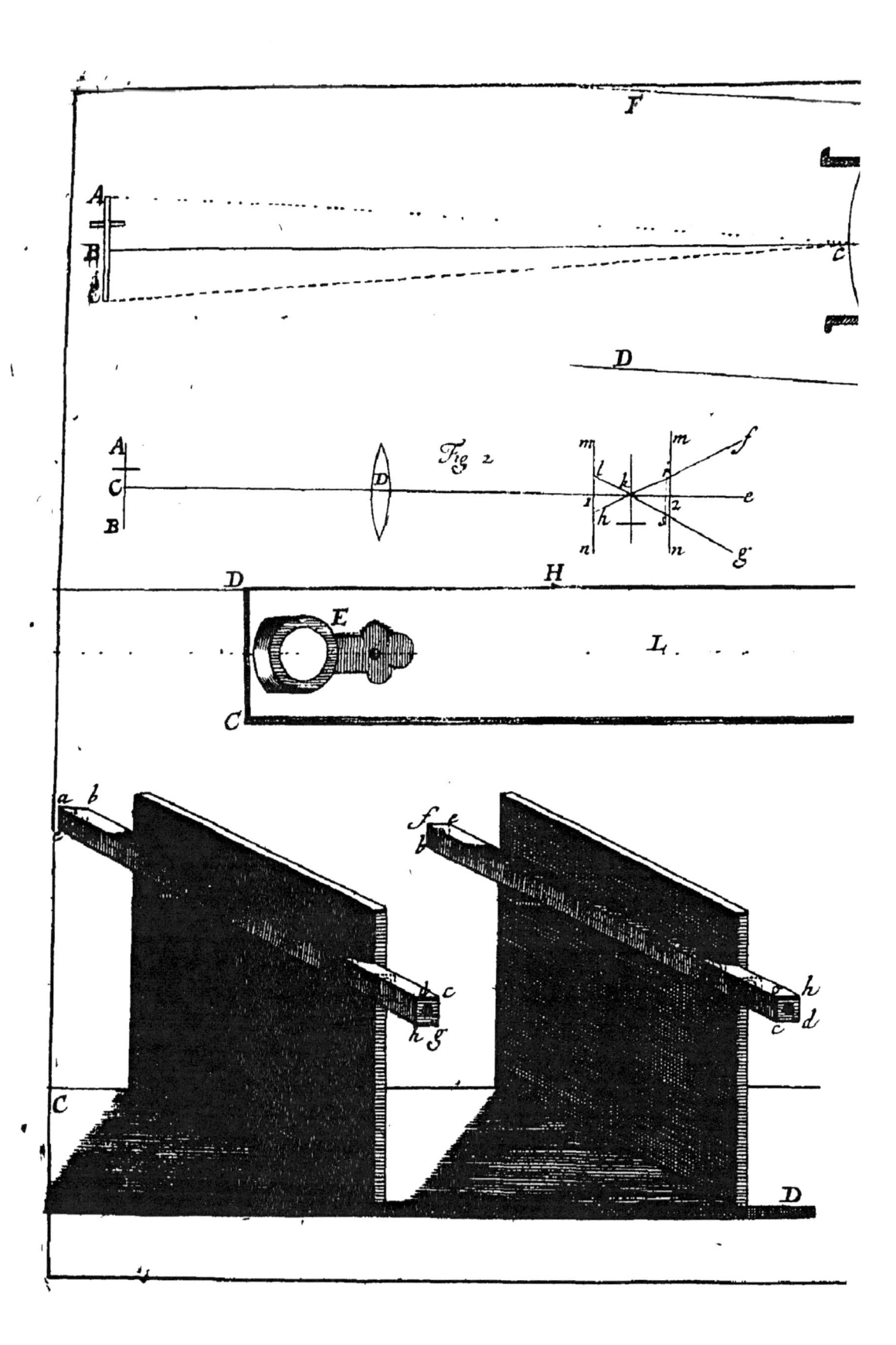

Tab 39 pag 271

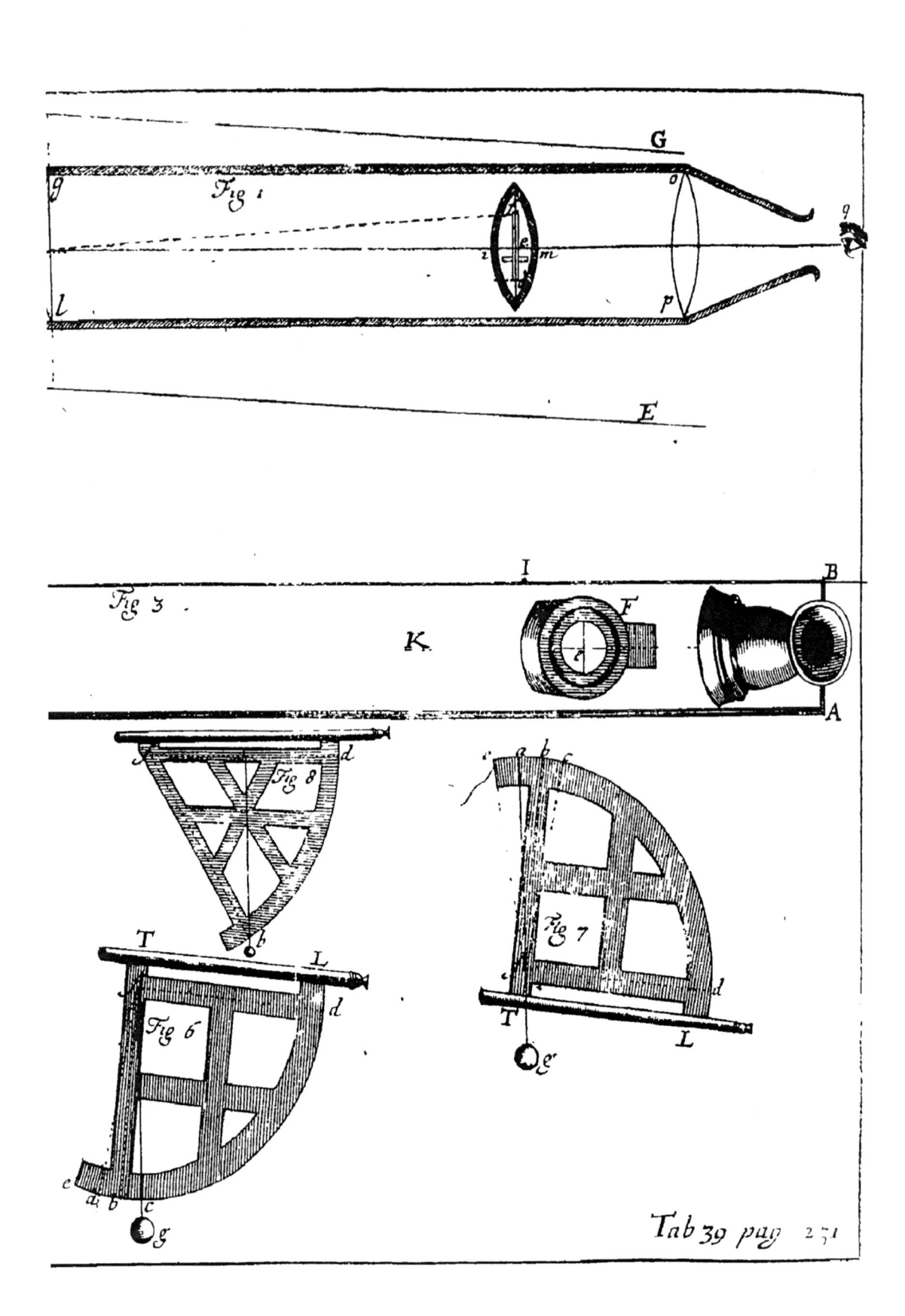

whereof, all those Objections would be answered, and would naturally vanish. This had been the right Method of proceeding amongst *Candid Philosophers*. Whilst vilifying his Instruments, and slighting his Performances with them as no better than those in the Age before him, did but exasperate the Noble old Man, and made him adhere more obstinately to his former Practice.

That *Hevelius* did not rightly apprehend the Nature of *Telescopick Sights*, is manifest by this Objection which he makes against them, from the *shortness* of the *Line* of *Collimation*, which he imagins no *longer*, than between the Eye or Eye-Glass, and cross Hairs; but is really as *long* as between the Object-Glass and cross Hairs. As shall be evident from what I shall now lay down.

Wherein I shall briefly explain their usual Fabrick or Contrivance; their adjusting to a plain Ruler, Cylindrick, or square Tube; their adjusting to Quadrants, Sextants, and other Instruments, and the Dioptrick Reason of their Performance and Exactness.

(3.) And first, the Fabrick or contrivance of these Telescopick Sights is briefly thus, *Tab.* 39. *Fig.* 1. Choosing an Object glass *g c l* and convex-Eye-glass *o p* proper for the length of the Ruler or Tube *g o p l* which we are to use. Let us take care that the Object-glass be pretty well *centred* (by Chap. 4. Sect. 4. of this part) but in this particular the greatest exactness is not requisite (whatever *Pere Cherubin* d'Orleans may say to the contrary, in the second Tome of his *Vision Parfait*. Paris 1681 *fol* in his description of Levels. *pag.* 23, 81, 106, 108, 109. &c. but chiefly *pag.* 107 wherein the Friar is most grosly mistaken) 'tis sufficient, if the Glass be pretty nigh the matter, as usually most Glasses are, immediately out of the Workmans hands. This Object-glass and Eye-glass are each to be fixed strongly on a brass Ring in the Ruler at their proper distance.

Their Fabrick or Contrivance T 39 F 1

True Centration of Glasses not absolutely requisite

And

And exactly in the Focus of the Object-glass $fmdi$ in another brass Ring are strain'd the finest cross-Hairs fd, im; This Ring is contrived to be moveable to the Right and Left hand, towards f, or towards d, and also (if the nature of the Instrument, to which we affix these Sights, require it) *upwards* and *downwards*; and to be steadily fixed in any posture by screws or otherwise. The Mechanick contrivance whereof is obvious enough, and needs not here be described, every one pleasing himself in his own way.

By the Doctrine in the first part 'tis manifest, that this Tube being thus disposed and presented before a Distant Object ABC, the Picture or Image of the Object is projected in the Focus of the Object-glass fed; and this Image in the distinct Base is at the plain of the Cross-hairs. Wherefore all the Rays that compose this Image, which escape, or do not fall on, the Cross-hairs, shall arrive at the Eye freely, and distinctly. But the Points in the Image, which are projected, and fall just on the Cross-hairs, are hid by the Cross-hairs from the Eye: and the Hairs themselves appear as if they were *really* stretch'd upon the *very Object*. For they are extended in the distinct Base, which, in this kind of Telescope, is the *Locus apparens* of the Object, by *prop* 50. *schol*. At the same time the Hairs themselves appear very distinctly to the Eye q in the outward Focus of the Eye-glass by *prop.* 32, 33. *schol.*

We may then conceive, that there is *some one* Point in the Object, as suppose B, which sending a Cone of Rays on the Object-glass, the Principal Ray of this Cone, or the Axis thereof, after passing the Object-glass, runs parallel in ce to the side of the Ruler or Tube lp. Wherefore, if the intersection of the Cross-hairs, e, without removing or stirring the Object glass in the Tube, be brought to meet with this Line, or to cover this Point B in the Object, and be there strongly fixed Whatever Point, in any Object, shall hereafter be found covered by this crossing of the

Hairs;

Hairs; we may be assured that this line of Collimation, *viz.* the line from the Eye to this point in the Object, or the line from this Intersection *e* to the point in the Object, runs parallel to the side of the Ruler or Tube, and therefore the side of the Ruler is directly pointed towards that mark in the Object. Respect being had to the Breadth of the Ruler.

In like manner, supposing the sides of the Tube were in the lines D E, F G; and the Object-glass fixed upon it in the posture expressed in the Figure. We may conceive some point A in the Object, the Axis of whose Cone of Rays *A c d* after passing the Object-glass, runs parallel to the sides D E, F G. If then the Intersection of the Cross-hairs *e*, without stirring the Object-glass in the Tube, be brought downwards to *d*, so that it may meet with the line *c d*, and cover the point A in the Object, and the Ring of the Cross-hairs be there fixed. Whatever point in an Object shall hereafter be found covered by this crossing of the Hairs, the line from the Intersection of the Hairs to this point in the Object runs parallel to the sides of the Tube or Ruler D E, F G. And therefore we may be sure, the sides of the Ruler are directly pointed towards the mark A in the distant Object. Respect being had to the Rulers Breadth.

For from whatever point on the inner surface of the Object-glass (how thick soever it be, or how *ill* soever *centred*) the Ray *c d* emerges; no other Ray can emerge from that same point, and fall on the point *d*, but it must necessarily be a principal Ray or Axis of some Cone, and must run parallel to the side of the Ruler D E. For whatever Optick Angle the length A B in any Object subtends; that length shall be projected by this Object-glass in *d e* subtending the same Angle *d c e*.

(4) Wherefore we now come to shew how to find out the Ray *c d*, that runs parallel to the side of the Ruler D E; or how to rectifie the Cross-hairs on the Ruler. *Adjusting them to plain Rulers or Tubes.*

H h And

[234]

Exactly determining the Focus of the Ob, ect-Glass.

And first for, adjusting the Cross-hairs at their *exact distance* from the Object-glass, that is, in its *exact Focus*. This is easily performed thus, Let us look at some Object distant 3 or 4 miles; and moving or shaking our Eye before the Eye-glass upwards and downwards, or to one and t'other hand, let us observe whether the Cross-hairs seem to *move*, or *dance*, upon the said Object: for if it do, then the Cross-hairs are *not* at their *exact distance* from the Object-glass; but they must be moved farther from or nigher to the Object-glass, till the Eye, looking at such a distant Object, and moving before the Eye-glass, perceives the Cross-hairs, as it were, *fixed* and *immoveable* on the Object.

(Note. *This is the way for exactly determining the Focal length of an Object glass, to which I have referred in* Chap. 4. Sec. 3.)

If in *raising* the Eye, the Object seems to *fall down* on the Cross-hairs, or if in *depressing* the Eye, the Object seems to *rise* on the Cross-hairs, then are the Cross-hairs *too nigh* the Object-glass: but if in *raising* the Eye, the Object seems to *rise* on the Cross-hairs; or in *depressing* the Eye, the Object seems to *sink* or *fall* on the Cross-hairs; then are the Cross-hairs *too far from* the Object-glass. All which will be evident from *Tab.* 39. *f.* 2. wherein let A B be a distant Object, whose middle point C is projected by the Object-glass, D at *k*. Let *m n* 1 be the Cross-hairs *too nigh* the Object glass and *m n* 2 the same *too far* from the Object-glass *e, f, g,* the Eye placed at three different stations. In the case of the first Cross-hairs, if the Eye *rise* from *e* to *f*, it perceives the point *k depressed* from 1 to *h*, or if the Eye *fall* from *e* to *g*, it perceives the point *k* raised from 1 to *l*: and here the Cross-hairs are *too nigh* the Object-glass. But in case of the second Cross-hairs; if the Eye *rise* from *e* to *f*, the point *k* seems to *rise* on the Cross-hairs from 2 to *r*; or if the Eye *fall* from *e* to *g*, it perceives the point *k fallen* from 2 to *s*: and in this case the Cross-hairs are *too far distant* from the Object-glass. But if the Cross hairs are exactly in the *Focus* at *k*, let the Eye *rise*

or

or *fall*, the Cross-hairs seem *fixed* and *steddy* on the Object. And this is the first thing requisite for adjusting these Sights.

This I have borrowed from my own *Sciathericum Telescopicum*, Published at *Dublin* 1686. *quarto*. And I hope, one may be allow'd to transcribe from himself without being called a *Plagiary*.

When this Affair is well adjusted; we may proceed to the second Rectification, which consists in making the *line of sight, mire,* or *collimation*, exactly *parallel* to the Sides of the Tube or Ruler, to which the Telescopick Sights are to be adapted. And for the easier obtaining of this, we are first to be ascertain'd, that even the *two sides* of the Ruler or Tube are exactly parallel. And hereof we may be informed after this manner. Tab. 39. Fig. 3. On an even board draw the right line D H I B, let A B C D be a Ruler, to which the Telescopick Sghts are to be fitted, E the Ring carrying the Object-glass, F the Ring carrying the Cross-hairs, G the Snout carrying the Eye-glass. To the line B D apply the side B D of the Ruler, and looking through the Glasses observe the point in an Object distant a mile or two whereon the Cross-hairs fall. Then remove the Ruler, and apply its other side A C to the line B D, and observe whether the Cross-hairs fall on the same point of the Object, as before. If they do so, then are the sides of the Ruler A C, B D, parallel; if not, then the sides are not parallel. The reason that so remote an Object must be chosen, is, that the Breadth of the Ruler may subtend an imperceptible *Angle* in a circle whose *Radius* is the distance of the Object from the Object-glass.

Or otherwise, In the plain Board strike two round brass-wire Pinns. Suppose H, I, which having their *roundness* from their *being drawn*, must needs have their sides parallel. To these Pins apply *one* and *t other* side of the Ruler, and observe as before.

Having thus *found*, or *made* the *two sides* of the Ruler (or four sides of the Tube, if need be) parallel; the next thing is to make the line of Collimation L K parallel to these sides; or to

Hh 2 bring

[236]

bring the Interfection of the Crofs-hairs *e* to meet with the Axis L K of fome of the *Radious Pencils*, which Axis, after paffing the Object-glafs, runs parallel to thefe Sides.

Tab 39
Fig 4, 5.
    To effect this (*Tab.* 39. *f.* 4, 5.) we are to raife the plain Board A B edgwife on the Board of a window or table C D, fo that we may reft or fuftain the Ruler or parallelipiped Tube *a b c d e f g h*, on the round Pins *i*, *k*. then looking through the hole in the end *g h d c* defigned for the Eye, let us obferve the point in a far diftant Object, which falls exactly on the Interfection of the Crofs-hairs. Afterwards, let us invert the Ruler or Tube (as we have it in *fig.* 5.) making the fide *a b c d*, which in *fig.* 4. was *uppermoft*, now undermoft in this *fig* 5 by which means, the fide of the Tube *a d h e*, which in *fig.* 4 was *fartheft* from the Board, in *fig.* 5. is *next* the Board. Then looking through the Tube, let us obferve, whether the Crofs-hairs fall now on the fame point in the Object, as in the firft pofture · If they *doe* agree exactly, then is the *line of collimation* parallel to the fides *a h*, *b g*; if they do *not*, but fall to the *right* hand apparently of the faid point in the Object, then are the Crofs-hairs to be removed (by whatever Contrivance they are made moveable) to the *Left* Hand (the contrary requiring the contrary), fo that the Tube continuing in this latter pofture, the crofs-Hairs may cover a Point in the Object, middle between the Point covered in the pofture of *Fig.* 4. and in the pofture of *Fig.* 5. at the firft fight. And thus by frequent Repetitions and Tryals, we at laft bring all to rights. After the fame manner that we have rectified the Line of *Collimation* to run *parallel* to any two parallel Sides of the Tube, we may rectifie it to a *Parallelifm* with the other two parallel Sides of the Tube (fuppofing the Ring that carries the crofs-Hairs to have all the Motions requifite to fuch Rectification). And fo we fix all ftrongly, chiefly the Object-Glafs and crofs-Hairs, and the Operation is compleat.

By

[237]

By this Method the *Line of Sight* of any Cylindrick or square Tube may be made to run parallel to its Sides, for many Operations and Observations Mathematical and Natural: Amongst others, for finding the *Declination* of the *Magnet*, according to the Methods lately proposed by Monſ. *Hautefeville*, and M *Sturmius* in the *Journal des Sçavans*, 23. *Aug*. 1683. And in the *Acta Eruditorum, Lipsiæ, Ann*. 1684 *Decemb*. And for want of this Method, what Monſ. *Sturmius* says in the foresaid *Act. Lipſ*. pag 579. is very *defective*. For thus he, *Sola Tubi locatio, ut Axis Visionis per medias Lentes excurrens Meridianæ Lineæ exactè respondeat, difficultatis quippiam habere videbatur; verum & huic infirmitati præsens, uti credo, inventum est Remedium, &c*. And the Remedy he tells us is, That the Tube be made a *Parallelipiped* of Wood or Brass, for then, *says he*, Applying the Side of your Tube to the *Meridian* Line, the Axis of Vision will be *parallel* to the said *Meridian Line*. But with the Leave of so Great a Man, *I deny this*, unless first it be *rectified*, so that this *Axis* runs *parallel* to the Side of the Tube. And let us take what care soever possible for truly centring the Object-Glass, and placing it, and the cross-Hairs exactly in the Tube, we must after all rectifie these Sights by some such Method as I have laid down, or else we may be egregiously deceived. And on this account, all the *Levels* and *Instruments*, to which *Pere Cherubin D'Orleans* has adapted Telescopick-Sights, and which he has so neatly and sumptuously described by curious Schemes, and a large Volume, *La Vision Parfait. Tome* II. *A Paris* 1681. *Fol*. are *deficient* and *useless*. For he places the whole *Rectification* of this *Line of Collimation* in the *true Centration* of the Glasses, *pag* 107. And rejects the Right Rectification by moving of the cross-Hairs as erroneous, *pag*. 107. But in this the Friar betrays his Ignorance, for tho the *true Centration* of the Object Glass be of good *Convenience* and *Advantage*, yet it does not *perfect* the Instrument

Sturmius Mistake.

Cherubins Gross Error.

without

without farther Rectification; as being impossible to be obtained to sufficient accuracy; and therefore we must have recourse to some such Method as foregoes.

I have hitherto mentioned only two of the finest cross-Hairs to be extended as a Mensurator in the Focus of the Object-Glass: But for some Uses, perhaps the *finest Silver*, or *Gold Wire*, is better; as not being disordered by *Heat* and *Cold*: Or else, the *Point* of the smallest and most curious *Needle*, on whose Extremity, the smallest Telescopick-Star may be visible.

See the end of this Chapter.

Constancy and Security of these Telescopick-Sights.

When these Telescopick Sights are rightly adjusted in the Tube, and strongly fixt in their due Posture by Screws, and all covered over from outward Injuries and Accidents, they are of all Sights the most constant and lasting, and the least subject to be disordered: So that, when one finds the *Great Hevelius* objecting against them, their *Aptness to be out of order*, one would think the most commodious Fabrick of them was never explained to him; tho I am sure, his Instructor Mr. *Hook* was as able, as any in the World, to inform him rightly in this Matter.

To *Quadrants*, *Sextants*, &c

(5.) I come now to the Rectification of these Sights on *Quadrants* and *Sextants*, for taking Angles. This is done either *before* or *after* the Divisions into Degrees, &c. are made on the Limb of the Quadrant. If it be done *before*, then we suppose the Telescope T L (*Tab.* 39. *Fig.* 6, 7.) fixt to the Quadrant, which we suppose continued a little farther than the Fourth part of a Circle. Choosing then an Object pretty near the Horizon; let us look through the Telescope, in the usual Posture of Observation, as *Fig.* 6. and observe the Point in the Object marked by the cross Hairs; and at the same time we are to note most nicely the Point *c*, which the Plumb-Line *f c g*, hung from the Centre *f* of the Quadrant, cuts on the Limb. Then we are to invert the Quadrant into the Posture of *Fig.* 7. (which is easily done by the usual Contri-

Tab 39 Fig 6,7

vances

vances for managing great Quadrants, by tooth'd Semicircles and endless Screws) keeping still the Telescope T L nighly upon the same height from the Ground, as before) unless the Object we look at, be so far distant, that the Breadth of the Quadrant subtends but an insensible Angle. But yet for certainty, 'tis better to keep the Telescope, as 'tis said, upon the same height from the Floor); then direct the Telescope T L, that the cross Hairs may cover exactly the same Point in the Object, as before in the Posture of *Fig.* 6. And hanging now the Plumb-Line *a f g* on the Limb of the Quadrant; let us remove it *to* and *fro*, till we find out the exact Point *a*, from which the Plumb-Line being hung, shall most nicely hang over the Centre of the Quadrant *f*. Then carefully marking the Point *a*, let us divide the Arch *c a* into two equal Parts in *b*; and drawing *b f*, the Point *b* is the Point from which we are to begin the Divisions of the Quadrant: And the *Line* of *Collimation* through the Telescopick-Sight, stands exactly at Right Angles to the Line *b f*. So that the Quadrant *b f d* being compleated and divided, the said Line of Sight through the Telescope runs exquisitely parallel to the Line *f d*.

In the next place, supposing the Quadrant *b f d* truly compleated and divided; and that we designed to fix thereto the Telescopick-Sight T L; so that the *Line* of *Sight* may run exactly at Right Angles to the Line *b f*, or parallel to the Line *d f*. We are to do as in the foregoing Praxis. And if in dividing the Arch *a c*, we find its half exactly coincident with the Point *b*, we have our desire. But if it differ from the Point *b*, and fall *between* *b* and *d*, then the *Line* of *Collimation* through the Telescope stands at an *obtuse* Angle with the Line *b f*, and the Instrument errs in *excess*: If this half Arch fall *without* *b* and *d*, then the *Line* of *Collimation* makes an *acute* Angle with the Line *b f*, and the Instrument errs in *defect*.

defect. And by often Tryals, we are to remove the crofs-Hairs within the Tube, fo much, as is requifite to correct this Error. And when we have thus rectified them to their due place, there they are to be ftrongly fixt. Or elfe, in Obfervations taken by this Inftrument, we are to *make allowance* for this Error; by *fubtracting from* (if it be in *excefs*) or by *adding to* (if it be in *defect*) each Obfervation fo much, as we find the Error to be.

The reafon of this Rectification is moft plain; for 'tis manifeft, that cfd (*Fig. 6.*) *wants* of a full Quadrant, as much as afd (*Fig. 7.*) *exceeds* a Quadrant. So the difference of the two Arches in the two Poftures being ac, half this difference bc added in *Fig. 6.* or ab *fubtracted* in *Fig. 7.* makes bd a compleat Quadrant.

If we find our Inftrument *err* in taking Angles, and we defire to know the Error *more nicely*, than perhaps the Divifions of the Inftrument it felf will fhew it: We are to do thus; Let us obferve diligently the Object pointed at, in the Pofture the Inftrument difcovers its Error, and the Object pointed at when the Inftrument lies *truly*. Then, with a large Telefcope and Micrometer (as is ufed in taking the Planets Diameters, as fhall be declared hereafter, *Sec. 7.*): Let us take the Angle fubtended at the Object-Glafs of the Quadrants Telefcope by the length between thefe two Objects, and we obtain the Error of our Inftrument moft *nicely*. Thus for Example; Suppofing the Quadrant bfd already accurately divided, and that the Plumb-Line, *Fig. 6.* plays over the Point c: And upon the Inverfion of the Inftrument, *Fig. 7.* we find that before we can get it to play exactly over the Centre f, we muft hang it over the Point e, fo that the Arch eb exceeds bc by the Arch ea; 'tis plain that the Angle efa is the Error of the Inftrument: For had the Plumb-Line hung over a, and over the Centre f in this latter Pofture, the In-
ftrumen

strument had been *exact*; because *a* is as much on one side *b*, as *c* is on t'other side *b*. Wherefore *e f a* being the Angle, by which our Instrument *errs* in observation: Let us turn the Instrument into the usual Posture of Observation, as in *Fig.* 6. and hanging the Plumb-Line on the Centre *f*; let us bring it to play nicely on the Point *e*, and observe what distant Object is covered by the cross-Hairs: Then let us bring it to play exactly on the Point *a*, and observe likewise what distant Object is pointed at by the Telescope Hairs. Lastly, by a large Telescope and Micrometer, let us measure the Angle between these *two Objects*, and we shall have the Angle of Error much more nicely, than 'tis possible the Angle *e f a* should be given by the Divisions on the Limb of the Quadrant *e a*. And thus much for adjusting a Quadrant.

A *Sextant* is rectifi'd in like manner; If we consider (*Tab.* 39. *Fig.* 8.) that if from the Centre *f* to the beginning of the Divisions *d* there be drawn the Radius *f d*; and it be divided equally in *c*; and from *c* there be supended the Plumb-Line *c b*: When the Plumb-Line hangs over the 60th Degree at *b*, then the Line *f d* lies horizontal: And consequently, if the Line of Collimation through the Tube be parallel to *f d*, this Line also lies horizontal. To try which, Whilst the Sextant stands in this Posture, observe the Object marked by the cross-Hairs, then invert the Sextant; and over the Point *b* hang the Plumb-Line; and when from the Point *b* the Plumb-Line hangs over the middle Point *c*, then again is the Line *f d* horizontal in this Posture. Mark then, whether the cross-Hairs cover the same Object as before: If they do, then the *Line of Collimation* is parallel to *f d*: If they do not, but the Point in the Object marked in this latter Posture be *higher* than the Point marked in the first Posture, the Instrument errs in *excess*, if it be *lower*, the Instrument errs in *defect*. And either we are to remove the cross-Hairs, till we

T 39 F 8 Rectification of a Sextant.

bring

bring all to rights, and there fix them: Or by the Methods before laid down in the *Rectification* of the *Quadrant*, we are to find the Quantity of this erroneous Angle, and to allow for it in Observation.

Rectification of a movable Sight. In Instruments furnished with two pair of Telescopick-Sights, one on a *fixt* Arm, and t'other on a *moveable* Arm (by the Ancients termed an *Alidade*); 'tis easie rectifying the Sights on the *moveable* Arm thus: After the Sights on the *fixt* Arm are rectifi'd by what foregoes; bring the Index of the moveable Arm to the beginning of the Divisions on the Limb of the Instrument, be it Quadrant or Sextant, &c. 'tis then manifest, that the *Line of Collimation* through the *movable* Telescope (if it be right) should lye *parallel* to the Line of *Collimation* through the *fixt* Telescope. Observe therefore, whether the cross-Hairs in *both* Telescopes do at the *same time* cut the *same* Star, or fall on the *same* Point in an Object distant three or four Miles. If they do, then the *movable* Telescope agreeing with the *fixt*, and the *fixt* being *supposed rectifi'd* to the Divisions on the Instrument, the *movable* is *right* likewise. But if the Hairs in the *movable* Telescope do *not* agree in marking the *same* Point with the cross-Hairs in the *fixt* Telescope; then the Hairs in this *movable* Telescope are to be *removed* (by whatever Contrivance there is for that purpose) and brought to *rights*, and there *fixt*.

There are other Methods propounded for rectifying Telescopick-Sights on other sorts of Instruments, by means of Observations towards the *Zenith*, as our former Methods have been imployed towards the *Horizon*. But 'tis sufficient here to lay down only what foregoes, as being of the greatest and most frequent use: Referring for the others to M. *Picard's* Treatise of the *Measure of a Degree of a great Circle of the Earth*; publish'd at the end of *Memoirs for a Natural History of Animals*, &c. By the *Academy Royal* at Paris; lately translated into English, and printed at *London*, 1688. *Fol.* Before

Before I quit this Point, it may not be amiss to intimate one *Use*, to which a plain Ruler furnished with Telescopick-Sights (such as is expressed *Tab. 39. Fig. 3.*) may be apply'd; and that is, not only for trying the exquisite *straitness* of either of its *own* Edges, and *parallelism* of its *own* two Sides; but also, for the ready Tryal of the same in any *other* Ruler: For 'tis but affixing (by a little Cement, or otherwise) this *Telescopick-Ruler* over the Ruler to be try'd, and resting the Edge of this latter against the Pins H, I, and gently sliding the Edge alongst these Pins, and always touching them; looking all the while through the Telescope, observe whether the cross-Hairs do steadily adhere to the same Point in an Object: For if the Edge of the Ruler have the least irregular Crookedness, the cross-Hairs will move from the Point first observed. And this shall detect the least Curvity in the Edge of a Ruler (especially if the Ruler be long, and the Distance of the Pins be considerable) that shall escape the most exquisite Eye of a Workman. The way of trying the Parallelism of the two Sides of this latter Ruler, is the same with what foregoes for the Telescopick-Ruler it self: For when the Telescopick-Ruler is adjoyned over the other, they may both be taken but as one Ruler with Telescope-Sights affix'd.

Further Use of a Telescopick-Ruler

(6.) I come now to the last thing proposed concerning Telescopick-Sights; and that is, To shew the *Dioptrick-Reason* of their Performance and Exactness. But herein there will be little requisite to be added to what foregoes, both in the First Part concerning Telescopes in general, and to what is laid down in this Chapter concerning Telescopick-Sights. 'Tis manifest by Experiments, that the *ordinary Power* of Man's Eye extends no farther than perceiving what subtends an Angle of about a Minute, or something less. But when an Eye is armed with a Telescope, it may discern an Angle

Dioptrick Reason of their Performance.

less than a Second. The Telescope that magnifies distinctly the Appearance of *Body*, magnifies also distinctly the Apppearance of *Extension*, *Space*, and *Motion* through this Space; so if the Minute-Hand of a Watch, which can but just be percieved to move, be looked upon with a Magnifying-Glass, we shall see it give a considerable Leap at every Stroak of the Balance. And thus likewise the slow diurnal Motion of the Sun or Stars, which is hardly perceivable by the bare Eye, unless assisted by an Instrument of a vast Radius, is most easily perceived through an ordinary Telescope of 18 Inches long: Insomuch that we may determine to the greatest Niceity and Exactness, when a Star passes just over the cross-Hairs, even to the single Beat of a Second-Pendulum. And let an Object in the Heavens rise never so little, the Image in the Distinct-Base falls correspondently at the cross-Hairs; and the Eye, by means of the Eye-Glass, perceives this Motion, be it never so small. Thus suppose (*Tab.* 39. *Fig.* 1.) that a Star *rise* from B to A, the Image *falls* at the cross-Hairs in the Distinct Base from *e* to *d*; then by means of the Eye-Glass *o p*, the Space *e d* is mightily magnified, and consequently the Angle B *c* A, equal to *e c d* by which the Star is risen, is made most sensible to the Eye *q*. By what foregoes in the First Part concerning the magnifying of this sort of Telescope.

Hevelius Mistake farther manifest

By this we may perceive, how the Noble *Hevelius* was mistaken in his Estimate of these Sights; when he imagin'd the *Line of Collimation* therein was no *longer* than between the cross-Hairs and Eye-Glass: Whereas this Distance is not at all to be consider'd in their Performance; the *Line of Collimation* being full as *long* as the Distance between the Object-Glass and cross-Hairs. I am perswaded, had he been rectifi'd in this particular, he would never have adhered so obstinately to the Use of *plain Sights* upon his most costly Instruments. Tho I must confess, 'tis difficult to wean a Man from the

Use

Use of what he has been accustomed to for so many Years; and upon the Exactness of which, the Accuracy of all his former Labors did depend.

As to all other Objections which he makes against them, *His other Objections answered.* as that they are easily disordered, that the Glasses are easily vitiated by the Breath of the Observer, &c. They are not of any the least moment. For 'tis manifest, they may be contrived so, as to be *more secure,* and *less* subject to Injuries, than any other plain Sights whatsoever: And in this particular, Telescope-Sights are so far from being obnoxious, that certainly they are preferable to the best contrived plain Sights, for what can be more simple and easier preserved, than the forementioned small (but strong) Brass Rings defended by a Tin or Brass Tube covering all? When once these are adjusted and fixt, nothing can possibly injure them. 'Tis true, the Breath of the Observer, if puft into the Telescope, will sully the Eye-Glass; but how easily is this avoided? Who is it goes purposely to make a *speaking-Trumpet* of a *Telescope*? The other most considerable Objection against their Use is, That in dark Nights, at the smaller Stars, the cross-Hairs in the Telescope require a little *enlightening,* or else they are *invisible,* and cannot be seen when the Star just applies to them. This is so easily remedi'd, by admitting to them, through a small opening purposely left in the side of the Tube, the least glimmering Light of a Lanthorn; or by placing a Lanthorn a little aside before the Object-Glass; that 'tis not worth mentioning as a Difficulty, much less is it to be made an Argument for their utter rejection. As to what he says of the Hairs being so gross as to cover the smaller Stars, this only relates to the Material we employ; and the finest Silk-Worms Clue will be found small enough almost to bisect the smallest Stars: If not, let us use the *finest Needle,* on whose slender Point we may distinctly receive the most minute Star.

And

Farther Uses of Telescopick-Sights.

And thus much concerning *Telescopick-Sights*; from whose application to Mathematick-Instruments, Astronomy, and Geography may expect their utmost Advancements. And even Natural Philosophy it self may hereby receive the greatest Help, when we consider how Telescopes may be apply'd to many Experiments therein; amongst others, to make the most nice *Hygroscope*; and has already been used for accurately determining the capricious *Variations* of the *Magnet*. *Telescopick-Sights* have been already successfully apply'd to most exquisite Levels; wherein Monsr. *Picard* in his Curious Treatise *Du Nivellement* has prevented any farther Explication: And I doubt not, but every Day will find new Uses for these Sights. Amongst others, I'll presume to mention my own *Telescopick-Dial* already publish'd, *Anno* 1686: A Contrivance, which, without Vanity I may say, has not displeased *at Home*, and has been well received *Abroad*.

Adapting the Micrometer to a Telescope.

(7.) The next Telescopick Instrument which I shall explain, is the *Micrometer*. Concerning the *Invention* of this Ingenious Instrument, I have only this to say, That for the Honour thereof, there are several Competitors: Monsr. *Petit*, Surveyor of the Fortifications in *France*, was the first that publish'd to the World the rough Draught hereof, 12. Mar. 1667. *Vid. Journal des Scavans*, 16. *May* 1667. After him Monsr. *Azout*, another Ingenious *Frenchman*, publish'd a Tract concerning the exact Mensuration of the Planets Diameters, wherein he seems to challenge the Invention of this Instrument to himself and Monsr. *Picard, Journ. des Scavans*, 28. *Juin*. 1667. and *Philosoph. Transact. Num.* 21. *pag.* 373. But last of all a Candid *Englishman* of our own, Mr. *Rich. Townley*, does vindicate the first Contrivance hereof to its *true* and *original* Author, Mr. *Gascoigne* an *English* Gentleman, who was kill'd in King *Charles* I. Service, *Vid. Philosoph. Transact. Num.* 25. *pag.* 457.

Inventor of the Micrometer.

wherein Mr. *Townley* (who is of undoubted Credit) asserts, that

that Mr. *Gascoigne* made and used this Instrument before the Civil Wars in *England*: And that Mr. *Townley* had then in his Custody two or three of these Instruments first devised by Mr. *Gascoigne*; to which Mr. *Townley* himself had added some considerable Improvments. All which, with the exact Fabrick, and fitting of the Body of the Instrument to a Telescope, we shall find accurately described in *Num. 29. p.* 541. *Philosoph. Transact.* to which I shall therefore refer the Reader; and shall hint only such things concerning it in this place; as may be *there wanting* for the clearer Instruction of the unexercised Beginner.

First therefore for a brief Description thereof (as much as is requisite to maintain the order of our Discourse); 'tis in short this. In the Focus of the Object-Glass of a Telescope, there are placed two fine parallel Hairs, or smooth Edges of Brass Plates; these are made by Screws to open or close at pleasure, as wide as the Telescope admits. The Turns of these Screws are reckon'd out by proper *Indices*; so that in opening the Edges of the Micrometer, the Indices do shew, how many *Revolutions* of the Screws, and Parts of a *Revolution* are compleated in that Opening. Suppose therefore the Screws to be of so fine a Thread, as to contain 30 Threads in an Inch length; then every Revolution of the Screw opens or closes the Edges of the Micrometer a thirtieth part of an Inch. By one Revolution of the Screw, the *Index* receives one Revolution: Then, the Circumference of the Plate, over which the *Index* moves (as the Hand of a Watch over the Hour-Plate) being divided into 100 Parts; when the *Index* moves one of these Parts, the Screw moves the Edges a three thousandth part of an Inch; (or the one thirty six thousandth part of a Foot; by which we find how easie 'tis to divide a Foot into thirty six or forty thousand Parts) And this Motion, tho every Minute, is made, by the Eye-Glass of the Telescope, perceivable.

The way of taking small Angles by this Instrument is thus; Suppose it were the Diameter of the Moon; Open the Micrometer till the two Edges do just clasp or touch the Moons Edges; then observe by the Indices how many Revolutions and parts of a Revolution were compleated to this opening; and by a proper Table (the way of composing which I shall shew presently), convert these Revolutions and Parts into Minutes and Seconds. In like manner, for observing small Angles on the Earth, the Diameters of the other Planets, the Distances of *Jupiter's Satellits* from his Body, or the Moons Spots, &c.

But now for making the Table, First we are to fix the Micrometer exactly in the *Focus* of the Object-Glass (by the Rules before given, *Chap.* 5. *Sect.* 4.) if it be at very distant Objects we design to use it: Or otherwise in the *respective Focus*, if it be designed for nigh Objects. We may then compose the Table two manner of ways: The first is more easie, tho not so very certain and accurate, yet exact enough for most Uses. Measure by Inches and Decimal Parts the Distance between the Object-Glass and Micrometer, taking into the Account two Thirds of the Object-Glass's Thickness: Let us suppose the Distance 10 Foot, or 120 Inches, or 120000 Parts; and we desire to know what Angle is shewn by the Micrometer, being open 2 Inches, or 2000 Parts. The Computation is plain (*Tab.* 35. *Fig.* 4) $ey = 120000$, $fd = 2000$, then $ed = ef = 1000$. And As ey : To Rad. :: So ed : To Tang. $\angle eyd = \angle eyf = 0°\ 28'\ 38''$, and therefore $\angle fyd$ is equal to $0°\ 57'\ 16''$. Then finding by accurate Admeasurement, how many Revolutions of the Screws or *Index*, are requisite to open the Edges 2 Inches; the same compleats the Angle $0°\ 57'\ 16''$. Suppose therefore 60 Revolutions open the Micrometer 2 Inches; then 60 Revolutions shew, that the Object, that just appears through the Edges

Edges at that opening, subtends an Angle of 0° 57′ 16″. Then 30 (*viz.* half 60) Revolutions give 28′ 38″, *viz.* half 57′ 16″. And one Revolution gives an Angle of 57″ 16‴; and the hundredth part of a Revolution gives 34‴ +. And thus the Table is composed to any Number of Parts and Revolutions requisite. But this Way, depending on the exact Admeasurement of the Distance of the Micrometer's Edges (which can hardly be obtained to sufficient Accuracy, unless we know most nicely what Number of Threads in the Screw there were in an Inch length; for then we know what Number of Revolutions compleat an Inch), 'tis not so accurate as what follows, which is,

The second way for composing the Table, is this: Having fixt the Micrometer at its due Distance from the Object-Glass; on the side of a Wall or House far distant mark out two conspicuous Objects, that may both at a time be received into the Telescope: Measure nicely the distance of these Objects from each other; and also the distance of either of them from the Object-Glass (which we suppose directly before the Point in the Wall middle between the two Objects). And by Trigonometry calculate the Angle, which the distance between these two Objects subtends before the Object Glass. Then looking through the Telescope, open the Micrometer, till the two Edges thereof exactly meet with or embrace these two Objects; and observe, how many Revolutions and parts of a Revolution are performed in this opening; for so many compleat the Angle before calculated. And having the Revolutions and Parts that compleat any one Angle, we may easily find all the rest, as aforesaid. For in these small Angles, the Angles and Revolutions are proportional, that is, if a *certain* Number of *Revolutions* give a *certain Angle*; half this *Number* gives *half* this *Angle*; and the hundredth part of this Number gives the hundredth part of the Angle, &c.

In the firſt Method that I propoſed for adapting the Micrometer, and compoſing the Table, I have allowed for the Object-Glaſſes Thickneſs in meaſuring its diſtance from the Micrometer. But this Nicety is hardly requiſite; unleſs it be in ſhort Tubes. For at the Radius of 10 Foot, 1 Inch is the Tangent of 28′ 38″; and at the Radius of 10 foot + one tenth of an Inch, 1 Inch is the Tangent of 28′ 37″; ſo there is but *one Second* difference; tho we ſhould err one tenth of an Inch in admeaſuring the diſtance between the Object-Glaſs and Micrometer.

Other Teleſcopick Inſtruments.

I might now mention the Application of a *Lattice of fine Hairs* in the Focus of the Object-Glaſs of a Teleſcope, as an help to draw diſtant Objects in *Perſpective*: And of applying there a pretty contrived Parallelogram for the ſame purpoſe. But the firſt is obvious enough by the leaſt intimation thereof; and the latter is ſo amply deſcribed by *Pere Cherubin d'Orleans* in his *Dioptrique Oculaire*; that 'tis needleſs to add any thing farther in this place.

Inſtead of croſs-Hairs.

I conclude this Chapter with a brief hint of what I have found very commodious for many purpoſes; that is; inſtead of the forementioned croſs-Hairs, I have often uſed a curious piece of clear, thin, flat Glaſs, whereon there are drawn two very fine croſs-Lines by the curious Point of a Diamond, ſmaller than the moſt fine Wyre or Hair; not eaſily diſturbed by a ſleight Touch (unleſs we break the Glaſs), nor alterable by Heat and Cold. Thus alſo may we make a Lattice.

CHAP.

Chap. VI.

Of the Invention, Discoveries made by, and other Applications, of Optick-Glasses.

(1.) *Optick-Glasses unknown to the Ancients.* (2.) *Pretended Passage in* Plautus. (3.) *An other Passage in* Pliny. (4.) *Probably invented about* 1300. (5.) *Friar Bacon's Pretence.* (6.) *Inventers of the Telescope.* (7.) *Optick-Glasses long known before the Telescope. Remark thereon.* (8.) *Celestial Discoveries by the Telescope.* (9.) *In the fixt Stars.* (10.) *In Saturn. Examination of Gallets Hypothesis.* (11.) *In Jupiter. Motion of his Satellits diligently prosecuted by* Cassini *and* Flamsteed. *Satellits all disappearing.* (12.) *Reflection on the Motions of Saturn's and Jupiter's Satellits.* (13.) *In Mars.* (14.) *In the Sun.* (15.) *In Venus and Mercury. Hence the Falsity of the* Ptolemaick *Hypothesis.* (16.) *In the Moon.* (17.) *Planets whether inhabited.* (18.) *Telescopes Use on Earth.* (19.) *Uses of the Celestial Discoveries of the Telescope.* (20.) *Microscopick Discoveries and Writers.* (21.) *Viewing nigh Objects with a Telescope. Use thereof in Miniature-Painting.* (22.) *Measuring Distances at one Station by the Telescope.*

(1.) That the *Ancients* had no knowledg of *Optick-Glasses*, is most evident from their universal silence in this Matter: Their most learned and inquisitive Philosophers makeing no mention, or the least hint thereof, in their Writings. And doubtless a Contrivance of that universal Use, beneficial to all old Men, both in Reading and Writing, could never have been so concealed, as that not the least Footsteps

Optick-Glasses unknown to the Ancients.

thereof should remain to Posterity. The only Reliefs they had for their decayed Sights were certain *Collyria* or *Eye Salves*; and when these fail'd them, they were left almost in the *dark* for *minute* and *close Objects*.

We hear indeed mighty Stories of *Archimedes* burning the Ships of *Marcellus*, at a great distance from the Walls of *Syracuse*. But whether the Matter of Fact be *true* or *false* (as I am very inclinable to believe it *false*), yet there is no mention of his performing this admirable Effect by *Optick-Glasses*. Perhaps, if there were any such thing done at all; it was performed by *Concave Speculums*: And no one denies the Ancients the knowledg of *Catoptricks*. For *Archimedes* himself writ a Book (as 'tis said) *De Speculis Ustoriis Parabolicis*; but it has never yet seen the Light.

And yet there are in the World a sort of Men, so devoted to the past Ages, that they will not allow any Improvements of Arts in the modern Generation, unknown to the Ages some Centuries before us. Of this Class was he, (whoever he was) that, rather than the Ancients should be ignorant of *Optick-Glasses*, would forge a Passage in *Plautus* (which really is not at all to be found in him), for Confirmation of his Opinion.

Pretended Passage in Plautus

(2.) *Pancirollus* (who surely was too candid a Person to be the first Author of this Fiction) in the Second Book *De Rebus Inventis*, Tit. 15. quotes this Passage from *Plautus*, *Cedò Vitrum, necesse est Conspicilio uti*: Which, says he, cannot possibly be meant of any other thing but of the Glasses which we call *Spectacles*. And his Commentator *Salmuth* takes some pains to cite *Christianus Becmannus* (I suppose in his *Oratio de Barbarie & Superstitione superiorum Temporum*) for clearing this Passage of *Plautus*: But yet he is so hard pressed with it, that by no Art, but by main strength he breaks through it, and says, That notwithstanding that Passage, yet certainly *Optick-Glasses* are a modern Invention. Whereas

Whereas, had he been aware, that that Quotation from *Plautus* is a mere *Fiction*; and that no such Passage can be found in all his Writings; he might easily have avoided its Force, without all that stir. For so we shall find it answered in the *Lettere Memorabili del Abbate Michele Giustiani Parte Terza, Let. 16.* [Passage out of Plautus forged]

(3.) Another place cited for the Antiquity of *Optick-Glasses*, is that of *Pliny, Lib. 7. Cap. 53. Hist. Nat.* wherein we find the word *Specillum*. To this Passage we have this Answer in the forementioned Letters of *Giustiani*; that *Specillum* cannot possibly be here meant of a *Spectacle*-Glass, seeing we find the Expression, *Inungit Specillum*; which, says he, cannot be understood of *Spectacles*, which we rather *wipe* and *cleanse*, than *anoint* and *grease*. But this Construction of the Learned Authors is much *forced* and *unnatural*: For the plain sense of that Passage in *Pliny* is this. *Pliny* in that Chapter is giving Instances of the *sudden Deaths* of many Men; and telling how they were seized, whilst they were doing *so* or *so*, and wholly thoughtless of that fatal moment. Amongst many other Examples, he has this; *Super omnes C. Julius Medicus dum inungit, Specillum per Oculum trahens.* The meaning whereof is no more, than that the *Physician* C. Julius *was on a sudden seized by Death, whilst he was applying an Unguent to his Patients Eye, and drawing his Probe (called Specillum) through it.* Whereas, to joyn *inungit* and *Specillum*, spoils the Grammatical Sense of the whole, and renders it unintelligible [Passage in Pliny. Specillum a Chyrurgeon's Probe]

'Tis evident therefore, that from neither of these Passages can we draw any Argument for the *Antiquity of Optick Glasses*. [Optick-Glasses probably invented about 1300.]

(4.) Wherefore seeing we must necessarily allow this Invention due to the Modern Age of the World, our next Enquiry shall be, Where first to fix it. But herein we shall find but faint Traces to direct us.

Monsi. *Menage,*

Monsieur Menage a learned and ingenious French-man, in his *Origini della Lingua Italiana, Geneva,* 1685, commenting on the Word *Occhiali del Galilæi,* discourses there of the Time of the invention of *Spectacles*: And after relating the known Story of *Frier Jordan,* (of which more anon) he has this notable Passage; That *Monsieur du Cange* had told the Author (*Monsieur Menage*) of a Greek Poem, the Manuscript whereof is now in the *French* King's Library, wherein the Poet, who lived *An.* 1150, Jesting on the Physicians of those Times, says of them to this Purport in *French, Qu'ils tatent le Poux, & qu'ils Regardent les Excremens du Malade aver une Verre.* That they *observe the Excrements of their Patients with a Glass.* But Monsi. *Menage* is of Opinion, that this was a Transparent Glass, whelm'd over the Vessel, more for the Relief of their Nose against the Stench, than of their Eyes.

Menage's Opinion

But however we may doubt of *Spectacles* being so ancient as 1150. We may be certain that about the Thirteenth Century, they were commonly known and used. For (beside what we shall say hereafter of our Country-man *Frier Bacon*) the most learned Monsi. *Spon* in his *Recherches Curieuses D'Antiquité, Dissert.* 16. inserts a Letter of Signior *Redi* to *Paulus Falconerius,* concerning the Time when *Spectacles* were invented; and this he fixes between 1280 and 1311. from the Testimony of a Manuscript Chronicle in Latin, in the Library of the *Friers Preachers* of St. *Katherine* at *Pisa,* Fol. 16. Wherein 'tis said, that *Frater Alexander de Spina, Vir modestus & bonus, quæcunque vidit aut audivit facta, scivit & facere. Ocularia ab aliquo primo facta, & communicare nolente, ipse fecit & communicavit corde hilari & volente.* And this *Alexander de Spina* was a Native of *Pisa,* and dyed there, *An.* 1313.

Spina's Pretense

Signior *Redi* has in his Library a Manuscript written *An.* 1299. *Di Governo della Famiglia de Scandro di Pipozzo.* In which there is this Passage; *Mi truovo cosi Gravoso di Anni che non arei Valenza*

Another Authority

lenza Di Leggere e Scrivere senza Vetri appellati Okiali, Truovati novellamente per Commodità delli Pouveri Veki, quando affebolano del Vedere. Thus in English, *I find my self so pressed by Age, that I can neither read or write without those Glasses they call* Spectacles, *lately invented, to the great Advantage of poor Old Men, when their Sight grows weak.*

The *Italian* Dictionary, *de la Crusca*, on the Word *Occhiale*, makes this remark, That *Frier Jordan de Rivalto*, who dyed at *Pisa, An.* 1311. in a Book of Sermons which he writ *An.* 1305. tells his Auditory in one of them, that it is not Twenty Years since the Art of making *Spectacles* was found out, and is indeed one of the best and most necessary Inventions in the World. Frier Jordans Authority.

About the same time *viz.* 1305. *Bernard Gordon* a famous Physician of *Montpelier*, in his *Lilium Medicinæ*, thus commends a certain *Eye-Salve*: *Et est tantæ Virtutis, quod decrepitum faceret legere Literas minutas absque Ocularibus.* And *An.* 1363. *Guido de Chauliac*, in his Book entituled *Grand Chirurgery*, after proposing several *Collyria*, saith; If these or the like will not do, you must make use of *Spectacles*. Gordon. Chauliac.

From all which we may be pretty certain, That *Spectacles* were well known in the 13th. Century, and not much before. But who the Happy Man was, that first hitt upon this lucky Thought, may yet be questioned. 'Tis true indeed, if we credit the forementioned Chronicle of the Convent at *Pisa*, Frier *Spina* makes as fair a Challenge to the Invention, as the first Author, who refused to communicate it. But I am apt to believe, That, whoever this close Man was that would not impart to *Spina*, He was a Frier; and that these Monkish Men, and *Jordan* amongst the rest, had this Invention whispered amongst themselves, before it was publick; and that they all had the *First Hint* thereof from our Country-Man Frier *Roger Bacon*.

Bacon's Pretence.

(5) That this learned *Frier Bacon* who dyed *An.* 1292. and lyes buryed at *Oxford*) did perfectly well understand all sorts of *Optick-Glasses*, shall be plainly made out, from the natural and easie sense of his own Words, in his Book of *Perspective*: Whereby we shall find, that he not only understood the Effects of single *Convex* and *Concave-Glasses*, but knew likewise the way of *combining* them, so as to compose some such Instrument as our *Telescope*. This perhaps will be looked upon as a *Great Paradox*, and as great Partiality in an *English* Author to his Country-Man, especially considering, how universally the contrary has prevail'd; the Votes of most learned Men having conferr'd the Honor of this Invention on other Pretenders. But if, from the unconstrain'd Words of his Books, we plainly make out this Assertion, I hope the Attempt may not be counted unreasonable or partial.

And First in his Book of *Perspective* Part III. Dis. 2. C. 3. he has these Words; *Si vero Corpora non sunt plana* (having treated of them before) *per quæ Visus videt, sed sphærica; tunc est magna Diversitas, nam vel Concavitas Corporis est versus oculum, vel Convexitas, &c.* By which 'tis manifest, he knew what a *Concave* and *Convex Glass* was. Moreover, in the same Place *Dis.* ult. he proceeds thus; *De Visione fractâ majora sunt, nam de facili patet, maxima posse apparere minima, & è contra; & longè distantia videbuntur propinquissimè, & è converso: Sic etiam faceremus Solem & Lunam & Stellas descendere secundum Apparentiam huc inferius, &c.* Thus in English, *Greater Wonders than all these are performed by refracted Vision*; For thereby, 'tis easily made appear, that the Greatest Object may be represented as very little, and contrarily. And so likewise, the most distant Objects as just at hand, and contrarily. Hereby also may we bring the Sun and Moon and Stars down here below in Appearance, &c. This, I think, is so express in the Point, that it leaves no room to doubt, but that he had some admirable Secret in Optick Glasses. Add

to

to this what he has in his Epistle *ad Parisiensem*, of the Secrets of *Art* and *Nature*, Cap. 5. *Possunt etiam sic figurari Perspicua, ut longissimè posita appareant propinquissima, & è contrario, Ita quod ex incredibili Distantia legeremus literas minutissimas, & numeraremus Res quantumcunque parvas, & stellas faceremus apparere quò vellemus.* Glasses or Diaphanous Bodies, says he, *may be so formed, that the most remote Objects may appear as just at hand, and contrarily, So that we may read the smallest Letters at an incredible Distance, and may number things though never so small, and may make the Stars appear as near as we please.*

And that these Things may not seem *incredible* of this *Great Man*, who, in that dark, ignorant Age could be master of these admirable Inventions; I shall refer the Reader, for a more compleat Account of him, to *Ant. a Wood Hist. & Antiquit. Universit. Oxoniensis*, Lib. 1. Pag. 136. and to Dr. *Plott's Nat. Hist. of Oxfordshire*, Cap 9. Sect. 2, 3, &c. and Sect. 39, 40, 41. Where we may find, how he was persecuted by the ignorant malicious *Friers* of his Order, as practising *Magick* and *Necromancy*: for which they cast him into Prison, and there detain'd him for a long time, some say to his Death, in the 78th. Year of his Age. There we shall find, how he was the first Promoter of the *Emendation of the Calendar*. compleated afterwards in the Time of Pope *Gregory* II, But above all, his Pretense to the first *Invention* of *Gunpowder* seems as well founded, as possible, on this Passage in his *Epistola ad Parisiensem*, Cap. 6. (a Hundred years before *Barthold. Swartz.* lived) *In omnem Distantiam quam volumus, possumus artificialiter componere Ignem comburentem, ex sale Petræ & Aliis*; (These *Alia*, in another Manuscript Copy, are, *Sulfur & Carbonum Pulvis*) And soon after he adds, *Præter hæc* (i.e. *Combustionem*) *sunt alia stupenda Naturæ, nam sont velut Tonitrus & Coruscationes possunt fieri in Aere, imò majore Horrore* [Bacon invented Gunpowder.]

quam

quam illa quæ fiunt per Naturam: Nam modica materia adapta, sc. ad Quantitatem unius Pollicis, sonum facit horribilem, & Coruscationem ostendit violentem, & hoc fit multis modis, quibus Civitas aut Exercitus destruatur.: Igne exsiliente cum Fragore inestimabili. Mira hæc sunt, si quis sciret uti, in debita Quantitate & Materia. By which last Passage we may guess, he had not the way of applying it to a Gun; though 'tis manifest, he was sensible that some such Use might be made of it. But the particular Manner did not offer it self to him at first.

Note I Confess, I have not by me at this time the Originals, from whence these Passages are quoted, the present Distractions of our miserable Country having separated me and my Books; and the Place, where I am, affords not the Copies: Therefore, if in these Quotations I am any wife mistaken, I must not be blamed, acknowledging that I have them *at second hand* from the forenamed Authors.

But to return to our *Optick Glasses*. 'Tis evident that *Bacon* was acquainted with them; and probably knew how to adapt them in a *Telescope*. But the long and close Imprisonment he suffer'd before his Death (for 'tis said no one was permitted to speak to him; and that all his Writings, Books and Instruments were seized and burnt, except only those few Fragments of his which we have saved accidentally) was the Reason, that we have no farther Advancements of his in this kind transmitted to Posterity. But 'tis very probable that the use of single Glasses in *Spectacles*, as being an Invention of immediate Advantage to Human Life, and in it self very easie and simple, might therefore be presently catched at by the World, and put into Practice: Whilst his other more curious Combinations of Glasses might be lost and forgot. And this I am the more inclinable to believe; First, because *Frier Bacon's* Time agrees so well with *Frier Jordans* forecited Testimony *An.* 1305. That it was not then twenty

years

years since the Invention of *Spectacles*: And secondly, because we find this sort of *Monkish Men* first take notice of the Invention, before all other Men, which shews, they had it delivered amongst themselves only, for a while before others.

(6.) And thus much concerning *Frier Bacon*'s Pretense. But that I may not seem altogether partial, I shall here add the Opinions of others, concerning *Other Inventors* of the *Telescope*. For I find no other Pretenders to the Invention of single *Convex* and *Concave* Glasses, but the forenamed. *Borellus* has written a small Tract purposely on this Subject, *De vero Telescopii Inventore*: Wherein, Cap. 12 he seems to give the Invention to *Zacharias Joannides* of *Middleburg* in *Zeland*, An. 1590. Another Candidate for this Discovery, he names *Johannes Lipperhoy*, or *La Prey*, An. 1609. A *Dutchman* also, whom *Surturus* calls *Lipperlem*. *Adrianus Metius* Mathematick Professor at *Franequer* says, his Brother *Jacobus Metius* of *Alkmaer* was certainly the first Inventor of the *Telescope*. And if we believe the *Italians*, we shall have the Honour of inventing this Instrument conferr'd on the incomparable *Galileo*. But he himself in his *Nuncius sidereus* confesses, that the first Intimation he received of this Instrument, was, that a *Dutchman* had then lately made one, which set him (*Galileo*) upon the thought how to effect it, which, he says, he successfully discover'd by the consideration of *Refraction*, and found that a *Concave* and a *Convex* Glass rightly adapted would perform what he only heard in general of the *Dutch* Invention.

But certainly the first Publick notice of this Contrivance came from some of the forementioned *Dutchmen* (for *Frier Bacon*'s Hint mentions not the particular Combination of the Glasses) and therefore the Instrument is deservedly called *Tubus Batavus*. Though we must confess at the same time, that *Galileo*, An. 1610. (see his *Nuncius sidereus*) did first apply this curious Instrument to Celestial Observations; and had then made such wonderful Discoveries in the Heavens thereby, that all his Philosophick Successors have ever since attempted to climb higher, by lengthening their *Ladders*, and advancing this Instrument by many Degrees. However I must not here conceal the Pretense of *Baptista Porta*, who, in his *Magia Naturalis*, Lib. 17. Cap. 10. Printed *An.* 1589. has these Words, *Si utramque* (*Lentem sc. Concavam & Convexam*) *rectè componere noveris, & longinqua & proxima, majora & clara videbis.* But *Porta's* Character is so well known, that we may easily imagine, he had got this Hint from *Holland*.

Franciscus Fontana a *Neapolitan*, in his *Observationes cœlestium: terrestriumque rerum*, contends that he himself *An.* 1608. first invented the *Telescope*, composed of a *Convex Object-Glass* and *Convex Eye-Glass*: For the *Tubus Batavus*, and *Galileo's* Tube was furnish'd with a *Concave Eye-Glass*, and *Fontana* confesses, it was before his; and that *An.* 1618. he first invented the double *Microscope*. *Rheita* in his *Oculus Enoch & Eliæ*, Lib. 4 towards the end, pretends to be the first Discoverer of the *erecting Telescope* of three Convex Eye-Glasses, as also of the *Telescope* for looking with both Eyes, called *Telescopium binoculum*: Of which latter, *Cherubin* has writ his whole Volume, *La Vision parfait*, &c.

Baptista Porta.

Fontana

Rheita

(7.) Thus we see, how long the Use of single Optick Glasses was common in the World (even about 300 years) before Men rightly understood their due Application, in the Composition of this admirable Instrument. They had them in their hands, they look'd through them, *now a Convex, then a Concave*, and admired their Effects, and the Help they gave to disorder'd Eyes; but still were ignorant of the vast Advantage the most *acute* Eye might receive by them, even to the Increase of its Power, some Thousands of Degrees beyond its natural Abilities. This was reserved for some lucky Chance in a future Age, to be discovered by him that should first

(7) *Optick Glasses long known before the Telescope.*

[261]

first be so fortunate, as to adapt these Glasses at their *due Distance*: for to some such happy Hitt, I imagine the Invention is due; and not to any profound Thought on the nature and properties of Glasses, that first suggested the Contrivance to the *Dutch Mechanick*, that was its Author.

And this does naturally suggest a Thought to us, of some incouragements in natural Enquiries, by the method of *experimental Philosophy*, that perhaps we are every day ingaged amongst some *particular Things*, which we commonly see, handle, use, and are conversant with, and which have in them some latent, hidden Properties, which, upon a right Application, (to be discovered perhaps by some lucky Hitt) may be of the most useful and surprising Effects. And that therefore, we should not despair of making the greatest Discoveries about even the *meanest* Things. Who could expect to see such Wonders from an easie Composition of three such plain, simple Bodies, *Niter*, *Sulfur*, and *Charcole*, as we daily see from *Gunpowder*? And the Property of the *Magnet's* drawing Iron was commonly known many generations, before it was so happily applyed to guiding a Ship. Who could have thought, by looking upon that dark unpromising stone, that future Ages should use it to such a stupendous and advantageous a Purpose, far exceeding the Virtues of the most illustrious Gemms? Hence may we learn, not to despise the Products of Nature, even of the meanest Appearance. And let us not say, that any Discovery is *useless*, since we know not what Time and Posterity may produce from the simplest Truth. And this naturally leads me to the discoveries made by *Optick* Glasses.

Remark thereon. Uses of Discoveries not immediately known

(8.) *Galileo* (as is noted before) is deservedly reputed the first that raised up this *Gigantick* Instrument, that ventures to climb Heaven and from thence brings down the Stars. He first, was surprised and struck with wonder, to see *four little Moons* dancing round *Jupiter*, that from their first Creation

(3.) Celebr D.C. coveries of Tele-scope

to

to the lucky Moment when he firſt diſcovered them, had never ſtruck the eye of any mortal Inhabitant of this Globe. Were theſe then made for the *Uſe* of *poor Man*, from whoſe Knowledg they were concealed for 5000 years together? Vain Man! that thus preſumes to confine the Deſigns of the *Almighty Creator* to miſerable Duſt and Aſhes; when his *infinite Power* can make Millions of *intelligent Beings*, and all intelligent after different ways, to ſerve and praiſe him. And theſe perhaps are the Inhabitants of theſe *diſtant Worlds*, and of thoſe again infinitely extended beyond theſe. 'Tis true indeed, now theſe little Planets are diſcovered, we have happily applyed them to an advantageous purpoſe (as ſhall be ſhew'd hereafter) But this we are to eſteem as a particular Benefit of Providence to theſe latter Generations, and reſpects not all the general Race of Mankind, that lived and were buſie for 5000 years together, and knew nothing of them. But in this ſtupendous Enquiry I ſtop, as not being able to reach it with the *longeſt Teleſcope*

Whether all for the uſe of Man

To keep therefore to our Subject: I ſhall take the Heavens in order, as they lie; conſidering firſt the *uppermoſt*, and ſo deſcend *down* to our Earth, and ſhall briefly declare the *Diſcoveries* made in each, and (as far as I can attain it) by *whom* and *when*; with farther References to thoſe Authors, where each particular may be found more fully treated of.

(9) In the fixt Stars

(9.) And Firſt, for the *Fixt Stars*. That whitiſh Band or Zone, the *Galaxia* or milky Way, that ſo irregularly incompaſſes a great ſcope in the Heavens, and of which the Ancients could give no tolerable Account, is found by the Teleſcope to be no other, than an heap of very minute Stars thickly ſet together, which, by their great Diſtance, Smalneſs and Cloſeneſs, appear to the naked Eye, as one united whitiſh Cloud. In like manner, the *Nebuloſa Orionis, Præſepe Cancri, &c.* are found to be a Congeries of ſmall Stars cloſely ſet together, but eaſily diſtinguiſhable by the *Teleſcope*. The *Pleiades* or
ſeven

seven Stars (tho scarce more than six appear) are found by an ordinary Glass to be nigh forty. And in the single Constellation of *Orion*, the Telescope discovers more Stars than the naked Eye can number in all the Heavens. On this Account, the Seed of *Abraham*, that was to be made *numerous* as the Stars in the Firmament, may yet (for ought we know) admit of Propagations through many future Generations, before it comes up to its Limits. And the number, which *Archimedes* demonstrated greater than that of the Grains of Sand composing this Globe of Earth, may perhaps fall short of the Stars in the Heavens: For hardly any Corner of the Firmament so dark; But the Telescope, turn'd towards it, descries Multitudes of *glittering Spangles* therein.

(10.) From the *fixt Stars* let us contract our Prospect, and in a vast, long, and almost immense Course homewards, we first meet with *Saturn*. By his slow Motion he takes State upon him, as carrying about him something more weighty than ordinary. But the short sight percieves nothing thereof, and sees only a plain round Globe, as the rest of the *Chorus* dancing round the Sun. All his Equipage and Attendants are hid from our View, till surveyed more closely by the Telescope: And then behold a mighty Ring parallel to the Equator, bright as the Planets own Face, encompassing round his Body; very thin, and separated in all Appearance on all sides from his Globe: sometimes appearing broader, sometimes narrower, and sometimes almost vanishing, then again returning by a regular Period, and resuming by Degrees its former Shape, which again by degrees it looses according to his own Periodical Motion. But this is not all his Equipage, for besides this Throne of Light, this Majestick Planet is constantly attended by a Guard of *five Satellits*, that follow his Motion and dance round him continually in a Circle.

(10) In *Saturn*

Galilæo.

Galileo.   *Galileo* was the first that observed any thing extraordinary in *Saturns* Appearance *An.* 1610. *Octob.* as he tells us in some of his *Italian* Letters: But his Glasses were too short to give the true Shape of this Planet. All that he descry'd was something appendent on each side of him, which he took to be two Globes much less than *Saturns* own Body; and therefore he first publish'd (and at the same time conceal'd) this Discovery, by transposing the Letters of this Sentence, *altissimum Planetam tergeminum observavi*. But when the Telescope was better advanced, (as what Invention is it, that receives not Advancements in Time?) the true and genuine Appearance of *Saturn* began to shew it self, and its regular Changes were taken notice of. But though several Authors writ Treatises of this surprising Appearance, and particularly the celebrated *He-*

Hevelius.   *velius (de nativa Saturni facie) Hodierna,* &c yet all their Observations were imperfect and deficient; and chiefly for want of ex-

Hugenii Systema Saturni-   cellent Glasses. Till the incomparable *Christ. Hugenius* has put

um.   the last hand to this Affair; and in his ingenious Treatise, *Systema Saturnium, Hag. Comit.* 1659. 4°. has publish'd to the World a compleat History of all Observations of this Planets Appearances with a most ingenious Theory for their Explication. In the beginning of the year 1655. his excellent Person first discovered the biggest of *Saturns Satellits* with a Telescope of 12 feet, charged with an Eye Glass of 3 Inches; afterwards, *An.* 1656. he doubled that Length, retaining the same Eye-Glass. The Satellit he discover'd, is the *Fourth* from *Saturn*, and in the fore-named Treatise, he gives us the *Epochæ* and *Tables* of its Motion; But our most ingenious Countryman, Mr. *Halley*, deservedly celebrated for his Astronomical Labours, discovered in the year 1682. that *Hugenius*'s Numbers were considerably run out; and therefore he set himself to correct the Period of this *Satellit*, which he has done accordingly, Num. 145. Pag. 82. *Philosoph. Transact.* And in Num. 187. Pag. 299.

we

we shall find Monf. *Caffini*'s Tables of the Motions of all *Saturns Satellites*, together with their diftances from *Saturn* correspondent to their Periodical Times: Of which more hereafter.

The other four *Satellites* were all difcovered by Monf. *Caffini* in the Order following. The third and fifth were firft feen by him, *An.* 1671, 72 and 73. by a 17 Foot Glafs of *Campani*, and 36 Foot Glafs of *Divini*, and by fuch another of *Borelli*. An Account whereof may be feen at large in Num. 92. of the *Philofoph. Tranfact.* But the innermoft or firft, and the fecond were not feen by him till the year 1684. at which time, having procured Glaffes of an extraordinary length, as 80, 100, 150 and 200 Feet; the vaft diftance and fmalnefs of thefe Planets could no longer conceal them from his fight. *Vid. Philofoph. Tranfact.* Num. 181. *Caffini's Difcoveries about Saturn.*

The laft thing I fhall take notice of, relating to this Planet, is, That Monf. *Gallet*, *Provoft* of S. *Symphorian* at *Avignon*, in the year 1684. has advanced an Hypothefis for folving its Appearances; which, as it relates to the Telefcope, may properly be here confidered. I fhall therefore briefly propofe fome of the chief difficulties, that feem to attend this Theory: And that I may not be prolix, I fhall fuppofe the Reader acquainted with what Monf. *Gallet* lays down in the *Journal des Scavans*, *An.* 1684. *May* 15. & *June* 12. and in Latin in the *Acta Lipfiæ*, *An.* 1684. *Septemb.* Pag. 421. *Examination of Gallet's Hypothefis.*

Firft therefore, he fuppofes *Saturn* and the other Planets, except the Moon, *polite Globes*, reflecting the Image of the Sun as a *Convex Speculum*. Which feems not at all to be founded on more than mere *Conjecture*: For we have no Reafon to think them different in this particular from the Moon; which is found of a rugged uneven Surface.

But fecondly, granting that they (and efpecially *Saturn*) may be *polite Spheres*, (for we will not confine the infinite Variety of the Creation,) and granting that *Saturn* reflects two

M m   forts

forts of Light; one whereby his whole Body becomes visible; and the other the bright Image of the Sun from his Convex Surface; as we see a Convex Speculum is it self visible, by the Rays it reflects disorderly from its whole Surface; (which so far partakes of a little Roughness) and at the same time reflects a bright and orderly Image of the Sun, from one certain part of this Surface to the Eye rightly posited: Yet this bright Image of the Sun, which is reflected from *Saturn*, (how far soever *Saturn* be removed) can never be projected by an Object-Glass, in its distinct Base, *greater* than the Projection of the whole Body of *Saturn* in the same distinct Base. And yet (if I mistake not) this is the Foundation of Monf. *Gallet*'s Theory. This is so evident to any one the least versed in *Dioptricks* and *Catoptricks*, that 'tis needless to insist upon it any longer. We may make a convincing Experiment hereof: Expose a reflecting Convex Speculum before the Sun, and by a Convex Glass project the Image of this Speculum on a Paper in a dark Room: we shall there see the Representation of the Speculum it self, and of the bright Image of the Sun on the Speculum. And indeed by the least Consideration of the matter, it will be evident to us, that 'tis impossible it should be otherwise: For the little Image of the Sun, reflected from the Convex Speculum, possesses but a very small part of the Speculum's Surface; and therefore cannot possibly be projected, by the Object-Glass in its distinct Base, *greater* than the Projection of the Convex Speculum itself. The same may we conceive of *Saturn*, by supposing him a Convex, polite, reflecting Speculum, for though he should then, besides the Figure of his own Body, reflect the bright Image of the Sun, from a small part of his Spherick Surface on the Object-Glass; yet the Object-Glass could never project, in its distinct Base, the Representation of this Image of the Sun *greater* than the Representation of the whole Body of

Saturn.

Tab 40 pag 267

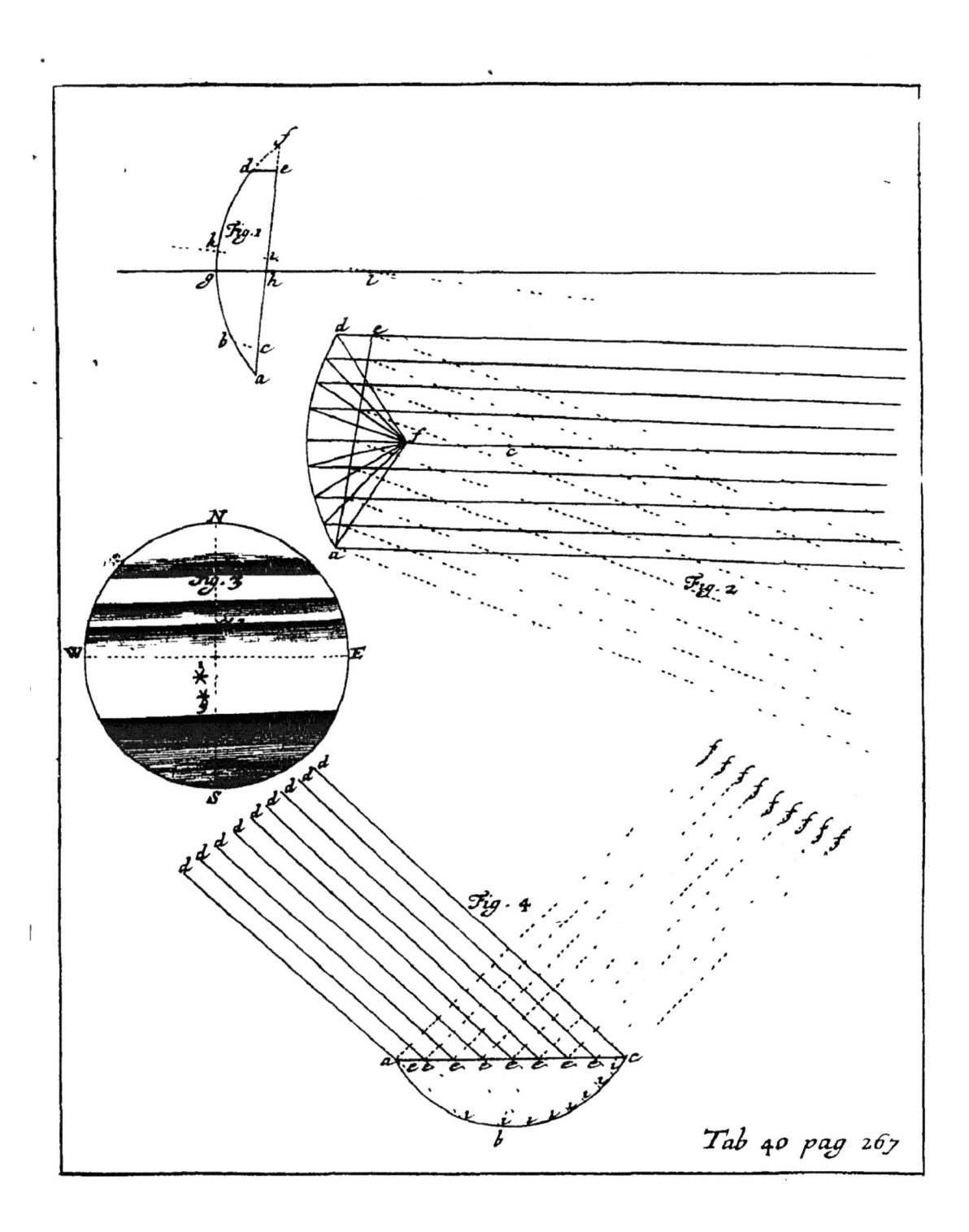

Saturn. And, notwithstanding the Evidence hereof, Monf. *Gallet* affirms, the Appearance of *Saturns Ring* or *Anfæ* proceed to-from hence; that the Object-Glafs projects, in its diftinct Bafe, the reprefentation of the bright Image of the Sun, reflected from *Saturn's Convex polite Surface,* greater than (or clearly *without*) the Reprefentation of his *Body* itfelf.

Thirdly, Monf. *Gallet* affirms, that the Reafon why *Jupiter, Mars,* &c. are not projected by an Object-Glafs, in its diftinct Bafe, with a *Ring* or *Anfæ,* is becaufe thefe Planets are *nearer* to us than *Saturn*: And therefore in the Projection of *Jupiter,* the bright Image of the Sun reflected from its polite Surface, is reprefented by the Object-Glafs in its diftinct Bafe, *equal* to the Reprefentation of *Jupiters* whole Body; in the Projection of *Mars* it is *lefs,* &c. But the Diftance of thefe Planets (even of the nigheft) is fo very great, (and as it were infinite) in refpect of the fmall Breadth of an Object-Glafs; that in comparifon to this fmall breadth of an Object-Glafs, we can make no difference between the Diftance of *Saturn* and even *Mercury.*

Laftly, the Experiments, on which Monf. *Gallet* founds his whole *Hypothefis,* feems not at all to confirm, or in the leaft wife to refpect what he builds thereon. The Phænomenon arifing from reflecting the Sun-Beams by an Object-Glafs on a Wall pofited *obliquely,* proceeds from the Object-Glafs being confider'd as a *Concave Reflecting Speculum,* having alfo another Surface either Plain or Convex befides the Concave, (as I have noted before, Chap. 4. Sec. 4.) and yet he fuperftructs hereon a Theory, for explaining the Appearances of *Convex Polite Surfaces,* fuch as he makes the Planets. This will be manifeft by *Tab.* 40. *Fig.* 4. wherein, for eafe fake, we take a Plano-Convex Glafs *a b c,* and expofing its plain fide *a e c* obliquely to the Suns Rays *d e, d e, d e,* fome of them fhall be reflected by the plain Surface *a e c* into *e f, e f, e f,* but others of them entring the Glass run on in *e i, e i, e i,* (we do not here consider the Refraction they suffer) and so falling on the Concave Surface *a i b i c* (for so I'll call it) are *reflected* by it, according to the Laws of *Spherick Catoptricks*: But the Reflections of these immerged Rays I have not expressed, for avoiding Confusion in the Scheme. I acknowledge, the *Physical Cause* of this latter Reflection, from the Surface of the Glass *a i b i c*, is perhaps not to be accounted for by Human Understanding; but the matter of Fact is certain. One should think, when the Rays are arrived at the extreme Points *i, i, i,* of the hindmost Surface of the Glass, they should, without any of them being reflected at all, emerge from the Glass: But 'tis manifest *some* of them are *reflected*, and that too, just in the same manner, as if the Surface *a i b i c* were a Polite, Opake, Concave Surface, and not covered by the Surface *a e c*. They that desire to enquire farther into the natural Cause hereof, may consult *Grimaldi Physico-Mathesis de Lumine & Coloribus, Bonon.* 1665. 4°.

'Tis then by the Reflection from this Concave Surface *a i b i c*, (give me leave so to call it) that the Similitude of *Saturns Ansæ* are represented in *Gallets* Experiment; and by the Reflection from the *Plain* Surface *a e e c*, that the Similitude of his Body is represented in the said Experiment. And how this can be accommodated to the Reflection, which *Saturn* himself makes from his own Body, and to his Appearance through a Telescope, I confess I cannot apprehend. Moreover *Gallet's* Hypothesis gives no Account of the two dark Spaces on each side the Globe of *Saturn*, between his Body and the *Ansæ*. For the Experiment, on which he founds his Fancy, shews no such Distinction, all being inlightened therein: As will be visible to those shall try it.

'Twere too tedious in this Place to consider particularly Monsf. *Gallet's* Scheme, and his *Particular System* of *Saturn*;

which

which might easily be shewn defective. But thus much I thought requisite to say in this Place; because the Theory he proposes is of a *Dioptrical* Consideration: Because it has never yet been taken notice of by any other: And because he advances it in Opposition to Monſ. *Hugens Syſtem*, which carries with it so much Probability.

(11) *Jupiter* next presents himself less incumbred than *Saturn*, yet not wanting a Courtly Train: For tho his Guards are but *four* in number, yet their size and brightness shew their *Strength*, and their quick Motion round him shews their Diligence.

Galileo was certainly the first Inhabitant of this Globe, that ever saw these *Satellites*, *Jan.* 7, 1610. And from that Moment to this, no more could ever be discovered about him: Though Vanity and desire of being the Author of some Novelty, made Frier *Ant. de Rheita* proceed so far, as to write a Tract of 5 more *Satellits* (9 in all) about *Jupiter*. But *Hevelius*, in the fourth Chap. of his *Selenography*, has demonstrated the *Frier* to be mistaken, and has shewn the small fixt Stars (only discoverable by the Telescope) that deceived him.

These *Satellites* are easily seen by a 3 Foot Glass, and I have just perceived them with one of 15 Inches. But to make exact Observations of their Motions, 'tis requisite, we use Tubes of 10 and 12 Feet and upwards. From the time of their Discovery, many curious Astronomers have attended their Motions round *Jupiter* with a diligent Eye; and have found, that sometimes falling into the Shadow of *Jupiters* Body, they disappear; and thence emerging, they again become visible: sometimes they are hid behind the very Globe of their great Lord, and sometimes being just in his Face, his Splendor overcomes theirs, and they become invisible, as a glimmering Lamp between the Eye and Sun.

Job.

Joh. Alfons Borellus has publish'd a Tract of the *Theoricks* of these *Medicea Sidera* (so named by *Galileo* in complement to his great Patron the *Duke* of *Tuscany*) *Theoricæ Mediceorum siderum, Florent.* 1666. 4°. But none have laboured more to reduce the Observations of these little Planets to something of Use and Advantage to the World, than the two celebrated Astronomers of the present Age, *Cassini* and *Flamsteed*: The former has taken great pains in Publishing Hypotheses, Tables, and Precepts for calculating their Appearances and Eclipses, (in his *Ephemerides Mediceorum siderum*, 1668. *Bonon.*) in order to setling the *Longitudes* of Places to a great Certainty. And the latter finding the Numbers of *Cassini*'s Tables not so *just* to the present Time, from most accurate Observations of his own, taken by the Telescope and Micrometer, has fixt new Numbers, that agree about this time most exactly to the *Phænomena*, but with the Liberty to himself of altering these Numbers, as by future Observations he shall find Occasion; For he is not so *positive* as to say, that what he settles (for 15 or 20 years) shall be *perpetual*. What he has hitherto published of this kind may be found dispersed in the *Philosoph. Transact.* wherein, he has given the World the Catalogues of these *Satellits Eclipses* for several years consecutively. In Num. 154. Pag. 404. he shews their Uses, and how (by their Help) the *difference* of *Longitude* betwixt any two Places on Earth, where they should be observed, might be determined: And *teaches* a Method of finding out, within what space on our Globe any of them are observable. These Directions he repeats in Latin, Num. 165. Pag. 760. for the use of Forreiners. In Num. 177 & 178. with the Catalogue of Eclipses for the year 1686. he describes a small Instrument; and shews how by the help of it, of the said Catalogue, and of the Tables of *Jupiters Geocentrick Places* and *Parallaxes*, the Appearances of the *Satellites* at any time in that year might be discovered, and delineated by Scale and

and Compass on Paper. But the Curiosities, which this excellent Astronomer has yet unpublished, relating to this useful Part of Astronomy, are very great and ingenious; which I hope, in time, he will impart to the World; as with much Freedom and Generosity, he now communicates them to his private Friends: In the Number of which I am very proud to reckon my self.

Before I quit this Article of the *Satellites*, I cannot omit taking notice of an Observation, which, by mere Accident, I made some years ago, of a *Total Disappearance* of all the *Satellites*. I had often attended their Motions with a good Telescope of 12 Foot, and often had them *all four* conspicuous at a time, very often *three*, frequently *two*, but never less than *one*, and this but very rarely; till *An.* 1681. *Novemb.* 2. *Hor.* 10. *p. m. Dublinii St. Vet.* there was *not one of them visible*; *Jupiter* there stood by himself, in all Appearance, without his Guards; and a bold *Lucian* might have pull'd him from his Throne without Resistance. Some years after, I obtain'd from my learned Friend Mr. *Flamsteed* his Tables of the Motions of these *Satellites*, And the Postures of these *Jovial Moons*, at that time, are found by them to be as is expressed in *Tab.* 40. *Fig.* 3. The first, third and fourth were *just in his Face*, and were therefore drown'd by his Light, and the second was *behind* his Body. The rarity of this Appearance (at least to me) makes me note it so particularly: perhaps those that are more frequently imploy'd in watching their Motions may meet sometimes with the like Conjunctions; but I believe 'tis very seldom. *Hevelius*, in his constant Attendance on them, for more than a year and half, hit not upon such an Appearance; as may be seen by the History of his Observations at the end of his *Selenographia*; Nor *Cassini*, as is manifest from his forementioned Ephemerides.

Satellites all disappearing

T 40 F 3

Besides these *four* little *Moons* about *Jupiter*, the Telescope discovers other Remarkables even in his Body. As first his

Jupiter's Belts

Face

Face is not all of a Colour; But there are in it *brighter* and *darker* Parts; and thefe are drawn athwart him, like broad *Zones* or *Belts* almoft parallel to the Ecliptick, as is expreffed in *Fig.* 3. *Tab.* 40.

T40 F3

Jupiter's Spot and Rotation

The laft thing that has been obferved in this Planet is a *Spot*, firft feen by our Ingenious Mr. *Hook* May 9. h. 9. p. m. 1665. By this *Spot* 'tis manifeft, that *Jupiter* turns round his own Axis in the fpace of lefs than 10 hours, or about 9^h. 56'.

Hence the Rotation of our Earth.

A very ftrong Argument to prove, that our Earth may do fo likewife; fince *Jupiter*, who is fo confiderably *bigger* than the *Earth*, has a Motion much more quick than ours in 24^h. *Kepler*, upon the Reftauration of the *Pythagorean* or *Copernican Hypothefis*, did conjecture, from the Motion of the Primary Planets about the Sun as their Centre, That the Sun *moved* about its own Axis; but could not evince it, till future Obfervations by the *Telefcope* difcovered *Spots* in the Sun, and by *them* demonftrated, that the Sun revolves on its own Axis, in $25\frac{1}{4}$ days. *Jupiter* has four *fecondary* Planets moving round him, and he himfelf in their Centre *turns* on his Axis: our *Earth* has a *fecondary* Planet, the *Moon*, that moves round her *once a Month*: is it not therefore highly *probable*, that the *Earth* alfo *revolves diurnally* on its Axis? For a farther account of this *Spot* in *Jupiter*, I refer to the *Philofoph. Tranfact.* N. 1. P. 3. N. 4. P. 75. N. 8. P. 143. N. 12. P. 209. N. 15. P. 246. N. 82. P. 4039.

(12.) Reflection on the Motions of Saturn's and Jupiter's Satellites, evincing the Order of the Creation.

(12.) But before I leave *Saturn* and *Jupiter*, I cannot but take notice of one admirable Property, for the Knowledge whereof, we are beholden to the Telefcope; and that is, the wonderful Agreement which is found in all the feveral Syftems of our Vortex; as well between the General *Syftem* of the Sun, and Primary Planets with the particular *Syftem* of *Saturn*'s or *Jupiter*'s Planets, as between the particular Syftems themfelves, in this fingle Property, *That the Periodical Times of the Planets Revolutions are in a fefquialtera Ratio of their Diftances from the Centre*

Centre of the Planet about which they revolve. That is, As the Square of the Period of the first *Satellite* (for instance): To the Square of the Period of the second :: So the Cube of the Distance of the first from *Jupiter*'s Centre. To the Cube of the Distance of the second from his Centre. This holds most exquisitely true in *Jupiter's Satellites*, as is noted by the admirably learned Mr. *Newton*, in his incomparable Treatise, *Philosophiæ Naturalis Principia Mathematica,* Lib. 3. Hypoth. 5. And the same *Law of Motion* is strictly observed by the five Primary Planets, and the Earth about the Sun. As he notes, Hypoth. 7, 8. This is also verifyed by Monsf. *Cassini* in the five *Satellites* of *Saturn*, as appears by his Account of them in the *Philosoph. Transact.* Num. 92. P. 5178. N. 133. P. 831. N. 181. P. 79.

And from hence may we justly fall into the deepest Admiration, that *one* and the *same Law* of Motion should be observed in Bodies so vastly distant from each other, and which seem to have no Dependence or Correspondence with each other. This does most evidently demonstrate, that they were all at first put into Motion, by *one* and the *same unerring Hand*, even the *infinite Power* and *Wisdom* of God, who has *fixt* this *Order* amongst them *all*, and has *establish'd* a *Law*, which they cannot *transgress*. *Chance* or *dull Matter* could never produce such an *Harmonious Regularity* in the Motion of Bodies so vastly distant: This plainly shews a *Design* and *Intention* in the *first Mover*. And with Submission to the Reverend and Learned *Divines*, I am apt to think, that one Argument drawn from the *Order*, *Beauty* and *Design* of Things, is more forcible against *Atheism*, than Multitudes of Notional Proofs drawn from *Ideas*, Apparitions of *Specters*, *Witches*, &c. (not that these should lose their due Strength) For besides the *Heavens*, even the *little Globe* we inhabit affords us infinite Variety in this kind: And for my own part, I must confess, I can read

Beauty Order and Design of natural Bodies strong Proofs of a Deity.

read more Divinity in Mr. *Charlton*'s admirable *Muſæum*, on a Box of beautiful *Shells*, of delicately painted *Plants*, curiouſly adorned *Inſects, Serpents, Birds*, or *Minerals*; than in large Volumes of Notional Writers. For *Animals, Plants*, and *Minerals* do yield us abundant Inſtances, which viſibly ſhew a *Deſign* or *End propoſed*; which, as it cannot poſſibly conſiſt with *Chance*, ſo neither can it be apprehended to have been ſo *ab æterno*: For 'tis abſolutely unconceivable, that a thing *deſigned* for ſome *End* or *Purpoſe*, ſhould not be ſo *deſigned* in *time*, by ſome *deſigning Being*. But I beg Pardon for this Digreſſion, in which I am thus ingaged before I was aware. To return therefore to our Subject.

(13) Mars

(13.) *Mars* offers himſelf next; who, truſting in his own Strength, is attended by no Guards; But the Prying Teleſcope diſcovers in his Face *Scars, Spots*, and *Ruggedneſs*, as we may find in the *Philoſoph. Tranſact.* Num. 14. P. 239. &c. By theſe

Rotation

Spots the acute *Caſſini* has determin'd, that he *turns* on his own *Axis* once in 24ʰ. 40′. tho others aſſign his Revolution performed in juſt half that time (a Miſtake eaſie enough) *vid. ibidem*. The fiery Face of this Planet requires a very good Teleſcope to view him, and a ſmall Aperture on the Object-Glaſs: or elſe this Glaring Light makes but a confuſed Appearance. But however furious his Beams are, he is beholden for them (as all the reſt of the Planets) to the great Fountain of Light and Heat the *Sun*. For what the great diſtance of *Saturn* and *Jupiter*, and their being ſo much *above* the *Sun* (as I may ſo

Increaſes and Decreaſes.

ſpeak) hinders us from ſeeing, *viz.* their *Increaſe* and *Decreaſe* in Light like our Moon, is very viſible in the Planet *Mars*; who, in his *Quadratures* with the Sun, and in his *Perigeon*, may be ſeen almoſt *biſſected*, but never *corniculated* or *falcated* as the other Inferiours, *Vid. Hevelii Selenograph.* Cap. 4. P. 66.

(14.) The Sun Sun's Spots

(14.) The glorious *Sun* does next preſent; in whoſe bright Face, we can hardly expect to find *dark Spots*. yet ſuch there are,

are, and *frequent* too. *Scheinerus* in his *Rosa Ursina* has published a large Book in *fol.* of nothing else; and *Hevelius*, at the end of his *Selenography*, has many Observations of these *Maculæ*, as also of some brighter Spots in the *Sun*, called *Faculæ*. The Way of observing them is taught at large, in the foresaid Authors; and is in short, either by admitting the Light of the Sun through a Telescope upon a white Paper, in a dark Room, or by arming the Eye with a small thin Glass *smoaked* over a Torch, Lamp, or Candle, and with it looking through a Telescope at the *Sun's* Body. The only Discovery that has been made by these *Maculæ*, is, that the Sun revolves round his own Axis, in the Space of about $25\frac{1}{4}$ days. But for a compleat and succinct Account of the Theory of these *Maculæ* and their Motions, I refer the Reader to the excellent Mathematician *Andrew Tacquet*, *Astronom.* Lib. 8. Tract. 3. Num. 7. 'Tis only to be noted, that for these several years past, the Appearance of these *Maculæ* has been much more rare, than when *Galileo* (who certainly first discovered them) *Scheinerus*, *Hevelius*, attended their Observations, viz. about 50 or more years ago. About that time, one should seldom see the *Sun's* Face (no more than now our brighter Beauties here below) free from one or more *black Patches*, but now (as if they were grown out of Fashion) he seldom wears any: One in 5 or 7 years hardly appearing. As if *now* he put them on, more of necessity, to cover an odd Pimple, that may otherwise disfigure his Countenance, than to adorn his Face. How far the *Fair Sex* should follow his Example, I dare not venture to determine. But from them we naturally fall to *Venus*.

Sun's Rotation.

Sun's Spots rare of late

(15.) *Venus*, the brightest Planet in the Heavens. She fears not sometimes even at Noon-day to display her Beauty; and in this Armour reposing an entire Confidence, performs her Course *alone*, and free from all other Attendants.

(15) *Venus and Mercury*

Mercury's Wit and Quickness secures him, therefore he has no Train, but generally shelters himself under the Beams of his potent Lord the Sun.

Increase and Decrease

But both these Inferiour Planets are found by the Telescope to *increase* and *decrease*, as our *Moon*. For sometimes they appear *corniculated*, sometimes *falcated*, sometimes *gibbous*, and sometimes *full* even on, or nigh to their Conjunctions with the Sun. By which last Phænomenon, 'tis manifest they move about the Sun, sometimes *farther* from us, sometimes *nigher* to us than he. and consequently the *Ptolemaick Hypothesis* is absolutely *false*. (whatever *Hyothesis* be true.) And for the Demonstriable Detection of this *Error*, we are beholden to the *Telescope*: And I doubt not but Posterity may, by the same Instrument, discover some *Hypothesis* as *positively true*: For the *Probabilities* of the *Copernican* System are already so strongly confirm'd thereby, that there seems no Room left for any farther Doubt, But Time and Labour will yet discover farther Proofs. How successfully Mr. *Hook* has applyed the Telescope to prove the *Motion* of the *Earth*, I leave the Reader to judge upon Perusal of his *Attempt*.

Falsity of the Ptolemaick Hypothesis

(16) *Discoveries in the Moon.*

(16.) And thus at last are we arrived at home to contemplate our Neighbour the *Moon*. Her may we properly call *our own*, as making us the Centre of her Periodical Motion. For, as the *Satellites* about *Saturn* or *Jupiter* move round *them*; so moves the *Moon* as a Satellite about our Earth. *Galileo* with his Telescope first discover'd great Ruggedness in the *Moons* Face, after him *Langrenus* the King of *Spain's* Cosmographer, attempted to draw her Picture. But the noble *Hevelius* in his curious and costly Work of *Selenography*, has perfected this Affair, perhaps beyond Amendment. There may we see the *Moons* Countenance distinguished in an admirable difference of Parts, both for Shape and Colour. We may there see greater Parts that resemble our Seas, Lakes, Rivers, Islands,

Peninsulas,

Peninsulas and Continents; other lesser Spots (almost infinite in number) that resemble our Mountains, Hills and Vallies. Of the *greater* Parts, those that are something *obscure*, may we reckon *Seas* and *Lakes*; and the brighter may we account *Land*. For just so does our Earth appear, when, from a distant Height we look upon a Mixture of Land and Water enlightened by the Sun. Of the *smaller* Spots, those that are *brightest* and *shine*, are Mountains and Rocks, and the *darker* Parts, which are usually encompassed with these *brighter* Verges, may we esteem *Vallies*.

Now that some Parts of the Moon are much higher than others, is as manifest by the Telescope, as that some Parts of our Earth are higher than others. For if we look upon it about the Quarter-days, we shall plainly see the Edge, towards the dark Part, broken and cragged, and many little bright Spots, that are clearly separated from the rest of the enlightned Part. Which is an evident Proof that these are the high Tops of Eminencies, which receive the Suns Light, before the Parts *below* them are enlightned. Moreover the Moons Spots cast their Shadows *opposite* to the Sun, that is, to the *Eastward*, whilst the Moon is *Increasing*, and to the *Westward*, on her *Decrease*. That these Mountains are very *high*, is manifest from the way of Measuring them, delivered in *Riccioli Almagest*. 1. Pag. 208. And *Tacquet Geom. Prac.* Cap. 8. Prob. 2. *Mountains in the Moon.*

For the better distinguishing these Spots, and making them more useful in the Observation of Lunar Eclipses, there are names imposed on them by Authours: *Hevelius* assigns to them the names of Places here on Earth: *Grimaldus* and *Ricciolus* give to them the names of famous Mathematicians and Astronomers. *Names imposed on the Spots.*

By means of these Spots, Lunar Eclipses are now much more accurately observed than formerly, to the great Advancement of Geography and Navigation, in setling the Longitudes *Eclipses accurately observed by them.*

gitudes of Places. For now the Immersions and Emersions of these Spots from the Shadow of the Earth are most nicely determined.

Moreover, by these Spots the Moon is discovered to have *various librating Motions,* from *East* to *West,* and from *West* to *East,* also from *North* to *South,* and from *South* to *North.* But hereof we cannot now enlarge, *vid. Bulhaldi Astrom. Philolaic. Lib.* 3. *Cap.* 13. *Hevelii Selenograph: Riccioli Almagest.* 1. *Lib.* 4. *Cap.* 9. Neither is it needful to insist on the Moons *Transits over,* and *Appulses to,* fixt Stars and Planets; which can never be accurately observed but by the Telescope. I cannot tell whether it be worth our while to take notice in this Place, that Monsr. *Isaac Vossius* has published a fantastical Conceit of his own, for explicating the Appearance of the Moons Spots; in his *Liber variarum Observationum.*

(17) Planets whether inhabited.

(17.) And now perhaps we may be allowed to sit down, and think awhile, whether all these Celestial Bodies, that thus dance round our Sun, may not be inhabited. But this Disquisition has been already so ingeniously managed by several, (particularly by the Reverend Dr. *Wilkins* Bishop of *Chester,* in his *World in the Moon;* and by Monsr. *Fontenel* his *Plurality of Worlds*) that there is little left to be said on the Subject. I shall only add, that there is nothing in *Nature, Morality* or *Religion,* that contradicts the *Affirmative* of this Opinion. And 'tis through a narrowness of Thought that some men *deny* it. They will not think on any other sort of Creatures, than what we see here on Earth; and presently begin to ask, how should *Men* possibly live in *Saturn's cold* Climates, or in the scorching *Heat* that affects *Mercury.* But shall we thus confine the *Great Creator* to our poor Conceptions? Cannot he that has made a Man, a Whale, an Elephant, a Fly, be able to create indefinite Varieties of Creatures, and all endowed with different Faculties, and various

Ways

Ways of Perception? Some adapted to one Planet, others to others? And all these may be ingaged in different Ways of Life and Thought, but should all be ingaged in Praising and Serving him that gave them all their *Beings*.

(18) But here I quit these remote Thoughts; and from viewing the admirable Extent, Beauty, Order and Variety of the Creation abroad, betake my self *home* to our own Globe. And here we shall not lay aside our *Telescope* as *useless*: We may imploy it on various Occasions and divers Concerns of Human Life. The Merchant may with this discern afar his rich-laden Vessels, whose Sides and Sails are swell'd, and look big with imported Wealth. The Seaman may discern his Friend or Foe. The wealthy Countryman may survey his distant Herds, Plantations, and Labourers, and Generals may observe their wide-spread Troops. But endless would it be to touch on all; the contriving Head will find it *useful*, and adapt it to his own particular Concerns on many Occasions, that cannot now be thought of. *(18.) Telescopes Use on Earth*

(19) And thus much shall suffice in short, concerning the *Discoveries* made with the *Telescope*. And now I hope it will not be asked, *Cui Bono*? To what *End* are all these Discoveries? What Advantage is there in them? For, if the Advancement of *Astronomy* have any good in it; if the furnishing us with a Contemplation from whence we may evince the *Power* and *Wisdom* of an *Almighty Creator* be any Good, If affording an Opportunity of admiring the vast Extent, Order and Beauty of the Creation be any Good, I am sure, hereby we reap all these *Goods* in an ample manner. But supposing that nothing of all these Advantages were at hand just at present, let not the inquisitive Philosopher therefore despond in his Enquiries. The consideration of the *Magnet* (as I have noted before) teaches us what Secret Virtues may lurk in the simplest Things. And what admirable Uses Posterity may raise *(19) Uses of the Telescopes Celestial Discoveries*

out

out of them. The *Torricellian Experiment* was long apply'd *only* to Disquisitions concerning a *Vacuum*, before our incomparable Philosopher the Honorable Mr. *Boyle*, one of the chief Glories of the *English* Nation, discovered its Usefulness in predicting the Weather, by which 'tis become one of the most pleasant Instruments in the World. But this I say, not so much to encourage men in the Prosecution of *useless* Enquiries (for doubtless he is *best* imployed that can propose the *best* Advantages to Mankind from his Studies) But to discourage some men from exclaiming against all Labours as absolutely *useless*, whose *immediate* Use they do not apprehend.

(20.) Of the Microscope.

(20.) And now that we are arrived at home, let us change our Instrument, and take into our hands a *Microscope*. And indeed with this, our Contemplations may be *endless*; all things affording such admirable Appearances, such curious Contexture of Parts, and such delicate vivid Colours; that the Contrivance of the *Almighty Creator* is as visible in the *meanest Insect* or *Plant*, as in the greatest *Leviathan* or strongest *Oak*. To touch upon all the Wonders this Instrument shews us, would be infinite, I shall therefore only refer to those, who have prosecuted Enquiries therewith to great Exactness.

Fontana

Franciscus Fontana in his *Observationes Cœlestium Terrestriumque Rerum* (wherein he challenges to himself the Invention of the *double Microscope, An.* 1618.) is the first (that I can learn) who published *Microscopical* Observations of some few Bodies. After

Borellus.

him *Borellus* at the end of his Tract, *De vero Telescopii Inventore, An.* 1650. does the same. Next a learned *Englishman* Dr. *Power, An.* 1664. did the like. But all these went no farther than verbal Description; they want those curious and lively Schemes,

Power

Hook

which the learned and ingenious Mr. *Hook* presents to the World in his *Micrographia, An.* 1665. a Book full of admirable Discoveries by the *Microscope*, and other curious Enquiries. The learned Dr. *Grew*, and the excellent *Bononian* Philosopher

Grew.

losopher *Marcel. Malpighius,* have laboured most successfully *Malpighius* in the *Anatomy* of *Plants* by the Microscope; and the latter has used it much in his Books, *de Ovo incubato, de Bombyce, de Viscerum structura, &c.* The *Heer Lewenhoeck* of *Delft* in *Holland,* *Lewenhoeck.* has lately apply'd himself with great Diligence to the use of Microscopes: of which Instrument he thinks he has a better kind than was ever yet known. When I visited this Gentleman at *Delft,* he shew'd me several that indeed were very curious; but nothing more than what I had ordinarily seen before; being composed only of one single, very minute Glass-Sphere or Hemisphere, placed between two very thin pierced *Laminæ*, or Plates of Brass, and the Object was brought to its due distance before the Glass by a fine Screw: But for his *best* sort, he beg'd our Excuse in concealing them. The Observations he has made with his Glasses are Printed in several Letters of his in *Dutch*, but for the most part, they are to be found dispers'd in the *Philosophical Transactions.* The last Author that has professedly treated of *Microscopick* Observations, is *Johan. Fran. Griendelius* in his *Micrographia nova Norimberg.* 1687. wherein he has taken a great deal of pains in giving the genuine Representations of his Objects as magnify'd. *Griendelius*

I have been often delighted with the curious Appearance of *Circulation of the Blood in Water-Newts* many Objects seen through the Microscope. But none ever surprised me more, than the visible *Circulation* of the Blood in Water-Newts (*Lacerta aquatica*) to be seen as plainly as Water running in a River, and proportionably much more rapid. Of this I have formerly given the Account at large to the *Royal Society.* And 'tis publish'd in the *Philosophical Transact.* Num. 177. P. 1236.

(21.) I shall conclude all, with two remaining Uses of *(21 Viewing nigh Objects with the Telescope.* the *Telescope.* The first is, *To view nigh Objects therewith.* The most apposite Telescope for our Purpose, is that consisting of a *Convex Object-Glass* and *Convex Eye-Glass.* But what is delivered

vered hereof, is easily accommodated to the Telescope with a Concave Eye Glass; but this latter, taking in but a narrow space of the Object, is not so proper for our Purpose.

Wherefore, suppose we have a Telescope, whose Object-Glass has its *Focal* Length for very *distant Objects* just 3 Foot, (how to find this exactly, I have shewn Chap. IV. Sect. 3.) This we'll call the *Solar Focus*. And suppose the Focus of the Eye-Glass be just 2 Inches; and that we were to view with this Telescope an Object 20 Foot distant from the Object-Glass. 'Tis required to find the *distinct Base* of this Object-Glass exposed now to this *nigh* Object 20 Foot distant, which in the First Part is called the *Respective Focus*.

And this is done by Prop. V. of the First Part: By this Analogy,

> As the difference between the *Distance* of the *Object* and *Glasses Focus*:
> To the *Glasses Focus* ::
> So the *Distance* of the *Object from the Glass*:
> To the *Distance* of the respective *Focus*, or *distinct Base from the Glass*.

In the Numbers of our Example thus,

204 . 36 :: 240 . 42,35 + = equal to the distinct Base of this Object-Glass exposed now to this nigh Object. So that the Distance of the Object-Glass from the Eye-Glass, which, for viewing *distant* Objects, was 36+2=38 Inches; must now be 42,35+2=44,35 Inches; and so much is the Telescope to be lengthened to view this Object distant only 20 Foot.

Viewing Pictures in Miniature. The use of this Theorem is very pretty; and they who draw Pictures in *Miniature*, may practise it to good Purpose. For the small Picture (being *inverted* that it may appear *erect*, and placed in a strong Light, and thus looked at with a Telescope) may

may be made to appear full as *bigg* as the natural Face, or *bigger* if we please. And by this means, the least Errors of the Painter may be easily discovered, which cannot be done so well by a single Convex-Glass, as will be manifest to those who shall try and compare both Ways. And this naturally leads me to the last Use of the Telescope I shall here mention; and 'tis as it were the *Converse* of this I have just spoke of. 'Tis,

(22.) *To Measure the Distance of an Object at one Station by a Telescope.*

<small>(22.) Measuring Distances by a Telescope.</small>

This is the great *Desideratum* in *Practical Geometry*; and always reputed *impossible*. Whatever Attempts have been made towards it have been always found to result at last to a *double Station*, tho some way or other disguised by the Contrivance. This is evidently shewn by *Tacquet* (*Geom. Pract.* Lib. 1. ad *Finem* Cap. 5.) concerning the Method proposed by *Clavius*. And may be shewn of any other, that I have ever yet heard of.

Towards the latter end of the year 1665. (as we may find Num. 7. P. 123. *Philosoph.Transact.*) Monsi. *Auzout* did propose to Mr. *Hook*, to exchange with him a Secret he had in Opticks, for another which Mr. *Hook* had. Monsi. *Auzout's* was, *Locorum Distantias ex unicâ statione, absque ullo Instrumento Mathematico metiri*. And therein he declares the Instrument, he uses for this Purpose, to be a *great Telescope*, with some necessary Tables. Adding withal, "That tho the Practice do not al-"together answer the *Theory* of his *Invention*, because that the "Length of the Telescope admits of some Latitude; yet one "comes *near enough*, and perhaps as *just*, as by most of the "Ways ordinarily used with Instruments. But tho Mr. *Hook* discovered the Secret which Monsi. *Auzout* desired from him, (which is that I mention at the End of Chap. IV.) yet Monsi. *Auzout* never (that I know) published any thing farther of this

<small>History of this Affair</small>

Invention

Invention of his own. And indeed I cannot see, how justly Monsf. *Azout* could say, that his Performance was, *absque ullo Instrumento Mathematico*; and at the same time tell us, that it was done by a *great Telescope*; which surely is a *Mathematick Instrument* in the highest sense: Perhaps he means, 'tis none of those *Mathematick Instruments* commonly used in this Practice.

Mr. *Oldenburg*, who then publish'd the *Philosoph. Transact.* adds Pag. 125. " That the Secret of measuring the Distance
" of Places by a Telescope fitted for that Purpose, and for one
" Station, is a Thing already known (if I am not misin-
" formed) to some Members of the *Royal Society*; who have
" been a good while since considering of it, and have contri-
" ved Ways for the doing of it. Whether the same with
" those of Monsf. *Azout*, I know not; nor have I (at the Di-
" stance that I am now from them) Opportunity of particular
" Information.

This is in short the History of this Affair. Wherein (for ought as ever I could learn) nothing more has been done hitherto. So that what I shall propose therein is my own Thought and Contrivance. Whereof I shall first declare the Method; and afterwards shall not conceal the Difficulties there-of: not doubting but more ingenious Heads may have Contrivances of the same kind far exceeding mine; tho nothing herein has ever yet been publish'd.

The Author's Proposal

Wherefore let the Distance of the Object from the Object-Glass be called d, the *Solar Focus* of the Object-Glass, or its *Focus* at very distant Objects f, the *respective Focus* or distinct Base at a nigh Object r.

By Prop. V. and the Rule immediately mentioned:

It shall be —— —— $d-f.f::d.r$
And Compounding—— $d.f::d+r.r$
Permute —— —— $r.f::r+d.d$
Divide —— —— $r-f.f::r.d$

Which

Which last Analogy is the Rule I give for finding the Distance of an Object by a Telescope, thus expressed in Words,

As the Difference between the Respective Focus *and* Solar Focus:
To the Solar Focus ::
So the Respective Focus:
To the Distance *of the Object from the Object-Glass.*

It now remains to shew how to obtain exactly the three first Terms of this Analogy; That thereby we may find the *fourth* required. And first for the *Solar Focal Length* of an Object-Glass, 'tis shewn before in Chap IV. Sec. 3. how to procure it exactly. Secondly for the *Respective Focus*, or distinct Base of any *nigh* Object we look at, I propose the Way to obtain it thus:

As the *Micrometer* is contrived to *open* and *close* in the Focus of the Object Glass, and the Indices give the exact Measure of this *Opening*: So may we adapt an Instrument, which may *advance* or *withdraw* the curious Point of a slender Needle *to* or *from* the Object Glass. And an *Index* (after the manner of the *Micrometer*) may shew how much the slender Point is withdrawn from the Object-Glass. Then looking through the Telescope at the Object, whose Distance we measure, let us withdraw the Needle, till by moving the Eye before the Eye-Glass, we perceive the Needle, as it were, *fixt* upon the Object: (as is taught Chap. V. Sect. 4.) Then is the Needle in the *Respective Focus*. And by observing the *Index* aforementioned, we have the Measure of this *Respective Focus* from the Object-Glass: And consequently the Difference between it and the *Solar Focus*. With which we are to work according to the Rule, and we obtain what was required, *viz*. the *Distance* of the Object. Thus suppose, in the foregoing Example, the Glasses Focus be = 36 Inches, and the Respective

spective Focus be measured 42.45 : The Analogy will then stand thus,

42.35 − 36 = 6.35 . 36 :: 42.35 . 240 = to the Distance of the Object from the Object-Glass. And thus may we make a *Table* to any *Telescope*, that upon the first Sight of the *Respective Focus* shall give the Distance of the Object.

Difficulties and Uncertainty thereof

But now I shall not conceal the Difficulties, that attend this Method of observing Distances. And first, The Eye can never be *justly* certain, when the Needle's Point is *exactly* in the Respective Focus; for tho the Way I propose of examining it (*viz.* by moving the Eye before the Eye-Glass, and observing whether or not the Needle seems to move on the Object) be the best Expedient, and most certain that I can think of at present: Yet we shall find, that it admits of some *Latitude*; and that the Needle may be moved a little more *forward* or *backward*, without shewing any visible Motion thereof on the Object; and this too most especially, the longer the Telescopes are that we use, and the wider the Aperture. But for the Remedy hereof, 'tis best to observe where the Needle (being *too nigh* the Object-Glass) *begins first* to move on the Object; as also to observe, where the Needle (being *too far* from the Object-Glass) *begins first* to appear to move on the Object; and to take the *middle* between these two Stations of the Needle for the true *Respective Focus*.

Secondly, where the Distance of the Object is *very great*, and vastly disproportional to the Solar Focal Length of the Object-Glass; the Observation will not be very accurate. And therefore it is that Monſ. *Auzout* in the forementioned Passage out of the *Philosoph. Transact.* confines his Practice to *great Telescopes*. For unless they be *so*, a considerable Alteration in the Distance of the Object makes no sensible Alteration in the *Respective Focus* of the *Object-Glass*.

But

Tab 41 pag 287

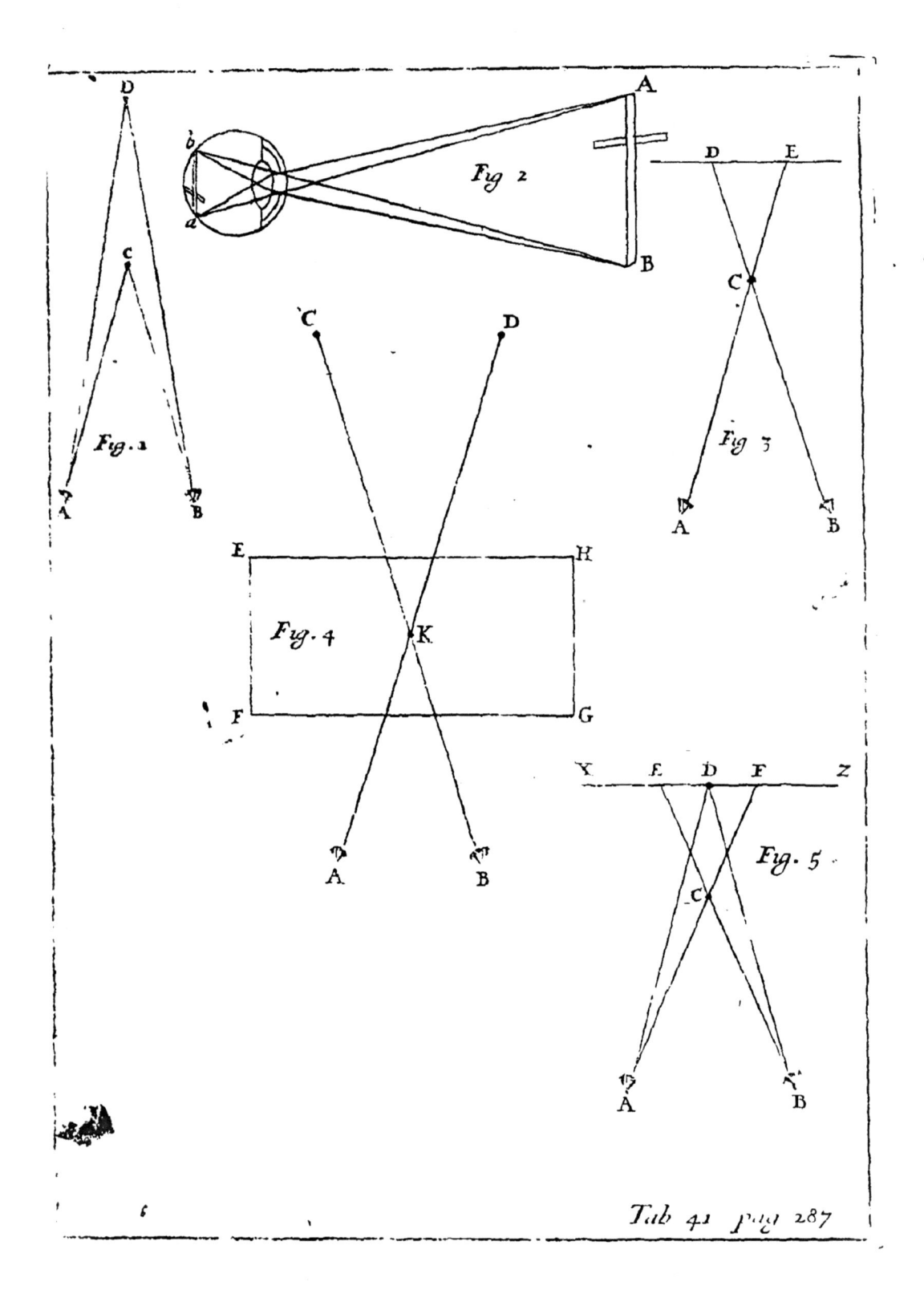

Tab. 42. Pag. Ult.

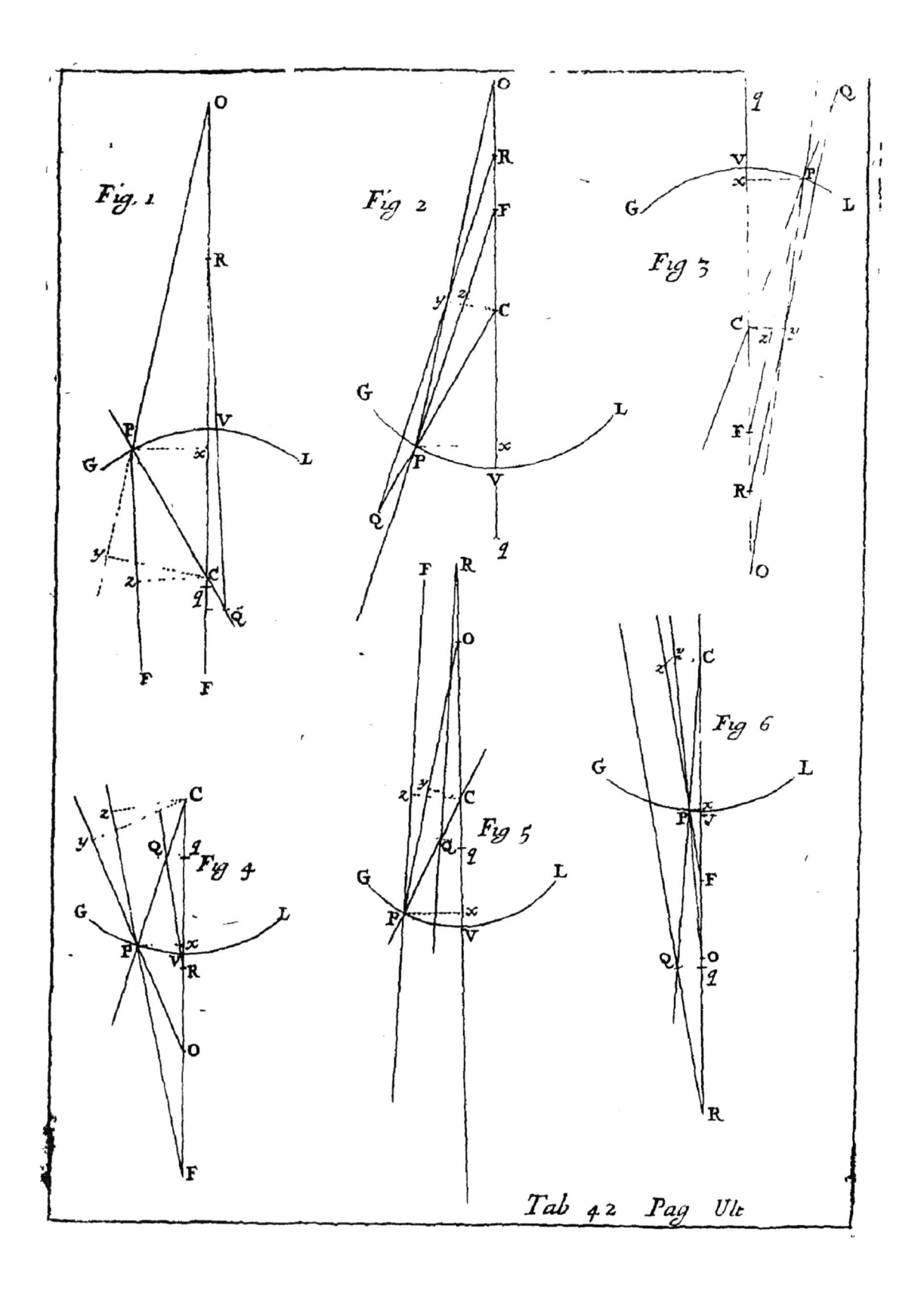

But if we believe the said Monsr. *Auzout*, by this Way, (if this Way which I propose be his, as I know not whether it be or not) one comes near enough to *Exactness*, and perhaps as just as by most of the Methods ordinarily used. However, tho the Practice, through some accidental Difficulties, do not so exactly answer the Theory. Yet it cannot be deny'd, that the Theory is true. And perhaps farther Improvements may bring it to Perfection.

Chap. VII.

An Optick Problem of Double Vision.

IN *Tab.* 41. *Fig.* 1. A B are the two Eyes, C the nigher Object, D the farther Object; If both Eyes open are fixt upon C, the Object D shall seem double, and then shutting the left Eye A, the left Image of D disappears; and shutting the Right Eye B, the right Image of D disappears.

But if both Eyes open are fixed on D, then C shall seem double, and if the left Eye A be shut, the right Image of C vanishes, if the Right Eye B be shut, the left Image of C vanishes.

This is the Declaration of the Phænomenon, which any one may experiment by placing two Candles, D 3 Foot, and C 1 Foot distant from the Eyes, and then standing so that the Nose and two Objects may lie in or near a right Line, he fixing his Eyes on either Object, alternately open and shut them. I choose two Candles, and at that Distance and Posture, because the Experiment thereby will be more sensibly evident; tho it hold in any two Objects at whatever Distance, till the Distance be so great, that the Interval between the two

Eyes,

[288]

Eyes bears no sensible proportion thereto, that is, till the Angle ACB (and much more ADB) is so very small, that the Lines AC, BC, may be taken to run as it were Parallel.

This being declared, I explicate the Reason of this Appearance, as follows.

In the first Case, both Eyes being fixed on C, if the Right Eye B be shut, the Object D will appear to the left hand of C, then shutting the Left Eye A, and opening the Right Eye B, and looking at C, D will appear to the Right Hand of C; therefore opening both A and B, and looking stedfastly on C, the Object D will appear on both sides C, that is, both to the Right and Left Hand of C, and therefore double. And 'tis manifest, the Right Eye B receives the Right Image of D, and the Left Eye A the Left Image of D; therefore in this Case, to the Right Eye being shut, the Right Image of D disappears, and to the Left Eye being shut, the Left Image of D disappears.

But in the second Case, fixing both Eyes on D, C seems double, for the Left Eye A being shut, C appears to B on the Left Hand of D; then the Right Eye being shut, the Left Eye A sees C on the Right Hand of D; so that in this Case, the Right Eye receives the Left Image of C, and the Left Eye the Right Image of C, and consequently the opening or shutting of either, does in this Case make the contrary Image of C disappear. And why C should seem double, is plain in this Case; for the Right Eye sees it on the Left Hand of D, and the Left Eye on the Right Hand of D; so that both Eyes see it on both Hands of D, and therefore double. But then in the first Case, the Object D, and not the Object C, seems double. And in the second Case, the Object C, and not the Object D, seems double. For in Vision, there is a Difference between *looking* and *seeing*; what-

ever

ever Object I *look* at with both Eyes appears *single*, and all others more remote or nigher, that I *see*, appear *double*; for upon the Object, I *look* at, the Optick Axes do concur, but not so on those I only *see*. And this is the Reason that at any time I can make all the Objects about me seem confused, only by turning the Optick Axes so, that they may concur in the free Air; as if there were a certain visible Object there before them, tho really there be none.

And that the Concurrence of the *Axes Optici* in a single Point or Object is sufficient to make that Object seem but one besides the Proof of the foregoing Experiments, I shall endeavour to evince, or at least to explicate, by an other known Affection of Vision; the Explanation whereof is allowed by all men as satisfactory, 'tis this, in *Tab.* 41. *Fig.* 2. the Image *a b* of the Object AB is painted on the *Retina* inverted, and yet the Eye (or rather the Soul by means of the Eye) sees the Object erect and in its natural Posture; Because the Mind takes no notice of what happens to the Rays in the Eye by Refraction or Decussation, but in its direction towards the Object; it follows streight alongst the Rays as they by their Impulse and in their plain Course lead it, and consequently following the Rays *a A*, it is directed strait to the upper part of the Object; and also following the Rays *b B*, it is directed to the lower part of the Object, and so of the rest: for suppose the Ball of the Eye taken out of its Socket, or Cavity in the Skull, and a Man receives in the Socket an impulse by a Stick coming in the posture of *B b*, and hitting him on the upper part of the Cavity, surely he would never look for the Original of this Blow at *A*, but would be certainly directed to hunt back as it were alongst the Stick *b B* towards the Place from whence the Stroak comes. So the mind does hunt back by means of each Pencil of Rays (which are as it were a Stick giving the *Retina* a certain Impulse)

P p

Impulse) to the Point from whence it comes, and is thereby directed strait thereto. To apply this to what I intend, I say then, that the Mind or visive Faculty (if I may have leave to use that Word for a thing we all understand and cannot better express) takes no notice that there are two *Axes Optici*, or two Pictures made by those *Axes Optici* on each *Retina*, but following back, and hunting *counter* alongst these Axes, it is directed to, and determined in *one single* Point, and therefore it sees it as *one*.

And seeing this Speculation does naturally lead me to the Consideration of an Opinion, first as I think started by the celebrated *Gassendus*, and since embraced by many, *viz.* that we see but with one Eye at once one and the same Point of an Object, *otiante alio*, (as they term it) whilst the other is idle and does nothing. I shall not think it improper to subjoyn to my former Discourse something relating to that Opinion, confining my self only to what may something illustrate my former Explanations, for to enumerate all the Experiments that prove we see with two Eyes, would swell this far beyond the limits I design it. Therefore to the Matter.

Against our seeing with two Eyes at once one and the same Point of an Object, it is commonly objected, that if it were so, every Object would seem in two places at once, *vide* Gassendi *Epist. 4. de Magnit. Solis humilis & sublimis, &* Taqueti *Opt. lib.* 1. *Prop.* 2. Thus in Tab. 41. Fig. 3. If the Eyes A, B, look at the Object C, and both see it at a time, A would see it on the opposite Wall suppose at E, and B at D.

I am so far from thinking this an Objection, that I assert first, that we do see all Objects in two places, and that this is not taken notice of by us upon these Accounts. First, the common Objects of our sight are large, and the Axes of our Eyes

directed

directed to but one Physical Point thereof at a time, and then we cannot be expected to see such in two places at once; for when I read on a flat broad Book, where is the opposite Wall for a single small Letter to be seen on at two places, the Letters themselves are fixt to the Surface that determines the Sight. What I Instance in Letters on a Book may be accommodated to most other Objects. Secondly, There are few Objects disposed fitly for shewing us that we see them in two places, for either their Bulk hinders the Experiment from appearing so plainly, or their distance from each other or from the Eyes. Thirdly, The Wall D E and the Parts thereof are seen so confusedly by the Eyes A, B, when fixed on C, that we cannot so clearly observe this Experiment; and this happens to all Objects more remote or nigher to us than C, when the Eyes are fixed on C, still supposing that it self be but in a moderate Distance from us, that is, in such a Distance from us, as may bear some considerable Proportion to the Distance of the two Eyes from each other. Fourthly, the chief Reason why we do not perceive so plainly the Object C to cover both D and E is, because, though D be cover'd by C from the Eye B, yet it is not covered from the Eye A, and therefore we think it not covered at all. Also though E be covered by C from the Eye A, yet it is not covered from the Eye B, and consequently because we see E, tho but with one Eye B, we imagine it not covered at all, so that both the Points D and E being open to both the Eyes A and B, *viz.* the Point D to the Eye A, and the Point E to the Eye B, we think neither of them covered, whereas really they are both obscur'd, each to its proper Eye, as will be evident by winking. And from hence is manifest the falsity of *Taquet*'s Assertion in the forecited Place, *viz.* that opening both Eyes A and B (*Fig.* 3.) and looking at C, it shall appear only to cover E (he imagining that most Men see generally with their left Eye) whereas I

P p 2

say

say it shall appear to obscure neither E nor D; tho to each Eye respectively it cover each. Fifthly, whereas the Bulk of Objects (as I have noted) does hinder the Experiment from being so sensibly evident; if by any Experiment I can shew how a large Object may be doubled, I think 'twill be sufficiently plain. Therefore in *Tab.* 41. *Fig.* 4. let A, B, be the two Eyes, before which at a convenient Distance place the two Candles C, D, then take a large piece of Paper E F G H K, in whose middle at K there is a small Hole. This Paper so place between the Eyes and Candles, that the Eye A may through the Hole K see the Candle D; and at the same time the Eye B may see through the Hole K the Candle C; the due Distance of the Paper that is requisite for this will be found by Tryals, and winking alternately with the Eyes. When all things are in this Posture, open both Eyes A and B, and direct them to look at either of the Candles, I say the Hole K shall seem double; and what is proved of the Point K is true of all other Points in the Paper, so the whole Paper appears double; but no Points thereof are so evidently doubled as the Point K, because they want the Advantage of Lights behind them to render the Experiment more sensible. And upon this Occasion I cannot but hint to all Persons that are desirous to make Experiments about Vision, that they always imploy the most luminous and vigorous Objects they can possibly, for many Experiments will be evident by them, that will not sensibly succeed with others.

But I assert secondly, that unless we saw with both Eyes, the two first mentioned Experiments would not succeed, and they may be reckoned amongst the greatest Arguments that can be produced for it. For suppose in *Fig.* 1. A and B to look stedfastly on C, I say they see C in two Places at once, for they see it both on the Right hand and Left hand of D. For tis the same thing to see C between two D's, as to see it at two Places at once. And this I'll declare more fully *Tab. 41. Fig. 5.* supposing the two Eyes A and B fixed on the Object C, I say C appears on the opposite Wall X Z in two Places, *viz.* at E and F (tho neither E nor F are obscur'd thereby for the foregoing Reason) for let us suppose the Object D of the first Figure to be placed duly on this Wall; shutting A, the Object C shall appear to B on the left hand of D by the Angle D B E: then shutting B, the Object C shall appear to A on the right hand of D, by the Angle D A F; wherefore to both open at a time and looking at it, it shall appear on both sides of D, to A on the right side, to B on the left side, and this happens by doubling of D; so that from hence this Paradoxical Corollary arises, *That an Object may be seen in two Places, and yet not seen double.*

They that assert that we see but with one Eye, whilst the other is idle and does nothing, assert likewise that all visual Spirits recede from the idle Eye, and only supply the Eye that sees; but I see no Reason why the Eyes A, B, looking at C, either of them should be said destitute of Spirits in respect of C, which they see single, and yet both replenished with Spirits in respect of D, which they see Double. The Images of C and D both are painted on the *Retina* of A as well as of B, and therefore A and B both being replenished with Spirits to see D, (even by the Concession of our Adversaries) why not to see C also, at which they stedfastly look?

To conclude, I propose it to the learned and ingenious Dr. *Briggs*, or to any other of the Philosophical Spirits of this Age to explain the foregoing Phænomena by the Doctor's Theory of Vision. And as a Conclusion to the whole shall only add one Experiment that Demonstrates we see with both

both Eyes at once; and 'tis, that which is commonly known and practised in all Tennis-Courts, that the best Player in the World Hoodwinking one Eye shall be beaten by the greatest Bungler that ever handled a Racket; unless he be used to the Trick, and then by Custom he gets an Habit of using one Eye only.

APPENDIX.

APPENDIX.

WHilst this Book was in the Press my Affairs were such, that I could not attend the Perusal and Correction thereof, but therein have made use of my Friend Mr. E. Halley, who was willing to do me that Service: He, after the first Part hereof was finished, sent me a Proposition of his own, which I took to be of that Consequence in Dioptricks, that I importuned him to permit it to be subjoyned by way of Appendix to my Treatise, it being of that Extent as to comprehend the whole Doctrine of the Foci of Spherical Glasses of all Sorts, exposed either to *Diverging*, *Converging*, or *Parallel Rays*. It is as follows.

PROPOSITION.

TO find the *Focus* of any Parcel of Rays *Diverging from*, or *Converging to* a given Point in the *Axis* of a *Spherical Lens*, and inclined thereto under the same Angle; the *ratio* of the Sines in Refraction being known.

Let G L *Tab*. 42. be the *Lens*, P any Point in its Surface, V the Pole thereof, C the Center of the Sphere whereof it is a Segment, O the Object or Point in the Axis, to or from which the Rays do proceed, O P a given Ray: and let the *ratio* of Refraction be as r to s; make C R to C O as s to r for the immersion of a Ray, or as r to s for the Emersion, (that is, as the Sines of the Angles in the Medium which the Ray enters, to their corresponding Sines in the Medium out of which it comes) and laying C R from C towards O, the Point R shall be the same for all the Rays of the Point O. Then draw the Radius P C if need be continued, and with the Centre R and Distance O P sweep a touch of an Arch intersecting P C in Q; the Line Q R

being

being drawn shall be parallel to the refracted Ray, and PF being made parallel thereto shall intersect the Axis in the Point F, which is the Focus sought Or make it as $CQ : CP :: CR : CF$ and CF shall be the Distance of the Focus from the Centre of the Sphere.

Demonstration.

Let fall the Perpendiculars Px on the Axis, Cy on the given Ray and Cz on the refracted Ray. By the Construction PF and QR are parallel, whence the △, QRC and PFC are similar, and CR to QR as CF to PF, that is, CR to OP as CF to PF. Now $CF : PF :: Cz : Px$ *ob similia Triang.* whence $CR : OP :: Cz : Px$, and $CR : Cz :: OP : Px$. Again CR is to CO as the Sines of Refraction, by construction, that is as s to r or r to s; and as CR to Cz, so $CO = \frac{\cdot}{\cdot}$ or $\frac{\cdot}{\cdot} CR$ to $\frac{\cdot}{\cdot}$ or $\frac{\cdot}{\cdot} Cz$, and so PO to Px: But as PO to Px, so CO to Cy. *Ergo* $Cy = \frac{\cdot}{\cdot}$ or $\frac{\cdot}{\cdot} Cz$, that is, Cy to Cz is as the Sines of Refraction, but Cy is the Sine of the Angle of Incidence, and Cz of the refracted Angle. *Ergo constat Propositio.*

The several Cases of Rays Diverging or Converging as they enter the curve Surface of a *Convex* or *Concave Lens*, are for the Readers Ease delineated in the first four Figures of *Tab.* 42. as are in *Fig.* 5 and 6 thereof, and in *Fig.* 1, 2. of *Tab.* 43. the like Cases of emerging Rays. All which are drawn with the same Letters to their respective Points, only in some the Point F falling far distant, is to be understood in the Intersection of the Line PF with the Axis.

This thus demonstrated in the most difficult Cases, will give all the Rules for the Foci of Rays parallel to the Axis as likewise for the principle Focus, where the Rays nearest the Axis do unite, all which Rules I shall collect in these following Corollaries.

Cor. 1. If OP be equal to CR, then the Points Q and C are coincident, and the Rays OP after Refraction run on parallel to the Axis.

Cor. 2.

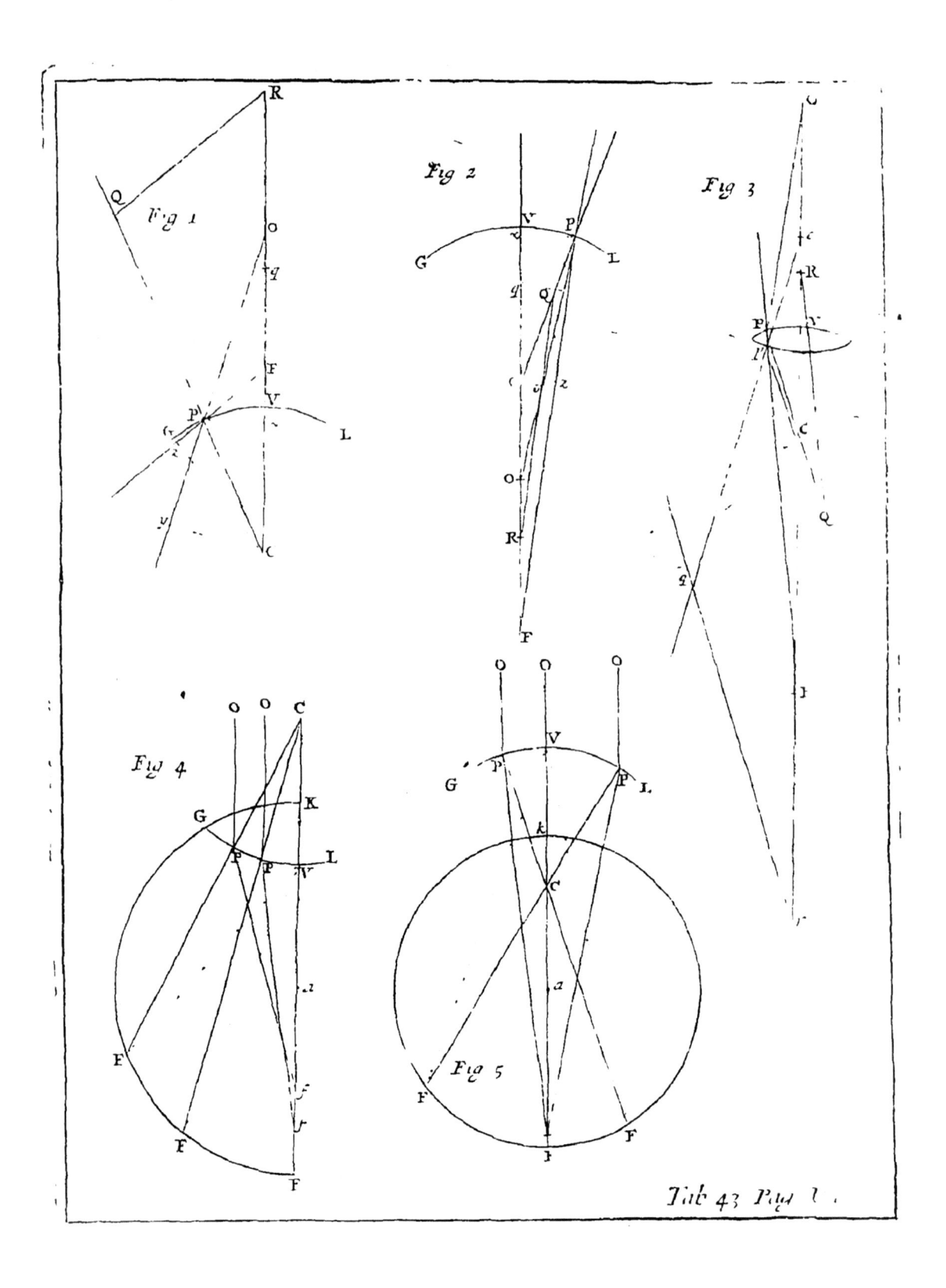

Fig. 1

Fig. 2

Fig. 3

Fig. 4

Fig. 5

Tab 43 Pag 1

Cor. 2. If the Point Q fall on the same side the Axis as is the Point P, then the Beams after Refraction do tend on, either diverging or converging as before: But if Q fall on the other side the Axis, as in *Fig.* 1. the diverging Rays are made to converge by a Convex, or the converging to diverge by a Concave Glass.

Cor. 3. If O P do exceed C R, the Focus is in all Cases on the same side of the Glass as is the Centre of the Sphere C. But contrarywise if O P be less than C R, the Focus falls on the other side of the Glass beyond the Vertex V.

Cor. 4. An Object may be so placed, that the Rays next the Axis of a Convex-Glass shall have an imaginary Focus, transmitting diverging Rays, when the more remote Parts thereof shall make them converge to a real Focus.

Cor. 5. If O V the Distance of the Object from the Pole or Vertex of the Glass, be taken instead of O P, then will C Q be the difference of O V and C R, and as that difference to C R, so the Radius C V to C F the Distance of the principal Focus from the Centre of the Sphere whereof the Glass is a Segment: or else as C Q to O P or R Q·: so P C to V F the focal distance from the Pole of the Glass. Whence follows a general Rule for the Foci of all Glasses, only according to *Corol.* 3. if O V do exceed C R, the Focus is on the same side of the Glass as is the Centre of the Sphere. But if C R be the greater, then the Focus is on the opposite side of the Glass, whence it will be determined whether the Focus be real or imaginary.

Cor. 6. What has hitherto been said of one Surface of a *Lens* is easily applicable to the other; taking F the *Focus* of the first Surface as an Object, and using it as O in the Figures for emerging Rays, whereby the *Focus* of both Surfaces will be determined, as in *Tab.* 43. *Fig.* 3. where I have given an Example.

Cor. 7. Hitherto we have considered only *oblique Rays* either *Diverging* or *Converging*; it now remains to add something concerning

cerning *Rays parallel* to the *Axis*: In this Case the Point O must be considered as infinitely distant, and consequently OP, OC, and CR are all infinite; and OP and OC are in this Case to be accounted as always equal, (since they differ but by a Part of the Radius of the Sphere GPVL, which is no part of either of them,) wherefore the *ratio* of CR to OP will be always the same, *viz.* as *s* to *r* for immerging Rays, and as *r* to *s* for those that emerge. And by this Proposition CF is to PF in the same *ratio*. It remains therefore to shew on the Base CP, to find all the Triangles CPF wherein CF is to PF in the *ratio* given by the degree of Refraction. This Problem has been very fully considered by the celebrated Dr. *Wallis* in his late Treatise of Algebra, pag. 258. to which I refer; but I must here repeat the Construction thereof, *Tab.* 43. *Fig.* 4, 5.

Let GPVL be a Lens, VC or PC the Radius of its Sphere, and let it be required to find all the Points *f, f*, such as *Cf*, may be to *Pf* in the given *ratio* of *s* to *r* for immerging Rays, or as *r* to *s* for the emerging. Divide CV in K, and continue CV to F, that CK may be to VK, and CF to VF in the proposed *ratio*: Then divide KF equally in the Point *a*, and with that Center sweep the Circle FKF; this Circle being drawn gives readily all the Foci of the Parallel Rays OP, OP. For having continued CP till it intersect the Circle in F, PF shall be always equal to *Vf* the Distance of the Focus of each respective Parcel of Rays OP, from the Vertex or Pole of the *Lens*.

To demonstrate this, draw the prickt line VF, and by what is delivered by Dr. *Wallis* in the aforecited Place, VF and CF, will be always in the same proposed *ratio*. Again *Vf* being made equal to PF, CF and *Cf* will be likewise equal, as are CP, VC; and the Angles PC*f*, VCF being *ad verticem* are also equal: Wherefore *Pf* will be equal to VF, and consequently *Cf* to *Pf* in the same *ratio* as CF to VF, whence
and

and by what foregoes, the Points f, f are the several respective Foci of the several Parcels of Rays, O P, O P. Q. E. D.

That C F is to P F in the *ratio* of the Refraction, in the case of parallel Rays, will be yet more evident, if it be consider'd, that the Angle at C is equal to the Angle of Incidence, and the Angle at P to the refracted Angle; wherefore P F the side opposite to the Angle at C, is as the Sine of the Angle of Incidence, and C F opposite to the Angle at P, is as the Sine of the respective refracted Angle; whence in all Cases of parallel Rays, C F is to P F in the same constant *ratio* of Refraction.

If it shall be desired to effect in Numbers what we have here done by Lines, it will be most easie to adapt a Calculus to the foregoing Geometrical Construction. For if in the Triangle P O C there be given the Radius C P equal to *Unity*, C O the distance of the Object from the Centre of the Sphere, and the Perpendicular $\mathcal{P} x$ equal to the Sine of the Angle P C O, the side P O = Q R will be equal to $\sqrt{CO^q + CP^q \pm 2CO}$ in $\sqrt{CP^q - \mathcal{P}x^q}$. Then as Q R or P O to $\mathcal{P}x$ :: so C R to the Sine of the Angle C Q R, and the Complement to 180 gr. of the sum of the Angles C P O and C Q R is the Angle C R Q = C F P; and as $\mathcal{P}x$ to P O so the Sine of the Angle C R Q to C Q; and as C Q to C P so C R to C F, which is the distance of the respective Focus of all the Rays P O from the Centre of the Sphere C.

But the Foci of Rays parallel to the *Axis* may be more readily computed, following the Footsteps of the Construction delivered in *Coroll.* 7. (*Tab.* 43. *Fig.* 4, 5.) for thereby it will appear, that the Radius of the Circle K F, *viz.* a F, is equal to $\frac{rs}{rr-ss}$ CP, and $Ca = \frac{rr}{rr-ss}$ CP, for emerging Rays, as in *Fig.* 4; but for immerging Rays, as in *Fig.* 5, Ca will be found to be $\frac{ss}{rr-ss}$ CP: and supposing the distance of the Ray from the

Axis $= Px$, in the Case of parallel Rays Emerging, the distance of the Focus will be found, $PF = \frac{rr}{rr-ss}\sqrt{CP^q - Px^q} + \sqrt{\frac{rs}{rr-ss}CP^q - \frac{rr}{rr-ss}Px^q} - CP$: that is, r to s being as 3 to 2, $PF = \frac{9}{5}\sqrt{CP^q - Px^q} + \sqrt{\frac{6}{5}CP^q - \frac{9}{5}Px^q} - CP$. And for immerging Rays, the Focal distance is found by a like Rule, $PF = \frac{ss}{rr-ss}\sqrt{CP^q - Px^q} + \sqrt{\frac{rs}{rr-ss}CP^q - \frac{ss}{rr-ss}Px^q} + CP$: that is r and s being as 3 to 2 as before, PF is equal to $\frac{4}{5}\sqrt{CP^q - Px^q} + \sqrt{\frac{6}{5}CP^q - \frac{4}{5}Px^q} + CP$. These Canons are so easily deduced from the Constructions, that I shall not need to trouble the Reader with their Demonstration; only I shall add two Tables which I computed from them, with little more work than a continual Addition; which may by way of Example, serve to instruct and exercise the young Student in this part of Mathematicks.

Suppose CP the Radius of the Sphere of Glass 2 Inches, and the *ratio* of Refraction as 3 to 2; at each tenth of an Inch distance from the Axis, the *Foci* are as follows.

For Emerging Rays.

Px	PF
0	$\sqrt{12,9600} + \sqrt{5,7600} - 2$
1	$\sqrt{12,9276} + \sqrt{5,7276} - 2$
2	$\sqrt{12,8304} + \sqrt{5,6304} - 2$
3	$\sqrt{12,6684} + \sqrt{5,4684} - 2$
4	$\sqrt{12,4416} + \sqrt{5,2416} - 2$
5	$\sqrt{12,1500} + \sqrt{4,9500} - 2$
6	$\sqrt{11,7936} + \sqrt{4,5936} - 2$
7	$\sqrt{11,3724} + \sqrt{4,1724} - 2$
8	$\sqrt{10,8864} + \sqrt{3,6864} - 2$
9	$\sqrt{10,3356} + \sqrt{3,1356} - 2$
10	$\sqrt{9,7200} + \sqrt{2,5200} - 2$

For Immerging Rays.

Px	PF
0	$\sqrt{2,5600} + \sqrt{5,7600} + 2$
1	$\sqrt{2,5536} + \sqrt{5,7536} + 2$
2	$\sqrt{2,5344} + \sqrt{5,7344} + 2$
3	$\sqrt{2,5024} + \sqrt{5,7024} + 2$
4	$\sqrt{2,4576} + \sqrt{5,6576} + 2$
5	$\sqrt{2,4000} + \sqrt{5,6000} + 2$
6	$\sqrt{2,3296} + \sqrt{5,5296} + 2$
7	$\sqrt{2,2464} + \sqrt{5,4464} + 2$
8	$\sqrt{2,1504} + \sqrt{5,3504} + 2$
9	$\sqrt{2,0416} + \sqrt{5,2416} + 2$
10	$\sqrt{1,9200} + \sqrt{5,1200} + 2$

But

But it is to be Noted, that these *Foci* for Immerging Rays, must not be taken for the Foci of a Plano-Convex, when the Convex Side is towards the Object, for the plane Side by its Refraction, does contract the Focal length by about a Semidiameter of the Sphere; These suppose the Body of Glass continued, as in the First Proposition of this Treatise.

FINIS.

ERRATA.

Page	Line	For	Read
3	26	V	IV
4	12	Propofitions	Proportions
50	23	6th	16th
57	17	Convexity	Concavity
58	5	Plano-Convex	Plano-Concave
67	8	4th	5th
141	24	Breadth of the Object	½ Breadth of the Object
143	6	*Dele* XV	
149	12	We cannot add	We are to add
150	4	Lemma	Lemma 1
193	4	CF or FZ + FD	CF (or FZ) + FD
219	13	$l\,h$ more than $l\,s$	$l\,h$ is greater than $l\,s$
219	14	$h\,g$ lefs	$h\,g$ is lefs
220	1	fhall be	as fhall be
264	2	his	this

ADVERTISEMENT.

ALL the above named Instruments as Telescopes of all Lengths, Microscopes single and double, Perspectives great and small, Reading Glasses of all sizes, Magnifying Glasses, Multiplying Glasses, Triangular Prisms, Speaking Trumpets, Spectacles fitted to all Ages, and all other Sorts of Glasses, both Concave and Convex are made and sold by JOHN YARWELL at the Archimedes and Three Golden Prospects, near the great North-Door in S. Paul's Church-Yard: London.

LaVergne, TN USA
05 April 2011
222903LV00006B/5/P